Praise for *The Embodied Teen*

"I am so happy that this book is coming out. In a strange way, I have awaited it since 1976 when I was living in Santa Fe, New Mexico. Circumstances had me joining a group of other parents to design a public alternative high school that would meet the needs of the many students who were not doing well in the only existing one. One of the procedures that we put in place was to make class attendance optional, a daring move with teenagers! I was asked to teach a class on experiential anatomy. I had to think very carefully about how to do it in a way that would make students actually attend. To my happy surprise they thronged to the class. Contrary to my fears, they were neither bored and distracted, or silly and embarrassed by the many sensing, moving, and touching exercises. They seemed to drink them in like wanderers in a desert coming upon a spring. That experience informed my desire to return to the university world and to create a graduate program that was a more scholarly version of what I designed for those teenagers, and not unlike some of what Susan Bauer details here. I hope that many schools will adopt the plan proposed by this important book. It will change things that have gone so far astray."

—DON HANLON JOHNSON, PhD, author and founder of the somatics program at California Institute of Integral Studies in San Francisco

"A much-needed approach for empowering adolescents! Susan Bauer's curriculum provides relief and remedy for challenges teens face in finding out what's true for them—and helps them discover the value of time spent in somatic experience. With this guide, teachers of adolescents can provide intelligent, body-based learning via a unique and thoughtful treasure chest of embodiment explorations."

—CARYN McHOSE, somatic movement educator and coauthor of *How Life Moves: Explorations in Meaning and Body Awareness*

"*The Embodied Teen* is an important source book for anyone in the field of dance education. Although it addresses youth, the material is valuable for any age level. For years I have referred to Mabel Todd's *The Thinking Body* for reference. Now I have a new book to refer to. Susan Bauer has written with clarity and interest in a way that any one of us as teachers can find new ideas and inspiration. I would not be without this book as a teacher or a student of dance."

—ANNA HALPRIN, PhD, author of *Moving Toward Life: Five Decades of Transformational Dance* and cofounder of the Tamalpa Institute

"*The Embodied Teen* is an enormously valuable curriculum and book for professionals who work with youth. It is an exceptional gathering of significant somatic understandings that will help teens establish a solid foundation for later developmental stages. Susan Bauer is enormously experienced and knowledgeable about somatics and adolescent development. This culmination of her life work is a gift to teens, professionals, and others."

—ELEANOR CRISWELL HANNA, EdD, editor of *Somatics Magazine* and director of the Novato Institute for Somatic Research and Training

"Susan Bauer's curricular manual is a rare beginning into an important world—how to empower teens to access their own body intelligence and build their resiliency, so needed in these times. As someone who has been working with socioemotional learning since the early 1990s, it is refreshing to be able to suggest this guide for educators who want to integrate somatic education within youth programming. Join this thoughtful call to get more holistically involved with our young people!"

—MARTHA EDDY, CMA, RSMT, EdD, author of *Mindful Movement: The Evolution of the Somatic Arts and Conscious Action*

"This book is a rich and detailed resource for anyone wishing to support teens in becoming more fully embodied, present, expressive, responsive, and resilient. These skills are absolutely essential in a world in which so many young people (and adults) are profoundly disconnected from their bodies, minds, and hearts. If your work and play is supporting young people in living more fully and expressing their gifts, *The Embodied Teen* is an essential resource."

—AMY SALTZMAN, MD, director of the Association for Mindfulness in Education and author of *A Still Quiet Place for Teens: A Mindfulness Workbook to Ease Stress and Difficult Emotions*

"Susan Bauer is a bold pioneer in somatic education. She has spent many years of study and experimentation developing the somatic, emotional and creative program presented in this book, based on her work with many experts in the field. The result is a program that will immensely enhance the education of our future adults and leaders. *The Embodied Teen* presents a rationale and a program more comprehensive and systematic than many past experimentations in adolescent curriculum. It is a must-read for all educators and more importantly a must-do for all administrators. Our world needs much more than academic competence and the development of job skills. It needs the sort of fully developed human beings that this program can go a long way toward realizing. Do not simply read this book, but act upon it in any way you can to make its vision a reality in the education of our youth."

—DEANE JUHAN, movement reeducation therapist and author of *Job's Body: A Handbook for Bodywork* and *Touched by the Goddess: The Physical, Psychological, and Spiritual Powers of Bodywork*

"Susan Bauer has written a curriculum that will lift the standard of what teens need for building a healthy relationship with themselves, which ultimately impacts having a healthy society. In the fast-paced world of technology and social media, *The Embodied Teen* provides the meaning, purpose, and action steps for somatic movement education. This book is an important and practical resource for integrating body and mind to increase self-awareness, empathy, compassion, and self esteem for our youth."

—JUDY GANTZ, MA, CMA, founder of the Center for Movement Education and Research

"*The Embodied Teen* is superb! It weaves together the rigor of science and years of clinical practice and classroom experience to offer a much-needed guide to somatic wisdom for teens. I highly recommend this book."

—SHAUNA SHAPIRO, PhD, professor of psychology and author *of The Art and Science of Mindfulness* and *Mindful Discipline: A Loving Approach to Setting Limits and Raising an Emotionally Intelligent Child*

"*The Embodied Teen* is a gift outright to all teachers who want their students to fully experience what it means to 'know thyself.' Equal parts educational philosophy, informational resource, and curricular guide, the book braids all three to make the case for embodiment as fundamental to a deeply experienced complete education. Susan Bauer provides a clear, richly developed, and scaffolded model for teachers that resonates across age groups, cultures, and communities of learners. The generosity and wisdom of her methods, wonderfully illustrated by examples drawn from years of teaching, leads students and teachers alike toward an empowering sense of embodied wholeness."

—DIANE FRANK, lecturer (dance), Department of Theater and Performance Studies at Stanford University

"Adolescence is a developmentally critical time, with vital transformations occurring in both body and brain, yet mainstream educational models offer teens very little constructive support in navigating these changes. This clear and accessible book provides an invaluable resource for anyone wanting to support teenagers in becoming more grounded, self-aware, emotionally literate, and relationally engaged. An excellent book! I cannot recommend it highly enough."

—RAE JOHNSON, PhD, RSMT, author of *Embodied Social Justice* and chair of somatic studies in the Depth Psychology program at Pacifica Graduate Institute

"*The Embodied Teen* is an invaluable resource for educators in an age when youth are so disconnected from their own bodies. The bottom-up perspective—supported by the latest research in neuroscience and mindfulness—approaches the body as the root of healthy social and emotional growth. These experiential somatic education lessons guide teens through a profound process of self-discovery: first by befriending their own bodies, then by learning to use body awareness to become more self-aware and cultivate resilience, and ultimately toward forming healthy connections with others. This book truly teaches teens a new way of being in the world."

—MARK PURCELL, clinical psychologist and coauthor of *Mindfulness for Teen Anger: A Workbook to Overcome Anger and Aggression Using MBSR and DBT Skills*

The Embodied Teen

The Embodied Teen

A Somatic Curriculum for Teaching Body-Mind Awareness, Kinesthetic Intelligence, and Social and Emotional Skills

Susan Bauer

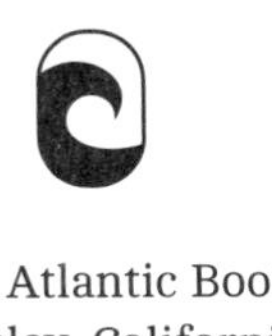

North Atlantic Books
Berkeley, California

Published by
North Atlantic Books
Berkeley, California

Cover design by Emma Cofod
Interior design by Happenstance Type-O-Rama
Printed in the United States of America

The Embodied Teen: A Somatic Curriculum for Teaching Body-Mind Awareness, Kinesthetic Intelligence, and Social and Emotional Skills is sponsored and published by the Society for the Study of Native Arts and Sciences (dba North Atlantic Books), an educational nonprofit based in Berkeley, California, that collaborates with partners to develop cross-cultural perspectives, nurture holistic views of art, science, the humanities, and healing, and seed personal and global transformation by publishing work on the relationship of body, spirit, and nature.

Some short portions of material in this book previously appeared in *Somatics Magazine-Journal* under the title "Somatic Education: A Body-Mind Approach to Movement Education for Adolescents," Part I and Part II, 1999/2000, by Susan Bauer, © Susan Bauer; reprinted with permission of *Somatics Magazine-Journal.* Body-Mind Centering® is a registered service mark, and BMC℠ is a service mark of Bonnie Bainbridge Cohen and is used with permission.

Please note that all student journal entries and drawings in the book are used with permission, with some students' names and slight details changed to protect their identities.

North Atlantic Books' publications are available through most bookstores. For further information, visit our website at www.northatlanticbooks.com or call 800-733-3000.

Library of Congress Cataloging-in-Publication Data

Names: Bauer, Susan, author.
Title: The embodied teen : a somatic curriculum for teaching body-mind awareness, kinesthetic intelligence, and social and emotional skills / Susan Bauer.
Description: Berkeley, California : North Atlantic Books, [2018] | Includes bibliographical references.
Identifiers: LCCN 2017050470 | ISBN 9781623171889 (trade paper)
Subjects: LCSH: Movement education—Study and teaching (Secondary) | Body-mind centering.
Classification: LCC GV452 .B38 20018 | DDC 372.86—dc23
LC record available at https://lccn.loc.gov/2017050470

1 2 3 4 5 6 7 8 9 Sheridan 23 22 21 20 19 18

Printed on recycled paper

North Atlantic Books is committed to the protection of our environment. We partner with FSC-certified printers using soy-based inks and print on recycled paper whenever possible.

To my students and teachers,
and to this generation and all those to follow

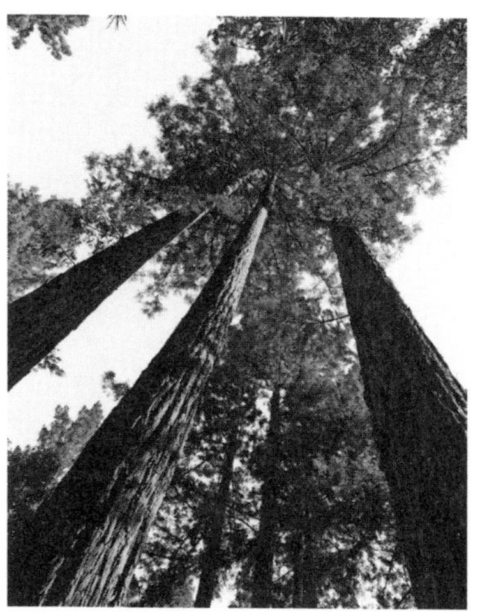

"One generation plants the trees;
another gets the shade."

Contents

PART IV: A CURRICULUM IN SME: EMBODIED ANATOMY FOR TEENS

EMBODIMENT FUNDAMENTALS–LEVEL II

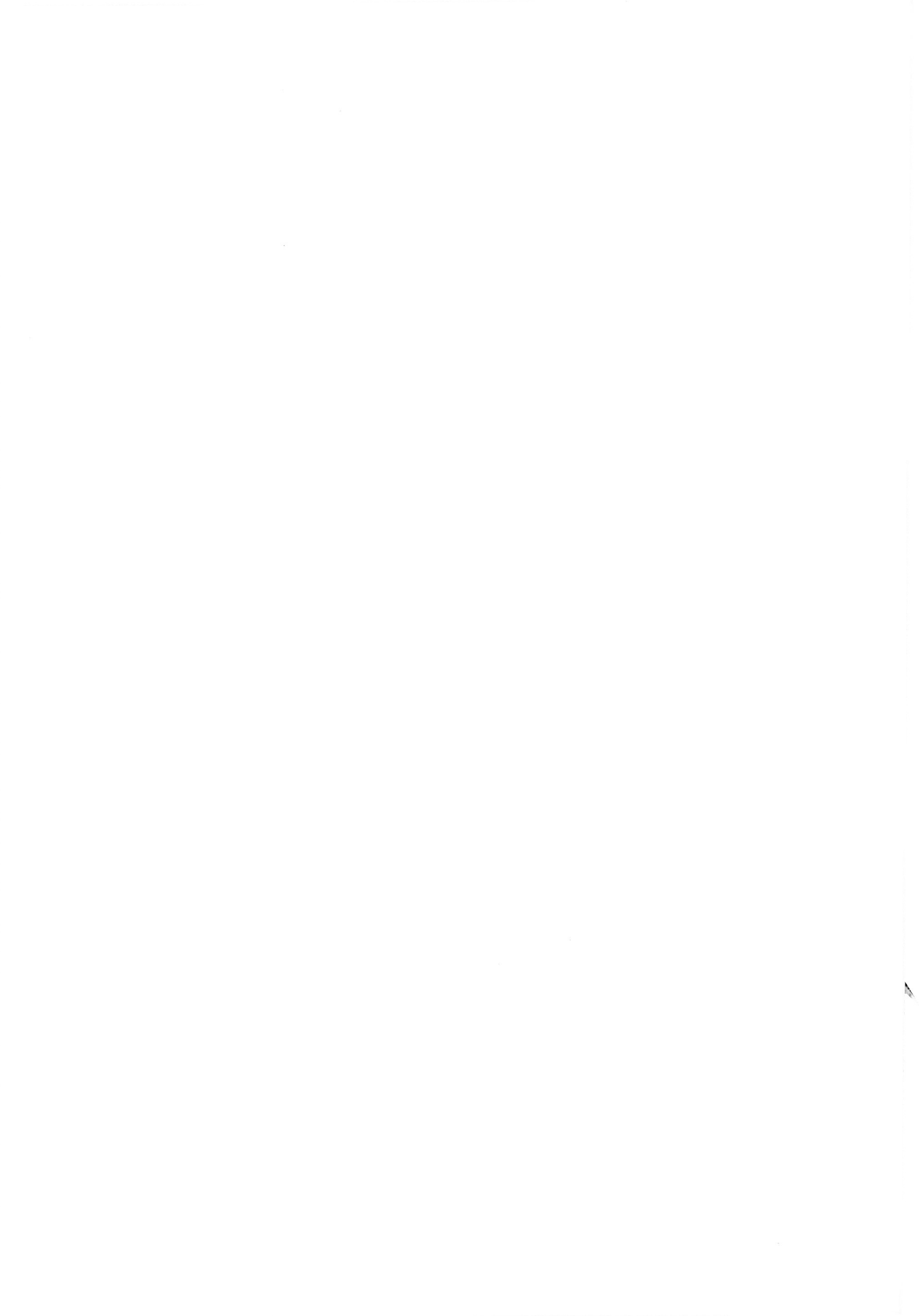

Acknowledgments

This book would not exist were it not for all of the dedicated and pioneering souls who have come before me. I've been blessed with many wise, warm, and giving teachers. I've done my best below to acknowledge and thank my primary teachers, though it may be impossible to go back far enough to truly do justice to the lineage of visionaries in dance and somatics who have paved the way for this contribution of mine, and of which I am so thankful to be a part. There are also many others to thank for their support that led to this creation, which has been more than thirty years in the making.

Although I documented my initial curriculum twenty-three years ago, at the time I could not convince a publisher that there would be an audience for this material. There was so much confusion: What is this? Is it science? Is it PE? Is it wellness? Is it movement? Yes, yes, yes, and *yes!* Who is your target audience? Is it for dance teachers? For PE teachers? For movement educators? For counselors? Again, yes! And then: Can teens really *do* this? Yes, they can! And although somatics has become much more well-acknowledged and integrated into many professional fields since then, the same was true ten years ago. Yet over the past five years, as I worked with several progressive schools and began to get a better "read" on the current educational climate, I came to believe that the time was ripe for somatic movement education in our schools and programs for our youth—with many aspects of the curriculum now backed up by recent research in both mindfulness and neuroscience related to adolescent development. Clearly, the time had come to try again.

Therefore, I would especially like to thank North Atlantic Books (NAB) for believing in my work and vision. I am particularly grateful to editor Hisae Matsuda and publisher Tim McKee at NAB for their immediate confidence in me and in the timeliness of this offering. After so many years, their enthusiasm was a breath of fresh air and a confirmation. Special thanks to my editors Erin Wiegand, Emily Boyd, and Ebonie Ledbetter for their care and dedication to help birth this book, and all those at NAB who also helped along the way.

Next, I am deeply thankful to the teens and young adults whom I have been privileged to work with. Teens are bold and daring, inspired and curious. Perhaps it is my hopeful vision for a more compassionate and consciously interrelated world that drew me to them, as the creators of our future. I thank all those who I have worked with over the years for teaching me so very much.

Very special thanks to the teens who enthusiastically came forward over this past year to participate in classes and be photographed for this book. Getting those first dozen replies—within *less than an hour* of putting out the word about classes in "body-mind awareness for teens"—helped keep me going on this project! Thank you to each of you, and to your parents, for your participation over many weekends: Cedar, Etta, Meera, Giuliana, Cameron, Cristiano, Cally, Jacob, Chloe, Jonathan, Sophia, Macey, CieArra, Abby, Ari, and Mateo; and to Shawl-Anderson Center and the many teens from my Experiential Anatomy classes for your participation and photo permission.

Thank you also to my students at the Williston-Northampton School and the MacDuffie School in Massachusetts and at the Moo Baan Dek School in Thailand, as well as those at Dominican University in California and Taitung University in Taiwan, some of whom are represented through anecdotes and stories in the book, for the insights you shared and the lessons we can learn from you all.

And next, a deep gratitude to my teachers, whose impassioned lives have changed my own. I would especially like to thank Bonnie Bainbridge Cohen, the founder of the School for Body-Mind Centering®, for her embodied teachings, and for our enduring friendship over these many years of learning and growing since 1984. Bonnie gave much time and care to this book, offering heartfelt support and discerning feedback. I thank her also for the inspiration of her work in embodiment and human consciousness, especially for acknowledging the innate wisdom and desire to learn present in every child. Her presence has deeply enriched my life.

I would also like to thank Caryn McHose for the gift of her embodied presence and her enthusiastic support over the years, and express my appreciation for her insightful comments during the writing process.

Andrea Olsen for the inspiration of her teaching and her prolific work as a writer about the ineffable world of movement, and for encouraging me to honor my intuition as a dancer, artist, and writer.

Irene Dowd for introducing me to Ideokinesis and methods of hands-on repatterning, particularly as applied to teaching dance, and for her sincere support and encouragement over many years.

Janet Adler for her support and devoted teaching in the Discipline of Authentic Movement, and the many lessons the process has afforded me and my adult students and clients, along with thanks to my first Authentic Movement teachers Joan Miller, Susan Schell, Alton Wasson, and Mary Ramsey whose wise and compassionate witnessing from years ago ever informs me.

Deane Juhan for his provocative writings that fueled my desire to advocate for somatics for our youth and to believe in the power of the written word to inspire, and for his support in reading sections of this manuscript.

Cynthia Jean Cohen Bull (AKA Cynthia Novack) for introducing me to dance anthropology and helping me to recognize that all forms of dance, and even our bodies, are cultural constructs. You are dearly missed.

Anna Halprin, Nancy Stark Smith, Simone Forti, Suprapto Suryodarmo, Sardono Kusumo, and Richard Bull for their friendship and support, and for sharing their love of improvisation as a mode of dance, teaching, performance, and as a joyous way of life.

I would also like to thank my Balinese teachers for their dedicated time and love to share the depth of their artistry with me over many years: Ibu Sang Ayu Muklen, Ida Bagus Oka, and I Ketut Kantor.

There are also many to thank for the production of this book. This took many hours and the commitment of a host of comrades. For photographs and illustrations, a special thank you to photographers Monica Xu and Danny Yugen, as well as Shinichi Iova-Koga, Yve St. John, and Kiera Chase for their photos that add so much vitality to the manuscript. Thank you to Mei-Chu Liu of the Somatic Education Society of Taiwan and to students at the Moo Baan Dek School in Thailand for photo permissions and our inspiring time together.

Thanks to illustrator and Body-Mind Centering teacher Marghe Mills-Thysen and BMC practitioner Michael Ridge for their lovely drawings; and huge bundles of love to Deirdre Spero for her generosity and patient care with editing, organizing, and preparing photos together over several months.

Thank you also to these individuals who have contributed their heartfelt support over the time of writing this book and beyond, enlivening my journey and allowing me to complete this manuscript: Jacques Talbot, for his thoughtful conversations and edits on the more philosophical chapters of the manuscript; Judy Gantz, Ann Vanderburgh, Ellen Tadd, Kimberly McKeever, and Sean Feit for reading specific brief sections of the manuscript during the editing process; Jaspen Amadeo and Jamie McHugh for providing moral support and synchronistic nature writing retreats at pivotal junctures in the writing process; Eleanor Criswell Hanna for her support and for permission to reprint material from my articles in *Somatics Journal* for this book.

For help with myriad other details of book production, thank you to Sanghi Choi, Andrea Olsen, Mo Miner, Basha Cohen, Len Cohen, Issa Cohen, Cindy Ma, and Ted Zeff. And special appreciation to BMC teacher Amelia Ender and practitioner Michael Ridge, for contributing suggestions and edits for the original masters thesis manuscript on which I based this book.

Warm thanks also to these friends and colleagues: Joanna Macy, Don Hanlon Johnson, Will Grant, Shannon Preto, John Genyo Sprague, David Rosenmiller,

Gill Wright-Miller, Greg Vennell, Effie Dilworth, Susie Richardson, Melanie Rios Glasner, Nancy Ng, Patricia Reedy, Penny Campbell, Peggy Schwartz, Lenore Grubinger, Sarah White, Galen Cranz, Chris Balme, Rae Johnson, Toni Smith, Margit Galanter, Amanda Williamson, Diane Butler, Mark Griffith, Xiuhtezcatl Martinez, Karen Risdon, and Terry Sendgraff. And special thanks to Carol Swann and Martha Eddy for their innovative work as founders of Moving on Center School in Oakland, California, and for their support of my first Somatics in Education program there.

Appreciation and thanks also to the devoted contribution of ISMETA and its Board, especially those board members with whom I served and who inspire our collective vision: Elisa Cotroneo, Mark Taylor, Teri Carter, Elisabeth Osgood-Campbell, Kimberly McKeever, Crystal Davis, and Tony Rezac.

Many of my students and clients, too numerous to name, have also been my inspiration and have provided enthusiastic support; thank you especially to all those who have participated in the Embodiment in Education workshops over the years. I have learned so much from all we have shared.

And finally, thank you to my mother and father, for encouraging me to follow my dreams, and for their love and inspiration as writers. And warm and loving thanks to my sister and others in my family, who have always believed in me, with special love to my nieces Rimley and Sitara, the two main teens in my own life.

Introduction

Everyone, no matter who, should learn as much as they can about their bodies—your body is with you forever!

—Sarah, seventeen-year-old high school senior

Most young people in the United States have twelve years or more of formal education, with an emphasis on learning to develop the intellect. While strong academics are important of course, the view of learning as a solely cognitive function, without any thought given to the role of the body, cumulatively perpetuates the body-mind split so detrimental to our well-being. Learning about our bodies as well as cultivating the capacity to be *fully* present—awake, attentive, and responsive to both our inner and outer worlds—can positively influence all aspects of our lives. As we learn to bring heightened awareness to our bodies and use that awareness to adapt in ways that promote well-being, we enhance our resilience to meet life's challenges.

This book represents an invitation to heal the body-mind dichotomy by presenting an avenue to help adolescents develop an *embodied self-awareness.* Embodiment is a fact of life. Yet *how* we embody ourselves—how we experience being a sensate physical individual and how we move and express that in the world—varies widely from person to person. Embodiment is also a process, one that evolves throughout our lifetimes in response to inner and outer circumstances.

As part of their core education, youth need to have opportunities to learn about their own bodies and, just as important, the relationship between their body and their mind—to develop inner resources and tap into their body intelligence on a regular basis. Somatic education practices, like those that form the basis of the curriculum in this book, provide a dynamic and engaging format for students to begin to participate in this lifelong process. The word "somatic," derived from the Greek word *sōmatikos,* means "pertaining to the body" and today encompasses a range of learning systems involving movement and sensory perception.

Whether or not you have a background in somatic education, the material presented in this book offers a pathway to understanding this evolving field and discovering the concrete benefits of introducing body-based curricula for youth to cultivate their somatic awareness. The material I am offering here serves as a guide and model for a somatic movement education curriculum designed specifically for teens, drawing on my own particular background and insights. This work is relevant to many educators; you may be an educator with an interest in progressive and student-centered education, working with teens and young adults. You may be a somatic movement educator or a teacher with a background in anatomy. You may teach sports, dance, theater, yoga, martial arts, or mindfulness to adolescents, and wish to increase your understanding of somatic awareness practices to complement your teaching.

When I first discuss my work in body-mind awareness for teens with other adults, even if they aren't sure exactly what it means, I usually receive a response like this: first a big sigh, followed by something like, "Wow, I could have used that!" or "I wish *I* had that as a teen; my life would have been so different if I'd had some tools earlier on!" A few have simply been incredulous, asking such questions as, "How do you ever get kids off their screens?" or my personal favorite, "How do you get teens to focus on their bodies—that's like teaching a cat to swim!" My experience has shown quite the opposite: teenagers yearn for more concrete information about their bodies and tools to help with their well-being. In fact when I offered my first class in this material to teens, within a year the class was full with a waiting list of more than thirty students! Teenagers know they need support, and with the many mental and physical health challenges that have their onset in adolescence, such as anxiety, depression, and eating disorders[1]—along with the ever-present distraction of screens and social media—we need to take the well-being of adolescents very seriously.

We've all heard the phrase "Know thyself." To promote their well-being, teens need a context in which they can slow down, settle into themselves, and pay attention to their inner reality. Without this inner awareness, as well as practical tools to manage their inner lives, young people often find that navigating their lives—not to mention learning, thriving, and living with purpose and vitality—can be a complex challenge. Traditional education is generally so driven by academic requirements, however, that there usually isn't room for the individual to self-locate, short-changing other aspects of self-development. What would it be like for teens to reawaken to their innate body intelligence, for instance, and learn how to integrate it in their busy lives?

As adults many of us have learned that when we feel stressed and anxious, our bodies tighten and our movement becomes constricted; when our bodies are tense, we may feel more anxious, perpetuating the problem. If we become more relaxed and flexible in our bodies and our movement, however, we also begin to feel more relaxed, adaptable, and "at home" in ourselves.

How might this feeling of being at home in their bodies impact teens' well-being as they struggle to cope with the stresses of adolescence and as they mature into adulthood? How can we help our youth to know this experience, along with the many other benefits of somatic practices?

We can each truly only begin from where we are. We begin with a simple process of coming back to basics to learn about our bodies and awaken more of our sensory awareness through movement. Movement is an expression of our life-force, and our bodies are the source of that expression. Through somatic movement education, students have an opportunity to learn about their bodies, to move, to lie down and be still, and to share their feelings and perceptions with each other. As they pay closer attention to what is within, they settle into themselves more deeply. This process of embodiment helps teens gain self-awareness, develop their kinesthetic intelligence, and establish a healthy body image. Students are also guided to discover both what they know about their bodies as well as the questions they may have. This approach provides a model in which students at any level of cognitive and physical ability can equally participate within a cohesive learning community.

Through the lessons in this curriculum, a student's own moving body becomes the lab through which to learn concrete anatomy, along with body awareness, self-care, injury prevention, and emotional resilience. From basics such as learning about their bones, muscles, organs, and proprioception to more advanced levels in which students apply this initial experiential learning to areas such as alignment and warm-up, these lessons encourage students to think *and move* to keep learning fun! These basic embodiment practices also establish the foundation for further skill development in sports, dance, and other leisure activities as teens gain both confidence and physical prowess. Having developed the curriculum over many years, I have long held the vision of the benefits of somatic education for our next generation.

A Case Study of Embodiment: My Own Path in Somatic Practices

Throughout my career, I have been privileged to work with children and adults as an educator in both community and academic settings in the United States and abroad, aspiring to support them as whole human beings—particularly in the transitional phases of adolescence and early adulthood. I've seen the amazing transformational effects that engaging in somatic movement education can have on individuals and communities alike, and experienced these in my own life as well, all of which has inspired me to develop this curriculum and to write this book.

In my early teens I discovered my passion for movement and dance and began weekly dance lessons. In the small town in New Jersey where I grew up, this meant classes in ballet, jazz, and tap. Soon I was dancing five or six days a week, and often cleaning the dance studio on Sundays to help pay for my classes. I also began to venture into New York City to study there as well. Even with my many years of intensive dance training, however, beyond being introduced to some anatomy in biology courses I had taken in my public high school, it was not until entering college that I received much education about my body—or encountered the concept of body wisdom for that matter.

As part of the dance program at Middlebury College, I was introduced to something called "experiential anatomy" through a course taught by Caryn McHose.[2] A major focus of the course was on participating in exercises described in Mabel Elsworth Todd's *The Thinking Body: A Study of the Balancing Forces of Dynamic Man,* first published in 1937. As a dancer and movement educator, Caryn had spent four years—much of it alone in a cabin in Vermont—working with Todd's book, along with an anatomy and physiology textbook, immersed in learning and integrating the material in her own body. This process afforded her the time necessary to begin to make the connection from words and images to deep, embodied sensory perception.[3] Throughout my course with her, she guided us to similarly deepen and personalize our learning—studying the anatomy and physiology of our own bodies through movement, journal writing, and by coloring anatomy drawings. We also used creative visualizations and other movement activities to learn how to move with less tension and develop new, freer movement—a method called *repatterning.*

My study of experiential anatomy with Caryn was reinforced in my modern dance classes with Andrea Olsen, who incorporated anatomy into her technique classes. For instance, for a month we would repeat the same warm-up phrase, but with a different focus each week—first feeling the support of our bones one week, then exploring the fullness of our organs, such as the lungs and heart, in our movement the next. As was true in my classes with Caryn, in exploring these variations I found that Andrea's own embodied expression also informed my own.

All of this experiential learning helped me to develop a much more realistic understanding of my body that helped me improve my range of motion, and move with more ease and vitality in my dancing. As an added benefit, I found that problems I had been having with my feet began to diminish as I spent time both in and out of class working on related activities and visualizations. This was especially significant in my case, as I had been born with a birth condition that affected my feet and ankles, and despite several operations before age fourteen to improve my movement function, I had continued to have occasional sprains and injuries. Shortly after my last operation, to my dismay I had even been told by a doctor specializing in dance medicine that I should stop dancing.

Spurred on by my love of dance, I instead continued to search for ways to expand my potential, and was inspired when I finally discovered an approach—experiential anatomy—that began to help me. Our final projects in the course were geared toward exploring a particular area of the body, and compiling a "body portfolio," about both the anatomy of that area and our personal relationship with our own bodies. My project, which I focused on my feet, helped me reflect on and integrate some of the challenges I'd faced; others in the class seemed to similarly dive into areas of personal significance, and emerge with fresh insight into themselves.

This more holistic approach to movement was very new to me as a dancer. Until then, I had spent hours working to control and mold my body, having been taught to view it as an object, the "tool" of my art form. My early dance experience had surely given me self-discipline, confidence, and technical skill. But my experience in these new classes opened up new worlds as they focused on the inner experience of movement, not just on replicating the outer form. Here I was able to explore and get to know myself in new ways, moving from within. This more sensory approach supported me to dance with less injury and to express myself in movement in a way that left me feeling much more present and empowered than before.

As I began to find out more about this field of inner body investigation, which I learned was a distinct area of study called "somatics," I discovered that several of the founders of particular somatic disciplines had similarly come to engage in personal research from a concern about their own body limitations that had not been adequately addressed through Western medicine alone. For example, F. M. Alexander, the founder of the Alexander Technique, was an Australian actor whose chronic laryngitis eventually caused doctors to suggest he find a new career. Instead, he began to observe his own body movement by looking in a mirror, and discovered that before speaking he would habitually move his head down and back. So he tried reversing that—moving his head forward and up before speaking, which also seemed to lengthen his spine—and soon found his bouts of laryngitis diminished and his voice improved. He later founded the Alexander Technique based on this principle, which he called inhibition, a process of consciously inhibiting a certain movement and substituting it with another, more integrated, movement pattern.[4] Other pioneers who founded specific somatic disciplines—such as Moshe Feldenkrais (the Feldenkrais Method®), Bonnie Bainbridge Cohen (Body-Mind Centering®), Emilie Conrad (Continuum Movement®), and Thomas Hanna (Hanna Somatics)—similarly discovered many of their insights and techniques through their own movement investigations.

After graduating from college, I dove deeper into studying somatics, primarily the experiential anatomy practices of Body-Mind Centering with Bonnie Bainbridge Cohen, which blossomed into an extensive study over many years. I also studied other somatic methods, namely Ideokinesis with Irene Dowd, along with the Feldenkrais Method and Bartenieff Fundamentals. Each of these somatic disciplines teaches unique embodiment methods, with myriad specific, practical applications to dance, movement, and other areas of life. (Interested readers can see chapter 2, "Somatic

Education and Other Influences: The Roots of the Curriculum," for more about the lineage and methods of somatic education.)

Developing a Curriculum for Teens and a Training for Educators

My teaching methods and the curriculum presented in this book have developed out of my own dance and somatics background, my ongoing experiential research with students and colleagues, and my own intuitive responses. Now many years after I first began teaching teens, I have found that the passionate vision I had of bringing somatic practices to youth is progressively being supported by recent research on adolescent development. This includes cutting-edge research in psychology and neuroscience that emphasizes the benefits of teaching aspects such as mindfulness and social and emotional intelligence, as will be explored further in chapter 1. Although these skill sets were not explicitly identified as central to education in the 1990s—independent courses didn't exist at that time to address topics such as mindful presence, self-awareness, self-regulation, and social awareness, for example—the experiential anatomy practices I draw upon naturally incorporated these elements already.

This may, in fact, be one of the reasons that somatic education proved so efficacious in my work with teens, as I discovered in my early days of teaching, when, upon graduating from college, I began working at several private middle and high schools in New England. There I quickly recognized the hunger students had to understand and feel more "at home" in their bodies, and started to bring these somatic methods into my work as a dance educator. I also developed a separate course in experiential anatomy that was offered outside of the dance curriculum—to bring the wealth of these somatic practices to *all* students, not just dancers. Whether or not someone has a particular interest in excelling in dance or sports, there is an inner world inside each of us that awaits our attention, one which, when given time to explore, can profoundly support our growth. Whether offered in a therapeutic or an educational context, this process of self-discovery is deeply personal, and needs both a clear, strong container and a wise, trustworthy guide to facilitate the process and respond to our unique challenges.

As I continued my work with teens, for instance, I soon began to see how their body image and self-esteem were profoundly impacted—often to their detriment—by the culture and media around them, such as advertising, movies, and video games. I began developing specific activities to help my students recognize inherent biases and judgments they hold that impact how they move, as well as how they view themselves and others, such as, for example, perceptions about posture. The resulting evolving awareness empowered them to see beyond their cultural conditioning and to begin to make more conscious choices, as well as to gain respect for themselves and their peers.

Over time it became clear that, in addition to being informative, my classes were creating a space for a warm and compassionate community to blossom among these teens. Here they could share their perspectives with their peers, learn about themselves and their bodies, and begin to truly flourish. Over an initial period of twelve years teaching at the middle and high school levels, I found that adolescents benefited enormously from these experiential approaches during this sensitive developmental phase when lifelong habits are being formed.

During that time, I offered the material in a variety of educational contexts. In the first school I taught at, I created a semester-long academic course for high school students in the Science and Humanities department. In another instance, my class was offered as a physical education unit for middle school students. When the athletic director began to notice how much the students in these classes were improving in their sports—better able to focus and less prone to injury during their seasonal matches—she invited me to offer the class as part of the preseason summer camp for the girls' field hockey team. The dancers in my technique classes also seemed to benefit from these approaches. Inspired by all of these experiences, I first formalized and documented a curriculum in somatic movement education in 1994 as my master's thesis for Wesleyan University, entitled "A Body/Mind Approach to Movement Education for Adolescents."

Since then I have spent many years teaching teens and young adults in schools and universities across the United States and in Asia, refining and augmenting the curriculum as I learn more about what my students need. I have come to see that while significant differences exist between cultures, adolescents nevertheless share some basic challenges related to movement and body image that appear to be more universal. When teaching teens in Thailand, for instance, my translator struggled to find words to express the concept of "body-mind"—since this Cartesian split is not part of Thai culture. Nevertheless, similar to their counterparts in the United States, the students I taught lacked concrete knowledge about their physical bodies and often experienced stress and self-consciousness. Across these cultural divides, however, teens also exhibit an innate curiosity about the body which, when nurtured, begins to slowly grow and enthusiastically prosper.

At the experimental school I taught at in Thailand,[5] for example, students are not required to attend any classes. Even so, at my first class an initial twelve curious teens showed up. The next day, they all returned and another dozen students also came. Each session involved both active movement explorations as well as inner-directed, meditative activities. The first day, for instance, I led an activity that I call "the Mind's Eye and the Body Systems," in which students are asked to lie down, close their eyes, and use their "mind's eye" to look inside their own bodies to discover what is there. I asked several questions to guide the visualization, such as: What can you see inside your body? How do you feel about what you see? What do you know about what's inside your body? What is a *mystery* to you? Later, students drew their perceptions and then gathered in small groups to discuss and share their drawings. They were also asked to make a list of any questions they had. Finally, we reconvened and students shared their drawings and some of their questions with the full group. Some of their questions included the following:

- How many bones are there in our bodies?
- Which is the largest bone in the body? The smallest?
- Do boys and girls have the same skeletal systems?
- What's in our blood?
- How does our digestive system work?
- How do we breathe?

In response to their questions, in the following sessions I was able to naturally progress to topics that interested them. Activities I led (each of which is included in this book) included "Bone Tracing" (in which students find the shape and location of the bones in their own bodies and learn their names), "Curves of the Spine" (in which students work in partners to count the vertebrae and discover the potential movements of the spine), and "How Do We Breathe?" (in which students locate the diaphragm and discover the relationship between the lungs in the thoracic cavity and the organs in the abdominal cavity to help them breathe more deeply). I also introduced corresponding readings on topics such as mindful breathing, written by the Vietnamese monk Thich Nhat Hahn, since many of the students were already familiar with his teachings. Students were fascinated to learn these simple techniques to begin to understand more about their own bodies, let go of some of their mental and physical tensions, and move with more ease. As students gained a more comprehensive understanding of their own bodies, they also came to respect individual differences and recognize their commonalities as human beings. Such profound yet simple realizations added to a growing sense of caring for themselves and others.

In 2008, I developed a training workshop for professional dance and movement educators called Embodiment in Education,[6] introducing my methods for teaching somatic practices with teens and young adults. I was very curious to see who else would be interested in such a topic, and was inspired to discover that over the next few years, participants from a variety of professional backgrounds from across the United States and six different countries attended: dance educators, outdoor educators, somatic psychologists, martial artists, yoga teachers, and environmental advocates, as well as educators and practitioners from many different somatic disciplines. What united us all was a shared passion for creating more pathways for our students to engage with the living body. Over the years the program has provided fertile ground to discuss the challenges of translating somatic education material into various cultural and educational contexts, and has become an inspiring incubator of fresh approaches. I have also often invited guest faculty such as Bonnie Bainbridge Cohen, Caryn McHose, and Deane Juhan to help expand our perspectives.

Through all of these experiences, I have come to recognize somatic movement education curriculum tailored to adolescents as an additional essential element to twenty-first-century educational models that prioritize students' inner lives, by helping teens gain tools to develop to their full potential, as I invite you to explore with me in this book.

An Overview of This Book

Part I, A Case for Somatic Movement Education for Teens, provides the rationale for including somatic movement education as an essential and imperative component of adolescent education. Responding to the question "Why teach teens about their bodies?" we'll look at the philosophical and theoretical basis of the curriculum, along with benefits of this work related to current educational practices, such as mindfulness and social and emotional learning. As many of the curricular goals relate to national education standards in many subjects, such as dance, physical education, science, and health and wellness, I will also address some of these correlations. Sections of chapter 1 take a slightly more academic angle than much of the rest of the book, as a means to build upon contemporary viewpoints germane to a discussion of education. This will assist readers who are seasoned educators but who may be new to a somatic approach to relate it with concepts and practices that may be more familiar, as well as to help somatic professionals to appreciate correlations between somatics and current best practices in education. Here I also discuss some of the specific challenges of teaching this material to teens, and ways in which I have shaped this curriculum to meet the particular needs of adolescents.

Chapter 2 provides a brief overview for readers who may be new to the field of somatics, including the realm of experiential or "embodied" anatomy that forms the primary basis of this curriculum. Readers already familiar with the history of somatics and its practices may be most interested in material at the end of this chapter, where I also touch briefly on the specific somatic disciplines and related fields of study, such as ecosomatics and dance anthropology, which have also informed my curriculum and may be of interest.

Part II, Getting Started: A Guide for Facilitators, will introduce readers to specifics of the curriculum, along with key considerations, such as teacher qualifications, characteristics of an appropriate "classroom," which activities are appropriate for different ages, and how and where it might be offered within or outside of a school context. It also discusses key points about curriculum design and implementation, like how to set up the space and introduce the class to students, along with supplemental supplies that may be needed.

Part II also provides guidance on how best to use this book, and key pedagogical principles to help prepare the way for understanding and implementing the activities presented in part III. Here you will find a discussion of eight essential pedagogy tips needed to adapt somatic movement education to meet the needs and sensitivities of adolescents. These teaching principles are vital to understanding the student-centered approaches presented in this book. This section also provides key concepts to consider when giving verbal instructions and speaking with your students, so that your use of language can effectively support embodied learning.

Finally, I address some of the complexity of including somatic movement education in schools and other programs for youth, beginning with the issue of touch and offering four specific guidelines for responsibly including touch-based activities within the program. While self-touch activities—such as using touch to locate the specific bones of the feet—are integral to the curriculum, activities in which students touch each other may be adapted or omitted as appropriate to a particular context. The chapter also covers some complex topics that need to be considered as well, such as stress, trauma, and sex and sexuality. All of these chapters will help prepare readers who may have the necessary background to teach the curriculum activities themselves, which are presented in parts III and IV.

Parts III and IV, A Curriculum in SME: Embodied Anatomy for Teens, comprise the heart of this book—the curriculum itself. The nine chapters from chapter 7 through 16 are divided into two levels: *Embodiment Basics—Level I* covers basics like body scanning and learning about body systems and proprioception, while *Embodiment Fundamentals—Level II* covers more advanced activities in which students apply this initial experiential learning to areas such as alignment, breathing, and warm-up. In each of these chapters, you will find basic anatomical information about each topic, along with specific introductory activities and anecdotal commentary about students' responses. Also included for your reference are myriad photos of teenagers engaging in many of the activities, to give you a practical sense of how these are done, along with examples of related student journal entries and drawings. You'll also find some photos of adult educators participating in them as well. There are also tips for facilitating the activities, and suggestions for further related activities like home practices or group projects. The last chapter of part IV offers some final comments, along with excerpts from students' journals to give further voice to their unique perspectives on engaging in these practices.

The final chapter, **Afterword: Envisioning the Future of Somatic Education**, briefly discusses the potential of creating a more body-based, somatically informed education for our teens, using examples from my own consulting and teaching, along with that of some of my students and colleagues, to make this more concrete and imaginable. Here readers will also find further academic discussion of the need to ensure greater diversity in and access to the field of somatic education as the profession moves forward, along with some suggestions in support of that goal.

Appendix A provides a summary sheet for easy reference of the eight pedagogy principles for teaching somatic movement education to adolescents, and **Appendix B** summarizes the four guidelines for introducing what I refer to as intentional touch.

A Note on Origins and Crediting

The activities in this book, which I call "explorations," draw from my background in movement and experiential anatomy, and may combine elements from several somatic disciplines. Many activities are explicitly my original design, such as several of the posture activities, the Breath of Life activity, or the Responsive Moving activity, for instance. In a few cases, explorations are more direct adaptations of activities used in a specific somatic discipline, or may be adapted from something designed by a particular teacher. In these cases, I have credited and referenced the origin of the activity, as well as directing the reader to the original version in the endnotes. This will help those readers who want to examine both versions to see how I have adapted my version for teenagers and young adults; in other cases I have stated that explicitly.

In this sense, I am not claiming that this curriculum is entirely my own creation. Rather, it is a combination of original and derived material to form an aggregate of approaches. While I have made every attempt to credit material where possible, as part of a lineage of movers and educators it can become difficult to trace the origins of some movement activities, particularly those drawing from dance and creative movement, and I apologize for any inadvertent omissions or misrepresentations.

Who Can Use This Book?

This book is for adults working with adolescents and young adults—particularly those with experience teaching some form of movement, social-emotional learning, health and wellness, meditation, mindfulness, drama, dance, physical education, and a variety of other movement forms like yoga, qi gong, or aikido. If you are active in any of these spheres, you recognize the importance of helping students develop inner awareness and related core life skills! Somatic movement educators and other movement teachers with an anatomy background and experience teaching adolescents will find this material especially relevant, and would likely be prime teachers of this material.

Sports coaches, camp staff, outdoor leadership facilitators, physical trainers, and physical and occupational therapists will find valuable material here as well. These professionals can augment their programs by adding aspects of these embodied movement practices to improve individuals' physical skills, as well as to build heightened awareness and compassion among group members. Others who work with teens—middle and high school teachers, counselors, therapists, social workers, conflict resolution and restorative justice leaders, administrators, home school educators, and consultants—can also benefit from learning about this somatic approach. Parents may find this book inspiring as a means of reflecting upon and understanding their own teen years and deepening their body-mind relationship; the curriculum may provide a model program that could be a beneficial addition to their child's school as well as to their family lives.

Finally, no matter what your particular background, I hope that this book will be an inspiration for you personally to reclaim an intimate fascination with your *own* body and bring a sense of newness to your experience. As I learned in my own journey, the body is an ever-transforming miracle of nature. Remembering this, we can each engage in a dynamic process of movement and body awareness as a means to become more resourced, self-aware, and fully alive. With all of the challenges facing us individually and as a global community, deepening our appreciation and awareness of our own bodies and our vital capacity for movement can be a profound reminder of the mystery of life that we are all a part of, and that we can continue to explore together. As educators begin to establish a context to bring this inspiring somatic inquiry process to our youth, it is my sincere belief that the benefits will expand exponentially through a next generation of more compassionate, whole, empowered, and embodied individuals.

PART I

A CASE FOR SOMATIC MOVEMENT EDUCATION FOR TEENS

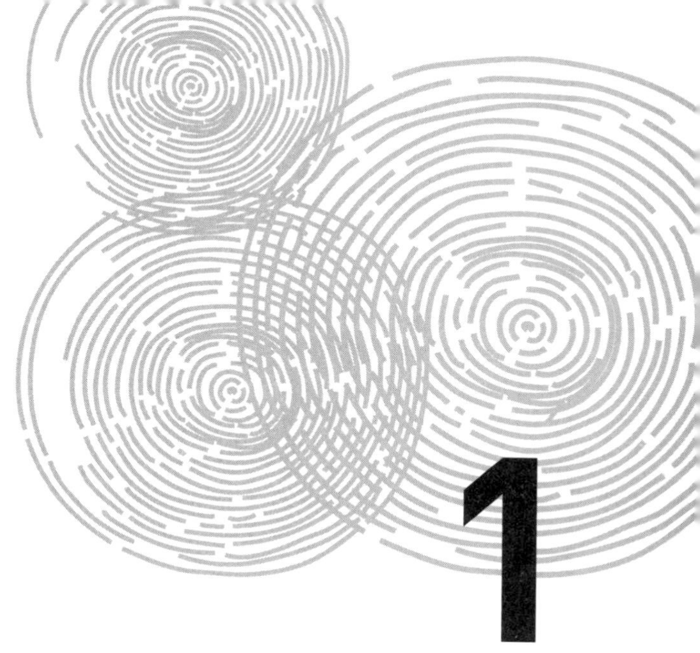

1

Why Teach Teens about Their Bodies?

The human body is not an instrument to be used, but a realm of one's being to be experienced, explored, enriched, and thereby, educated.

—Thomas Hanna

Adolescence is a pivotal stage of life: our teenage years can be a time of self-discovery, allowing us to explore our potential, develop our unique gifts, and set a healthy trajectory for the rest of our lives. Yet even in the best-case scenario, adolescence—loosely defined as the period of life when a child develops into an adult—can also prove to be a tumultuous period of adaptation. Teens face myriad inner and outer challenges, ranging from increasing changes in their brain chemistry and hormones, to pressures at school, at home, and from their peers. They struggle with complex lifestyle decisions that affect their well-being, regarding diet, sleep, exercise, sex, drugs, alcohol, and relationships. Increasingly, social media is both a distraction and a way of life for teens, with pop culture images and messages from a plethora of media sources affecting their self-image and self-esteem. Education reform presents another stressful challenge for today's teenagers, as standardized testing acquires greater importance at each new grade level. There has also been a rise of disturbing issues plaguing our schools, such as bullying, teen suicide, and incidents of school violence. As the complexity of modern life increases, it becomes more difficult to shield our youth from the stresses that lead to many of these issues.

Teens also confront momentous choices to do with their future, from the stress of their first job or applying to and deciding on college, to adapting to the workforce or college life, and integrating into their community as a young adult. Further, the pressures of current world events and environmental disasters are ever-present in their lives, as they are for all of us, presenting yet another source of stress, anxiety, and deep concern. And while nature can be a soothing balm in our otherwise hectic lives, many teens, as well as adults, have become alarmingly disconnected from the natural world around them—and have in many ways lost touch with both their inner *and* outer resources. All of these factors contribute to the pressing need to help adolescents successfully manage one of the most complicated—and potentially empowering—stages of life.

What resources do teens have to navigate these many volatile physical, emotional, and psychological challenges? Fortunately, educators and parents alike have begun to recognize that students need more than academics to thrive; they also need to develop essential life skills that fall outside the boundaries of purely cognitive learning. These skills, often referred to as "soft skills" and "non-cognitive skills," encourage self-reflection and a focus on students' inner lives as a means to develop as strong individuals and engaged learners. Such skills are increasingly valued in education today, and represent a shift from a focus on mere skill acquisition to also helping teens cultivate qualities or *capacities* that will support them throughout their lives.[1] This can be seen in the growing number of schools that dedicate time to independent classroom programs in areas such as mindfulness and social and emotional learning (SEL). SEL programs, many of them inspired by Daniel Goleman's book *Emotional Intelligence,* help students develop core competencies like self-awareness, self-management, and social awareness. Mindfulness programs, based on the work of Jon Kabat-Zinn, Thich Nhat Hanh, and others are also being widely introduced into schools worldwide to help teens use meditation and related practices to become more self-aware and deal with stress and anxiety.

While twenty years ago such programs were virtually nonexistent, there are now a growing number of curricular models in both mindfulness and SEL that can help students develop such essential life skills. For example, ten different countries and fifteen states in the U.S. now have independent programs that offer mindfulness in schools,[2] and SEL is offered in various districts in at least seven different states.[3] Project-based learning is another approach also increasingly being adopted in schools to encourage engaged, experiential education. Clearly this is a revolutionary time in education, and—within the many complex sociopolitical challenges of the times—adults are working hard to innovate and augment strong academics to serve the deeper, holistic needs of our youth to prepare them for an ever-changing world.

Yet even with all this well-intentioned revolutionary fervor, a crucial avenue has yet to be fully explored in adolescent education: the essential role of the *body* and *movement* in well-being. Sadly, like many adults, today's teens often know more about their cell phones than they do about their own bodies! On the other hand, teens are intensely focused on their bodies—often in unhealthy ways. They think about their appearance, weight, physical skill in sports and athletics, and especially about how they are perceived by their peers. With all this mental and emotional focus on their bodies, actual study of the body is mostly omitted from school curricula, except when offered marginally in biology or health class.

In her book *BodyStories,* Andrea Olsen notes, "the lack of information about the human body in our years of education is startling since it is our home for an entire lifetime." Silence around the body is of particular concern for teens, since the body is a major source of self-esteem, both positive and negative. As adolescents bloom into their sexuality, they may find that parents and teachers alike largely avoid the body as too volatile or taboo a subject to be dealt with openly. Frankly, the adolescent body is the elephant in the room, and too few schools have done anything to help students deal with this huge beast!

Although programs in dance and movement education are somewhat common in curricula for young children, movement curricula for adolescents have mainly consisted of Physical Education (PE) programs in sports and athletics, and, only occasionally, in dance.[4] And while some school districts today may be more progressive in their offerings, many programs still focus largely on particular physical skills being developed, such as being able to throw a ball or jump a hurdle—a measure of physical prowess, but not necessarily a measure of health or well-being. Despite the many benefits of athletics and team sports, these programs can end up alienating students who don't succeed in such skill-based approaches, and then often develop a negative body image and a negative relationship to movement and physical activity in general.

Outside of PE, the role of movement has been marginalized—and its benefits often overlooked—with students spending hours on end sitting at desks, such that being quiet and immobile has long been equated with being a "good student." Even when movement is encouraged, such as in PE or recess times between classes, it is often regarded as a "break" that is supposed to "refresh" students for further academic learning, rather than being recognized for having intrinsic value for the development of the individual. This is particularly evident now, with budget cuts limiting or eliminating programs in PE, arts, sports teams, and after-school programming in many states across the country. Compounding the problem, as technology becomes increasingly complex and central to modern living, the urge to keep overvaluing information and data over knowledge and *experience,* continues to increase. In fact Nielsen ratings note that in the United States both children and adults spend an average of six hours a day sitting still in front of some kind of screen or monitor.[5] Simultaneously, childhood obesity is a dire issue, with the Centers for Disease Control and Prevention reporting that one in five children in the U.S. qualifies as obese,[6] and further studies predicting the problem to be dangerously on the rise.[7]

Youth need more than just an opportunity to get up and move in PE class, however; teens need an entirely new framework for understanding their bodies and the relationship between their physical and emotional well-being. Adolescents need structured and experiential means to develop a level of comfort with their own bodies. This includes a clear context to learn about their bodies and develop a healthy body image and self-perception. They also need to be seen and appreciated for *who they are,* not just for what they can accomplish. A body-based, somatic approach gives teens the time and space to learn more about themselves, while gaining concrete information about their bodies that helps them become more confident, grounded, and empowered individuals. In fact, without accurate information about their bodies, teenagers will generally substitute whatever ideas they are exposed to from media, the internet, and those around them.

Consider these fascinating misperceptions. Did you know that most teens imagine their spines to be *straight* rather than *curved,* from having been told repeatedly to "stand up straight" or "not slouch"? Many have been so imbued with this delusion that when asked to draw their spines, they will generally draw a "straight pole" image—a perception that actually causes unnecessary tension in their bodies. Many teens also believe the abdominal area should move *inward* when they inhale (maintaining the "flat abs" ideal), which causes shallow breathing by impeding the natural descent of the diaphragm necessary for full breathing. These are just two of the most startling examples from many I have encountered over my years of working with youth. Likewise, many adults—who have also had little education about their own bodies—hold these same erroneous notions. Many of us have held such perceptions throughout our lives, without realizing the impact they have on our well-being and our enjoyment in being alive.

The Body in Education

How is it that we have so little education related to our living bodies? While beyond the scope of this book to explore the extensive roots of the historical repression of our bodies in American culture, several factors are worthy of note. As neuroscientist Stephen W. Porges notes, this marginalization of the body goes back to Descartes's dictum, "I think therefore I am," which has led to equating "smartness" with cognitive skill.[8] The impact of prioritizing cognitive intelligence should not be underestimated. As Porges laments, "despite this enhanced level of smartness, we have become literally ignorant about what our bodies really need to feel good."[9] In our education at large, when study of the body *is* included, the body is generally studied as an object, rather than by personalizing our learning to include our own body awareness.

In human biology for instance, you learn through readings, pictures, and plastic models. Rarely do we refer to, touch, or move our own body in studying the human structure or the mechanics of movement. Bonnie Bainbridge Cohen, founder of the School for Body-Mind Centering, notes with astonishment that our inner body awareness has been virtually omitted from the traditionally named five senses, and that "as all sciences are reflections of the socio-politico-religious ideas of their time, it is appropriate that the historical repression of bodily sensation in Western culture has been transmitted as a matter of scientific fact."[10] In physical education and many approaches to dance, the body is similarly objectified, primarily considered as a tool to be refined and controlled for the achievement of specific physical goals. There is much more to consider than physical prowess, however, in creating a holistic and more inclusive body-based education.

In the 1980s Howard Gardner, a developmental psychologist at Harvard University, paved the way toward recognizing the importance of the body and movement in education by including "bodily/kinesthetic awareness" in his theory of multiple intelligences. Gardner defined seven categories of interrelated "intelligences": linguistic, musical, logical, spatial, kinesthetic/bodily, interpersonal, and intrapersonal, and thereby succeeded in bringing the term *kinesthetic intelligence* into the national discussion of educational reform.[11] However, even Gardner objectified the body, referring to "control of one's bodily motions and the capacity to handle objects skillfully," such as that exhibited by a tennis player or violinist, as the core of bodily intelligence.[12] As noted by the pioneering dance therapist Mary Whitehouse, there is a difference between moving for the purpose of developing *specific movement skills* and moving for the experience of *deepened psychophysical awareness,*

> Physical activities are helpful ... at least they help us to move.... But they don't connect us with ourselves, because they still have a motive external to the experience of ourselves. They still put us in the position of moving our bodies for a purpose, instead of becoming aware of ourselves.[13]

In Gardner's model of kinesthetic intelligence, a kind of top-down approach is encouraged in which the mind informs the body and directs our movement toward an outer goal that we aspire to excel in. This is one approach to developing movement skill—and is one measure of kinesthetic intelligence. Yet as somatic educator Jamie McHugh notes, this "is truly not body wisdom, no more than someone who excels at taking a test is wise."[14] We may achieve the goal, but at what cost? Often such physical striving necessitates neglecting inconvenient messages from our bodies, such as fatigue or soreness, to reach our intended goals. Despite the self-discipline and other strengths this approach may afford, it can also lead to strains, injury, or even a sense of inadequacy from feeling that our personal value is being based on our level of physical competency.

Coupled with the copious distractions of modern life, this skill-based model can encourage the perception of the body as somehow separate from the self, yet nothing could be further from the truth. As somatic educator and bodyworker Deane Juhan explains,

> How completely I sense my body and how I feel about it has everything to do with the particular course of events going on within it. Attitudes, postures, patterns of behavior, and physiological functions are inextricably fused together in our organisms, and it is primarily my conscious awareness of their interrelationship which gives me some measure of control over my well-being … the only facts about myself that are altogether real to me are those that have come through my own attentiveness.[15]

An approach to developing kinesthetic intelligence that includes attention to students' subjective experience—their inner sensations, emotions, and perceptions—is therefore essential if it is to truly improve well-being and have any real value or meaning for teens. Yet the subjective reality of a teenager is so often precisely what adults don't want to deal with, creating a cycle of frustration for teens, whose primary reality is often deemed as inadmissible evidence![16] In her book *The Awakened Family,* clinical psychologist Shefali Tsabary writes about the dire ramifications of such interactions:

> When children aren't given the space to assert their authentic voice, but are drowned out by the roar of our … agendas, they grow up anxious and depressed. Many of our young people are so deprived of our acceptance—of simply being *seen for who they are*—that they self-harm in a variety of ways. Getting drunk, taking drugs, engaging in inappropriate sexual relations … all of these are cries for our acceptance. They are manifestations of a deep yearning to be seen, validated, and known.[17]

The causes of such behaviors clearly can have many complex psychophysical and socioeconomic roots as well; yet in any case such self-abusive behaviors can become dire problems with both short- and potentially long-term negative consequences.

As educators, we can support teenagers by both offering them a context in which to be seen and appreciated—making space for their personal expression—through many avenues, with a process of learning about themselves and their bodies being one of them. An experiential body-based and student-centered approach, especially in adolescence, when self-image and autonomy are of such major concern, can help students develop a sense of agency and increase their self-awareness. With this foundation, teens regain an essential self-respect and appreciation for the sacredness of life itself—instilling an increased respect for their own bodies that can lead to healthier behaviors.

Using a Somatic Education Approach to Support Adolescent Development

In this book, I propose an educational approach that is both cross-curricular and body-based to address these more *psychophysical* needs of adolescents and more fully support the whole person. While there are many elements involved in a well-balanced and in-depth education, I believe that having a basic understanding of the anatomy and physiology of one's own body—an understanding that is both personalized and physicalized—is a core competency. Somatic education can provide this type of learning, while expanding the definition of kinesthetic intelligence to include a deeper kinesthetic awareness available to *all* students—not just specialists—and which becomes a healthy foundation for learning complex gross motor skills and takes a more holistic approach.

In contrast to the "top-down" approach, a somatic approach to kinesthetic learning encourages a "bottom-up" approach in which the mind receives feedback from the body, activating more of a back and forth dialogue loop. For instance, many somatic movement activities are done initially only on one side of the body, affording us an opportunity to notice any changes that may have occurred in the process and compare that to our "normal" state, and then are repeated on the other side. Somatic movement is not just about *what* we are doing, but also considers *how* we are moving—where we are placing our attention or initiating our movement—as well as how the movement impacts us physically, mentally, and emotionally. Learning to *listen* as well as direct, we can move fluidly between top-down and bottom-up processing, as appropriate in each moment. Through a somatic approach we invite and contact more aspects of ourselves and can reconnect with our innate body wisdom. Applying this awareness, we learn to better care for ourselves. We might even call this *"somatic intelligence,"* which combines both kinesthetic intelligence and intrapersonal intelligence, and can actually be seen as the psychophysical basis for all other types of learning.

In his book *Intelligence in the Flesh,* Guy Claxton discusses the extensive research basis for claiming the central importance of "embodied intelligence," which rather than stemming primarily from the brain, resides in the integrated and systemic processes throughout the body.[18] In referring to Gardner's theories of multiple intelligences, Claxton offers a conclusion similar to my own:

> The view from the new science of embodiment ... suggests that these intelligences are not separate, and they are not of equal value ... practical embodied intelligence is the deepest, oldest, most fundamental and most important of the lot; and others are facets or outgrowths of this basic somatic capability. Emotional intelligence is an *aspect* of bodily intelligence.... To identify "bodily-kinaesthetic"

> intelligence just with what artisans have is to miss the fact that, at a deeper level, this one intelligence is in fact the root system on which all others depend.[19]

Movement is not something we should outgrow as we move on to "higher" levels of learning; rather, movement and the cultivation of enhanced body awareness should remain central to our education at every stage of life. The principles of neuroplasticity attest to this, as encapsulated in the famous phrase "use it or lose it" originated by neuroscientist Marion Diamond,[20] which indicates that neurological pathways, like muscles, strengthen through experience and atrophy when unused. Moreover, Claxton further emphasizes that the habitual diminishing of our bodily processes, whether through inattention or muscular tension, has been proven to have a powerfully negative effect on both social-emotional intelligence and cognition.[21] Recent studies have also demonstrated that people with higher levels of body awareness exhibit greater resilience, as they tend to recognize physical signs of stress earlier on and take steps to alleviate it, rather than allowing it to build up to the point of strain and illness.[22]

This is especially important in modern culture, which pushes us to achieve at all costs, as in the old adage, "all work and no play." Sitting for too long in schools and offices, training too hard in sports and athletics, and draining our energy with mental activity not balanced with physical activity are all signs of imbalance—beginning at a body level—that lead to injury, disease, and a range of mental health issues. A healthy paradigm for including the body in education would include helping young people to learn to engage their somatic awareness in a way that respects the rhythms of life: rhythms of the body, of nature, and of the inherent interdependence of all living things. When we learn to listen to our body, we begin to honor our need to pause, as well as to act. This leads to a more balanced life.

This deeper psychophysical learning process that somatics affords can therefore be a positive addition in our schools and youth programs to support physical, social-emotional, and academic learning. In fact a plethora of recent scientific research, examining the correlation between movement and academic achievement in youth, demonstrate that movement supports cognition. The proven physiological benefits of movement range from promoting clarity of mind by increasing blood flow to increasing levels of endorphins that lead to reduced stress and better mood and ability to focus, as well as increased growth factors that promote new nerve cells and enhance neuroplasticity.[23] The father of the progressive education movement himself, John Dewey, believed strongly in psychophysical learning as a foundation for abstract thinking and reasoning. Among other things, Dewey studied the Alexander Technique for realigning posture and decreasing muscular and mental tension. He appreciated the inherent value in somatic practice as a support and basis for learning in many aspects of education.[24]

Somatic Movement Education as a Complement to Dance, Physical Education, Science, and Health and Wellness Curricula

To introduce this more somatic approach, this curriculum draws on experiential anatomy, an aspect of somatic movement education in which one's own body becomes the "lab" through which one learns—through movement, touch, drawing, journal writing, and discussion. This process is both a scientific and humanistic approach, integrating many subject areas that encompass interpersonal, intrapersonal, cognitive, and kinesthetic learning. Because the material is cross-curricular—blending science, movement, mindfulness, and social-emotional learning—the curriculum easily aligns with many of the goals of current national and state standards for middle and high school students in areas such as dance, physical education, science, and health and wellness.

The benefits of somatic movement education are many. By helping students cultivate their kinesthetic intelligence, it can serve as a support for programs in dance and sports, and yet is also accessible to students with or without an interest in a particular movement form—providing another means of "physical education." Adding curriculum in experiential anatomy to the existing movement programs offered to adolescents also serves to balance the current focus on skill-based gross motor learning more prevalent in our schools with a more sensory-based experience accessible to students at all levels of ability. Based in scientific study of anatomy and physiology, the curriculum also provides a dynamic, personalized, and body-based complement to science curricula, such as biology and life sciences.

Further, students are provided with an opportunity to focus on themselves and the interconnection of body and mind at a time when this is particularly relevant to their self-development. Many of the skills that are cultivated relate to topics covered in health education, such as articulated in the National Health Standards for adolescents, like understanding the role of individual responsibility for enhancing health, describing ways to reduce or prevent injuries, and demonstrating healthy practices and behaviors that will maintain or improve health.[25]

The activities in this curriculum also help teens become aware of their cultural conditioning, with its myriad repercussions—on their bodies, their sense of self, and their expression in the world. By becoming more aware of their unconscious patterns and assumptions, students ultimately gain more choice and the possibility of consciously directing their development as individuals. This also begins to create a respectful community among teens in which to learn and interact. State and national health standards similarly include curricular goals to encourage adolescents to learn about these aspects: such as how culture and media influence their perceptions of body image and gender roles, the influence of technology on physical activity and personal health, and ways to support and encourage safe, respectful, and responsible relationships[26]—all topics explored in this curriculum.

When teens are searching for their identity, being given time to slow down and pay attention to these various interrelated topics of body and mind is essential to their self-development and well-being. Engaging in this kind of learning in a community of their peers also offers important opportunities to develop greater compassion and appreciation for diversity. Many of these areas related to both self-responsibility and community engagement are also explored in programs in social and emotional learning and mindfulness.

Somatic Movement Education as a Complement to Programs in Social and Emotional Learning and Mindfulness

Contemporary research on adolescent development increasingly emphasizes the need to help students skillfully engage in life by developing their inner resources. Including a curriculum in somatic movement education for adolescents can build on existing programs in both social and emotional learning and in mindfulness that are increasingly offered in schools today.

SME AND SOCIAL-EMOTIONAL LEARNING

For example, the framework offered by the Collaborative for Academic, Social, and Emotional Learning or CASEL, an organizing network for SEL programs and educators worldwide, promotes intrapersonal, interpersonal, and cognitive competence based in five core areas:

- **Self-awareness:** identifying emotions, accurate self-perception, recognizing strengths, self-confidence;
- **Self-management:** stress management, self-discipline, self-motivation, impulse control;
- **Social awareness:** perspective taking, empathy, appreciating diversity, respect for others;
- **Relationship skills:** communication, social engagement, relationship building, teamwork;
- **Responsible decision making:** reflecting, ethical responsibility, analyzing situations, evaluating.[27]

Somatic movement education incorporates many of these skills, with the learning integrated into the fabric of the educational situation, rather than being presented as a separate course of study as in many schools that offer stand-alone SEL programs.

Of these skills, which aspects should we prioritize? While some research indicates that many of these non-cognitive skills are so interrelated that there is no "silver bullet" to support all domains,[28] in his 2014 book *Age of Opportunity: Lessons from the New Science of Adolescence,* Laurence Steinberg defines self-management or *self-regulation* as a core resource with which teens can succeed in school and beyond: "Self-regulation and the traits it influences, like determination, comprise one of the strongest predictors of many different types of success: achievement in school, success at work, more satisfying … relationships, and better physical and mental health."[29] He notes several approaches, from mindfulness to yoga, martial arts, and aerobic exercise, which develop greater self-regulation by encouraging a combination of physical activity, mindfulness, and self-discipline.[30]

Somatic education can augment such offerings—further cultivating the baseline skill of mindful somatic awareness necessary for engaging in the type of movement practices he suggests. Self-regulation is essentially the ability to control and adapt our emotions, thoughts, and ultimately our behavior to meet the demands of the situation. Yet neurobiology tells us that we can only control what we can perceive. In other words, if I can't sense my current state of being, I can't begin to skillfully control or regulate that state, physically or emotionally. Once we can clearly sense our bodies and the physical processes going on within, we have much more information with which to manage ourselves, as well as to adapt to the world around us.[31] In this deeper sense, true self-regulation is based in the kind of sensory awareness developed through somatic education. As we become more aware of our sensations, our capacity for self-regulation increases; as we gain skill in self-regulation, we become better at adapting to the ever-changing world both within and around us.

Establishing the capacity for ongoing sensory awareness is particularly relevant for adolescents. With underdeveloped self-awareness and self-regulation skills, teens may make poor choices that can impact many aspects of their lives. For example, without internal awareness, they might exercise to the point of injury; they might begin to feel anxious after sitting for hours, not realizing that they need to get up and move around a bit; or they might become impatient with others when their blood sugar drops and they need to eat; or they may find they can't make sense of what they are reading and get discouraged, when actually they may be tired and need to go to bed. With increased internal awareness, teenagers can begin to become more conscious of the complex relationship between body and mind, such as the relationships between emotions and digestion, sleep and concentration, and physical stress and health. As they gain more accurate perceptions of their bodies, they have the potential to apply this awareness to actively improve their health. With knowledge and awareness comes *choice.*

On many levels, our bodies function whether we understand them or not. As Maurice Merleau-Ponty proposed with his "body-subject" model of embodiment, the experience of being alive is not dependent upon knowledge of anatomy and physiology.[32] Yet having accurate information about how our bodies move and function can be an important aspect of our development. Developing our knowledge of how our own bodies function and gaining sensitivity to the complex interrelationship of body and mind have enormous potential to impact our well-being. As Jon Kabat-Zinn, the founder of Mindfulness-Based Stress Reduction (MBSR), has said, "the biggest distractor is not your iPhone—it's your own mind."[33] With increased awareness, teens can make better choices that help, rather than hinder, their growth as they learn to draw upon their innate body intelligence. Establishing basic body-mind skills during the teen years provides an essential foundation for lifelong personal investigation toward ongoing health, vitality, and well-being. Adolescents can learn to adapt in ways that support their development across their lives: physically, socially, emotionally, and academically. As Steinberg espouses, "developing self-regulation [is] the central task of adolescence, and the goal that we should be pursuing as parents, educators, and health care professionals."[34]

Since these SEL competencies such as self-regulation can be taught in many ways in a variety of settings, there are numerous diverse CASEL-approved programs in place throughout the United States. SEL programs are also offered worldwide by other organizations, such as the Mind and Life Institute, which was founded by His Holiness the Dalai Lama and distinguished scientists and educators as a means to bridge scientific inquiry and contemplative practices.[35] Somatic movement education can enrich these inspiring SEL offerings through complementary programs with an experiential and body-based approach.

SME AND MINDFULNESS

Mindfulness programs offer a similar student-centered approach, and many SEL programs include elements of mindfulness training in their curricula. Both mindfulness and the embodiment practices of somatic education are essentially awareness practices that share a focus on developing inner presence to improve well-being.[36] These practices bring a particular quality of mindful awareness, which, Jon Kabat-Zinn notes, is "cultivated by paying attention in a sustained and particular way: on purpose, in the present moment, and non-judgmentally."[37] In fact, having a mindfulness practice can make somatic awareness much easier, and the reverse is also true: somatic practices can help the body soften and the mind calm down, making it easier to focus and sit comfortably in meditation, for example—a practice often taught in mindfulness programs.[38] There is also evidence that movement can be improved via a mindfulness practice; one such study demonstrated that mindful attention can affect postural control and balance, supporting the idea that both somatic awareness and mindfulness can affect physical performance.[39]

Mindfulness and somatic education are thus interrelated, yet there are also distinct differences between mindfulness as it is being taught in schools and the type of embodiment fostered in somatic education. First, mindfulness practices are often done in stillness—while sitting and focusing on one's breath—or in simple activities like walking or eating. Some mindfulness programs also include "mindful movement" practices, which commonly draw on yoga poses and other simple stretches. In yet other mindfulness programs, particularly those for young children, students are specifically taught how to "put on [their] mindful bodies," which teaches them to become as still and quiet as possible, and not to move their arms and legs.[40] In all of these approaches, the emphasis is on regulating emotions and developing an associated state of calm. In somatic practices, while some activities are done in stillness and similarly aspire to promote calmness, other activities intentionally invite a *wide range* of movement and psychophysical expression, thereby expanding our abilities, our comfort zone, and our resilience. Through a somatic process of embodiment, we begin to learn that we can also *move* our mindful body in myriad ways.

Somatic education therefore teaches us to develop a mindful awareness of our body, both in stillness and in motion, increasing our kinesthetic awareness. As we develop this awareness further, our bodies *themselves* develop mindfulness, or an alive presence in the moment. We can then begin to let go of any need for a more conscious mental focusing on our body. And while embodiment is a process—an ongoing investigation, rather than an arrival point—we can reach a state where, as with mindfulness, we are able to access our fullest embodiment more often and more easily in our daily lives. Somatic educator Christine Caldwell discusses our lack of understanding of this concept thus: "It's curious that in English we don't have a distinct word to express a state of being present and aware in the body—a deep state of somatic wakefulness—a state of profound occupation of the present moment, as it becomes explicit in flesh and nerve and bone."[41] Somatic movement is a potent pathway to accessing and establishing this inner wakefulness. Somatic movement education—and movement programs that take a more somatic approach—can be a complement to mindfulness programs by prioritizing kinesthetic learning.

Mindfulness programs for youth also often teach students detailed information about the brain from neuroscience—the research basis for many mindfulness programs—such as about the amygdala and its role in stress and the fear response, to help them understand and deal with stress.[42] Through programs in somatic movement education, students can also learn about other aspects of the body—like bones and organs—and be taught about how their proprioceptive senses relate to learning movement skills or to noticing and alleviating tension in their bodies, all of which has practical applications to their development and everyday life. Somatic movement education introduces such learning without a dichotomy of body and mind or a hierarchical view, and can be a further foundation that inspires youth to learn even more about the body.

As an example, both mindfulness and SEL curricula generally include meditation focused on one's breath to help students relax and become more present. During these activities, information about the actual physical body—the lungs, diaphragm, rib cage, and so on—often goes unmentioned.[43] Somatic training can help students learn to deepen their breathing through a better understanding of the practical basics of anatomy and physiology. For example, although we may intend to take "a deep breath," many people imagine this to mean expanding their upper chest as they breathe in, and do this habitually. Even when asked to place a hand on their belly to encourage deeper breathing, many students will often still resort to their habitual pattern of "chest breathing." Somatic educators can perceive students' *actual* physical response—such as this more shallow breathing instead of deep—and can teach students to perceive this difference on their own, while supporting them to learn and cultivate a healthier response.

Adapting Somatic Movement Education Specifically for Teens

If somatic learning can be so helpful for teens, then how should such a curriculum be structured to meet their needs? Further research on adolescent development shows that teens do best in an educational context in which they 1) are actively engaged in learning and practicing new skills within a cooperative community of peers,[44] 2) experience agency in choosing what is being studied,[45] and 3) believe they can improve in the subject area.[46] In other words, they need to believe that the process they are involved in both relates to them and involves a *malleable*, rather than fixed, attribute—referred to in education as having a "growth mindset."[47] Simply put, they need to believe that they can improve through their own effort. The curriculum presented here inherently encompasses all three of these best practices. While each of these will be described in more detail throughout the book, here's a brief summary.

To begin with, in the experiential nature of the curriculum, a student's own moving body becomes the learning lab, through a series of movement activities and subsequent discussions, so they are inevitably actively involved in their own learning. In this way, sharing their experiences in a peer group setting is also an integral characteristic of the process. Second, drawing on pedagogical principles described in chapter 4, the facilitator invites student input into choosing the topics that are being studied and thereby providing students with agency in determining course content. Third, by helping students learn the physiological basis of movement—how kinesthetic learning happens in our bodies—they come to see it as a malleable skill that anyone can improve upon regardless of their starting point.

This last issue is especially important, since by the time children reach the teenage years, they have often self-identified as either a "talented" mover (such as athletic or coordinated), or "klutzy"—believing this to be a lifelong sentence. Other teens may have experienced themselves as coordinated as youngsters or pre-teens, and then reached an awkward and more uncoordinated stage in adolescence as their bodies underwent rapid changes. In any case, as students recognize that their kinesthetic abilities can improve with ease, they develop greater self-confidence and are less apt to become discouraged if they don't immediately succeed in specific physical activities. With increased somatic awareness, they also gain an improved baseline upon which to build as they engage in physical activities that develop gross motor skills. Anyone can expand their kinesthetic or bodily awareness—regardless of physical prowess in a certain discipline or physical disabilities—based on their current starting point.

By supporting the whole person, somatic movement education approaches would appear to be primed for educating teenagers. Yet as I have discovered, most somatic disciplines have been developed for *adults* and have not yet been widely offered to adolescents. Adapting these approaches for teens can present some significant challenges. In fact, when I first began implementing embodied anatomy in schools, I discovered that many of the methods of exploration with which I was familiar—the pedagogy—didn't work very well with my teen students. There were several reasons for this, including three that seemed most immediately obvious.

First, many of the modes of exploring were too open-ended and improvisatory for them. Getting too much freedom to explore their movement can be a scary prospect for teens, as so many of the familiar modes of assessing their success are missing (such as how fast they run, how well they throw a ball, or how many pushups they can do). Teens may also associate such free-form movement with the type of play they engaged in earlier during childhood, and may perceive this kind of activity as beneath them.

Second, as research has consistently shown (and anyone working with teens has discovered), adolescents typically have a much shorter attention span than most adults. They also have a harder time shifting gears from their normal physically active state to the slower, more focused one that the program requires and need a trustworthy bridge into this inner realm.

Third, although teens do best when working collaboratively, this is easier said than done, and there are some particular challenges in getting teenagers to trust in and benefit from the group aspect of the curriculum. Working with adults, my experience has been that engaging in embodiment practices in a group has a way of building a palpable sense of community and mutual concern among the participants quite easily.

By contrast, and as recent research bears out, teens are particularly attuned to adults who try to create a false sense of community right away.[48] Simply put, trust must be *earned,* and teens are acutely attuned to any attempts to circumvent that. Adolescents are particularly sensitive to the opinions of their peers and, though less likely to admit it, of the adults around them, so getting them to relax and enjoy these activities in a group of their peers takes skillful facilitation. Once established, however, a safe and compassionate learning community provides a solid foundation for engaging teens in these somatic practices.

Taking all of this into consideration, I began to make significant changes to the structure and the content of my classes in order to meet the needs of the teens with whom I was working. I introduce these adaptations in the pedagogy section in chapter 4, "Eight Key Pedagogy Principles for Teaching SME with Teens," and I explain them in greater detail throughout the book.

ᔓᔕ

Offering more body-based, somatic learning helps our youth to become engaged and deepens and enlivens their education. When given an opportunity to experience and reflect upon the body as an *ecosystem*—sensitive to inner emotions, thoughts, and physical processes—they develop a renewed sense of appreciation for their bodies. Giving youth tangible avenues to appreciate their bodies can help them develop the kind of deep personal understanding needed to bring about kindness and caring for themselves.

We take care of what we love. But to develop love we need to make a personal connection. The way we treat ourselves is also intricately related to how we treat others—and the environment around us. As we come to respect our own bodies and understand our inherent interconnection with elements of nature, we become more resourced in ourselves, more compassionate with others, and more respectful in caring for our planet.

Although there are many mysteries in the workings of the body, there is much that can be known, felt, and understood. Keeping students as the focus of the learning experience, with their own interests, discoveries, and insights guiding the curriculum, is essential. As we create opportunities for students to learn about themselves and find their authentic expression, we can support the growth of the whole person in adolescence—the embodied teen.

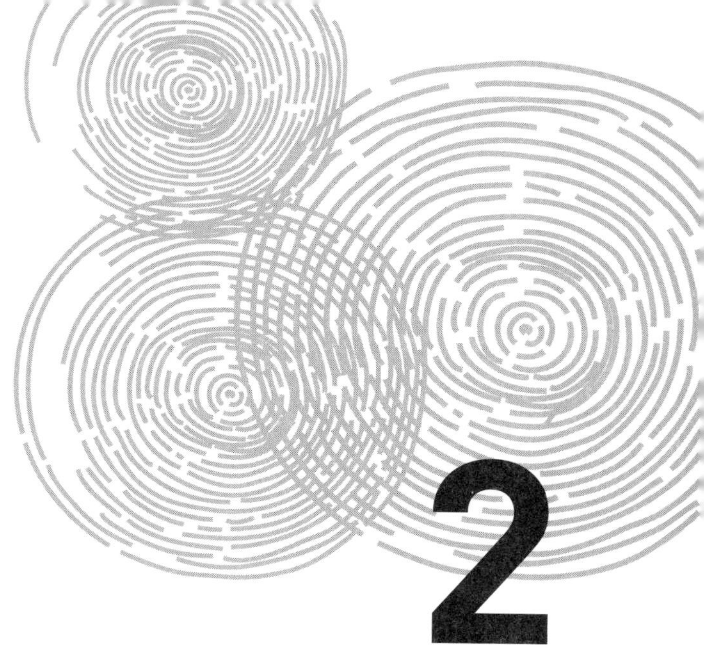

2

Somatic Education and Other Influences

The Roots of the Curriculum

Somatics is the field which studies the soma: namely, the body as it is perceived from within the first-person perception.

—Thomas Hanna

Somatic Education, also referred to simply as somatics, is a field of formal research that emerged in the mid-twentieth century. Somatics represents a variety of body-mind approaches developed primarily in Europe and the United States. These approaches have gone under various names you might be familiar with, including bodywork, body therapies, and movement repatterning. In the 1970s, philosopher Thomas Hanna coined the term *somatics* from the Greek, *sōmatikos,* meaning "pertaining to the physical body," to name the field. In doing so, he also distinguished between the "body," or the physical form, and the "soma," referring to one's *lived experience* of the body, or the body experienced from within. Similarly, all somatic disciplines share a common focus on the relationship between the body and the many aspects of the self.[1]

A somatic or first-person perspective is meant to enliven and empower—helping us to value our own psychophysical experience. Somatic psychologist Don Hanlon Johnson refers to this in his concept of "bodily authority," maintaining that we have been systematically alienated from our personal autonomy, and have become dependent on experts.[2] As such, many of us need guidance to learn how to reconnect with our own bodies, as well as education in how to use our sensory awareness to support our well-being. Within a somatic model of research and learning, personal experience is seen as a primary method of knowing, with body-mind awareness as the path to knowledge.

The term *somatic* is widely used in many contexts throughout many professions. Some basic definitions may help readers to clarify the use of terms within the professional field in general and in this book in particular:

- **Somatic** (adjective, meaning pertaining to the body, with the precise meaning varying according to the context as discussed above).
- **Somatics** (noun, the professional field related to primarily Western practices developed in the twentieth century as defined above).
- **Somatic Education** (referring to disciplines in the field of somatics that include an educational component [as opposed to methods like massage for instance] with distinct bodies of work, such as Body-Mind Centering, referred to as *somatic disciplines*, and specific activities within them referred to using terms such as *somatic practices, methods, or techniques*).
- **Somatic Movement Education** (a professional field related to those somatic disciplines that include movement as a primary somatic technique).
- **Experiential or Embodied Anatomy** (a subset of somatic movement education describing disciplines that include movement and embodiment of body systems as a primary somatic technique).

The subset of somatics known as somatic movement education (SME), then, is a field that prioritizes *movement* as a key dynamic dimension in developing well-being and self-understanding. This particular delineation of somatics is related to educational approaches based in embodied anatomy, which forms the basis of this curriculum.

Somatic Movement Education

Many of the founders of somatic disciplines came from a variety of different movement backgrounds, inspiring them to develop their particular approaches. Pioneers in this field include Mabel Elsworth Todd (physical education), Moshe Feldenkrais (judo), Rudolph Laban (dance), F. M. Alexander (theater), and Ida Rolf (yoga), along with dancer and physical educator Margaret H'Doubler. Developing their work through their research, teaching, and writing in the first half of the twentieth century, each created a systematized approach to working with the body and movement.

A characteristic of all of these approaches is that we learn by *doing*, rather than having something *done to us.* We also learn by experimenting, rather than following a preestablished protocol, helping us to cultivate practices that can extend into many aspects of our lives. These educators thus paved the way for this evolving field that honors the innate body wisdom we have within, while challenging us to expand our perceptual awareness.

For example, somatic movement education practices may include learning to notice and repattern habitual ways of moving that may be causing strain, stress, injury, or a range of other physical and emotional issues; sometimes the process may include hands-on repatterning of movement by a trained educator. The role of the somatic educator is to teach and empower us toward greater self-care, rather than to correct or fix. This process of somatic learning requires a trust-worthy container in which self-exploration and reflection can emerge in its own time, based on individual readiness. Depending upon the person and the context, the goals of such approaches can cover a wide spectrum, from an increased ease and range of movement, the prevention of injury, and improved physical performance, to increased health and wellness, expanded creative expression, the integration of body and mind, and personal transformation.[3]

A next generation of founders of specific somatic movement disciplines working initially in the 1930s to the 1970s includes such innovators as Irmgard Bartenieff (Bartenieff Fundamentals), Bonnie Bainbridge Cohen (Body-Mind Centering), Thomas Hanna (Hanna Somatics), Marion Rosen (Rosen Method), and Emilie Conrad (Continuum). These visionary leaders have each applied their somatic methods to myriad areas of health and wellness. For example, Irmgard Bartenieff worked with polio patients, Bainbridge Cohen applied her study of developmental movement to working with infants with neurological challenges, while Conrad developed a protocol for spinal cord injury and participated as a Movement Specialist at UCLA. Thomas Hanna, along with somatic educator Eleanor Criswell Hanna, started *Somatics Journal* in 1976 to provide information on their programs in Hanna Somatics, as well as to encourage further dialogue in the field at large.

As the field of somatics grew, somatic movement education emerged as its own professional field with the establishment of the International Somatic Movement Education and Therapy Association (ISMETA) in 1988, an organization that created both a defined scope of practice and set of professional standards. Currently ISMETA maintains a registry of more than thirty approved training programs worldwide and a listing of all the individual practitioners who have been approved as Registered Somatic Movement Educators and Therapists (RSME/T). Many such practitioners have integrated several different somatic approaches through their studies—with particular individuals having been instrumental in contributing yet further bodies of work from their own embodied research.

Through the work of practitioners and organizations such as ISMETA, the field has grown in influence within many professions such as psychology, physical and occupational therapy, medicine, fitness, and dance education. To speak about their work, some somatic educators use terms like *somatic movement, embodiment,* and *mindful movement* somewhat interchangeably, as is evident in many of the book titles on somatics by noted authors in the field. In books such as *Bone, Breath, and Gesture: Practices of Embodiment* (1995) and *Groundworks: Narratives of Embodiment* (1997), somatic psychologist Don Hanlon Johnson has been instrumental in documenting some of the most prominent contributions in both somatic psychology—another subset of somatics—and of these somatic movement pioneers. In her book *Mindful Movement: The Evolution of the Somatic Arts and Conscious Action* (2016), Martha Eddy details her extensive research to provide an overview of this contemporary field, highlighting the complex interweaving of dance, somatic, and indigenous practices that led to many of the current somatic lineages.

Many somatic principles have roots in indigenous wisdom, and many indigenous cultures have practices that, by today's definitions, would be considered "somatic." Myriad somatic pioneers have been deeply influenced by certain indigenous forms of movement practice. Moshe Feldenkrais earned a black belt in judo;[4] Irmgard Bartenieff studied qi gong;[5] and Bonnie Bainbridge Cohen studied aikido and t'ai chi.[6] In this sense, somatic movement education practices have drawn on multiple cultural influences and practices, with many forms of martial arts considered by some to be somatic practices in and of themselves, with concrete physiological benefits—such as increasing one's proprioceptive awareness, balance, and sensory-motor development. In establishing his physical education programs, Seymour Kleinman, creator of a world-renowned PhD program in somatic studies at Ohio State University, made a point to include movement practices such as yoga and t'ai chi to encourage body connectivity, grounding, and centering, in contrast to the externally focused movement of competitive sports.[7]

Somatic movement education disciplines that were newly developed in the West, however, maintain a distinct scope of practice in which sensory awareness and movement integration—rather than skill-building in a particular movement form—is the primary goal. This is quite different, for instance, from training in dance or sports, or even from a regular "exercise" mode, in which you repeat movement sequences toward a particular physical outcome, such as doing a set of sit-ups to strengthen the abdominal muscles. Somatic movement practices are meant to elicit enhanced awareness, which can then be applied in many aspects of our lives. Letting go of our tensions and blockages, we can rediscover a core integrity and support within ourselves—activating and learning to trust more of our own innate body intelligence. This begins a process of self-inquiry and learning that empowers us toward more ongoing, sustainable self-care, creativity, and expression.

Experiential Anatomy

The aspect of somatic movement education we call experiential or embodied anatomy encourages experiential learning about body structure and function through active physical participation. In this process, embodying anatomical structures is one of the primary somatic techniques used to bring about change in the body-mind.[8] Although anatomical information is included, rather than merely using our mind to memorize it, we use our entire bodies in this learning process. As Bonnie Bainbridge Cohen relates, "Our education is so much about remembering with our nervous system. And this is about forgetting with our nervous system and remembering with our cellular life force."[9] The two embodied anatomy approaches with which I am most familiar, Ideokinesis and Body-Mind Centering, have informed the approaches presented in this book in specific and significant ways.

Ideokinesis

Lulu Edith Sweigard, a student of Mabel Elsworth Todd, coined the term *Ideokinesis* in 1973 to represent a method of training the nervous system through the use of imagery. Through Ideokinesis, you become aware of habitual patterns and then learn to establish new, more efficient patterns through both movement and imagery. Using visualizations, we can initiate or inhibit certain neurological pathways to the various muscles; such visualizations become a first step in the process of repatterning our movement.[10] These principles have made their way into popular culture as well. Sports training utilizes imagery to enhance performance, such as "rehearsing" the perfect tennis swing in your mind before the game, and in fact recent research in brain science has demonstrated that the same regions in the brain are used whether one is mentally practicing a movement or engaged in the actual movement itself. [11]

In *The Thinking Body,* Todd's seminal book, a primary principle was the idea of developing balance of both body and mind to maximize one's movement potential. Balance of the body relates to skeletal alignment and balancing muscle action around the joints, which minimizes the muscular energy needed to maintain the body in an upright position. As we gain a more balanced alignment, more energy is available for movement. More efficient movement also minimizes the risk of injury or chronic strains.[12] Balance of the mind involves quieting inner dialogue. While there are a variety of relaxation and meditation techniques to achieve this balanced mind, visualization is especially effective in letting go of previous thought patterns by providing an image on which to focus.

Ideokinesis helps us recognize habitual patterns of movement and begin to make changes in our bodies. The visualization techniques also help us to clear the mind of self-criticism and develop greater concentration, essential skills we can use throughout our lives.

Body-Mind Centering

The 1970s were a fertile time for somatic education in the United States. In 1973, Bonnie Bainbridge Cohen founded the School for Body-Mind Centering in New York City. In addition to studying dance, dance therapy, martial arts, yoga, and voice, Bainbridge Cohen is an occupational therapist and a neurodevelopmental therapist; her innovative techniques integrate her experience in traditional and alternative approaches to movement and healing. Body-Mind Centering (BMC) is an experiential process of inquiry and study based on the embodiment and application of anatomical, physiological, psychophysical, and developmental movement principles.[13]

The BMC paradigm provides a comprehensive body-based language for describing movement and exploring the body-mind relationship, while the creative and innovative pedagogical techniques of BMC—for example, using warm water-filled balloons to represent our bodies' organs—bring anatomy study alive. Practitioners and teachers of Body-Mind Centering are applying BMC principles in many disciplines such as dance, yoga, athletics, bodywork, physical, occupational, and speech therapies, psychotherapy, medicine, child development, education, and the arts in the United States and abroad.[14]

One of the unique contributions Bonnie Bainbridge Cohen has made to the field of somatic education is the exploration of each of the body systems through movement, based in the revolutionary concept that we can actually *initiate* movement from any system in our bodies. By doing so, we can personally embody and integrate each system—to access both a movement quality and a particular state of "mind" associated with that system. While we often think of "mind" as referring to the brain, and therefore the intellect or thought processes, here it refers more to an overall *state of being.* For example, moving from the bones evokes a state of clarity and directness, whereas moving from the muscles evokes vitality and power, and moving from the organs evokes emotions and fullness.[15]

As Body-Mind Centering teacher Linda Hartley has noted, the idea that mental functions, emotions, and bodily processes are interconnected—what many of us know intuitively—is now backed up by current neuroscience research. By tracking chemical messengers called neuropeptides and their receptor sites in the brain and throughout the body, researchers have demonstrated that there are inherent connections between the brain and other systems, such as the immune and endocrine systems.[16] This has also been proven by research into the importance of the enteric nervous system, often referred to as the second brain or "gut brain," with a system of neurons throughout the gastrointestinal tract.[17] Body-Mind Centering reflects this more holistic perspective through an embodied approach to movement, the body, and consciousness.

Body-Mind Centering approaches teach us to engage direct sensory perception based on anatomical structure. This process provides us with a tangible relationship —developed from within—to our own body and our states of consciousness, as a comprehensive framework for exploring the body. The psychophysical aspect, of relating movement qualities, emotions, and states of mind, also helps us to become more self-aware, resourceful, and resilient.

Related Fields and Movement Practices

A few other related fields that have influenced this curriculum are worthy of note, though they are beyond the scope of this book to discuss at length. The first of these is ecosomatics, a new field of somatic education developing parallel to that of ecopsychology.

Ecosomatics

Ecosomatics emphasizes direct sensory experience and perception of the body as part of—not separate from—the natural environment. As we come to recognize that our breath, bones, and fluids are in fact parts of the natural world around us, we realize our deep interconnection with one another and are inspired toward creativity and heartfelt stewardship of our planet.

Dance educator Rebecca Enghauser was one of the first to coin this term in 2007,[18] and since that time pioneering dance and somatic educators who have been instrumental in developing curricula related to ecosomatics include Andrea Olsen (author of *Body and Earth*), and Caryn McHose and Kevin Frank (coauthors of *How Life Moves*). Much of the work of Anna Halprin, whose outdoor dance deck in Northern California has been a site for movement for over half a century, is ecosomatic, along with the work of Jamie McHugh, a faculty member with Halprin at Tamalpa Institute, who teaches outdoor workshops to explore the relationship between the inner and outer ecosystems that he calls Somatic Expression®.[19] Emilie Conrad's Continuum work, described in her book *Life on Land,* further emphasizes movement from the "fluid body" that reflects our emergence as primordial beings from the waters of the planet,[20] while author and environmental activist Joanna Macy's "Work that Reconnects," based in deep ecology, has long echoed ecosomatic philosophies.[21]

Feeling a kinship with these contributing colleagues, I've developed a series of ecosomatic activities, a few of which are included in this book. I believe that ecosomatic practices—going beyond mere theory to offer personal, experiential knowing—have great potential to positively impact our next generation, encouraging them toward more sustainable living practices.

Dance Anthropology, Cultural Studies, and Social Somatics

My graduate study in the fields of dance anthropology and cultural studies also inspired me to create several of the activities in this book, by introducing me to what I call the "anthropological lens."[22] This perspective helps us to recognize cultural conditioning and more closely examine our more unconscious beliefs, biases, and assumptions. Through this process, we gain greater self-awareness and also begin to perceive with more objectivity—helping us to become less reactive and judgmental. When I began to explicitly integrate this cultural aspect in my classes in the 1990s, it was generally not part of somatic education. More recently this type of approach—that takes into account context, culture, and relationships as an inherent part of somatic education—has been called "social somatics."[23] Depending upon how it is facilitated, social somatics can also be seen as a form of embodied activism that develops an awareness of complex social dynamics, such as contexts of privilege and oppression, as a means to transform cycles of injustice and create new paradigms of mutual respect.[24] I believe that this social aspect is an essential and potent aspect of somatic education for teens, as they develop personal perspectives and worldviews that will impact them throughout their lives.

Dance, Contact Improvisation, and Authentic Movement

Particular movement forms in my own background—creative movement, modern dance, Contact Improvisation, and Authentic Movement—also inform the curriculum. My experience as a dancer inspired me to craft an approach to somatic education that keeps *active full-bodied movement* as an integral part of the learning process. Like many of us, teens need time to integrate their experiences in a progressive and engaging way that movement can provide. For example, I draw on many forms of creative improvisation to add an aspect of playfulness and spontaneous social interaction to the class.

Another practice I draw upon, called Contact Improvisation, was developed by Steve Paxton in 1972 as a duet form in which dancers improvise their movement while playing with a dialogue of touch, momentum, and shared body weight. Contact Improvisation teaches us to rely on our reflexes for quick responsiveness. We also learn to use gravity and momentum to establish a connection with the earth, as opposed to resisting gravity, such as in classical ballet training. The techniques of Contact Improvisation continue to evolve through experience and experiment and often integrate somatic practices. Studying Contact Improvisation was one way in which I learned how to integrate various somatic practices into teaching movement. In this curriculum I draw on principles taught in Contact Improvisation in specific activities, such as teaching students about counterbalance as a means to help them develop more of an ability to ground through the pelvis and legs and move from their pelvic center, as is often taught in martial arts. The overall philosophy of Contact Improvisation—that equally values all students' ability as movers—has also influenced my philosophies; growing out of the 1960s counterculture movement, the form was rooted in the belief in the movement potential of all people and rejected the view that to be a dancer one had to undergo years of training in a specific technique.[25]

I also draw on principles of Authentic Movement from practicing and teaching it over many years beginning in 1984. Authentic Movement is a term that was used by dance therapist Janet Adler to describe a method of self-directed movement she studied with Mary Starks Whitehouse in the 1960s.[26] The practice of Authentic Movement involves a mover and a trained witness, in a timed session in which the mover moves with eyes closed, allowing inner impulses from the body to guide the movement. The witness provides a nonjudgmental presence and compassionate support for the mover, while observing both the mover and their own internal responses to the movement. After the movement session, the two speak about the experience. The form is based on the belief that when we listen within, we will know what we need.

The practice of Authentic Movement also allows the mover to observe thoughts in the mind, much as one does in the beginning stages of many forms of meditation. Over time, the mover internalizes the presence of the discerning, yet nonjudgmental witness.[27] Authentic Movement develops mindfulness in body and mind, and as such, I and other practitioners often compare it to meditation and other forms of mindfulness practice.[28]

These basic principles—of paying attention within and establishing a less judgmental inner 'observer'—inform the curriculum in general, and are also evident in the form and philosophy of a practice of warming-up I call "Responsive Moving," which I describe further in chapter 16.[29] Authentic Movement also reminds us of the importance of a reliable witness for inner work, and the need to establish a safe and trustworthy container for our students, philosophies that have also influenced my pedagogy suggestions presented in chapter 4.

Ritual: Offerings and Dedications

Finally, from years of living in Bali, Indonesia, and studying Balinese dance and ritual there, I learned to appreciate the many dimensions that movement can express, spanning physical and emotional realms, as well as serving as both an individual and communal offering. This deepened my belief in the power of dance and movement to positively impact our lives, and inspired me to bring forward the perspective of movement as an offering more consciously in my work as a dancer and educator. One way this manifests in the curriculum is in the form of dedications, a way of setting an intention to offer one's movement practice toward a goal, an outcome, or even an ideal (see chapter 8), using a style I've adapted for teenagers.

ᔕ

Essentially, all somatic methods provide a pathway for us to come home to ourselves and to experience being alive. Contrary to the digital world, which provides quick and immediate access to an overflow of copious information, the body—and the natural world of which we are a part—has its own, often slower, pace and perhaps more subtle language. While much in contemporary culture encourages an outer focus, getting from point A to point B—and hopefully as quickly as possible—somatic practices encourage us to go within, s l o w d o w n, breathe, and arrive. I invite you to take a moment now to practice this for yourself, before reading on. This gives you time and space to prepare the way for new information and experience.

PART II

GETTING STARTED: A GUIDE FOR FACILITATORS

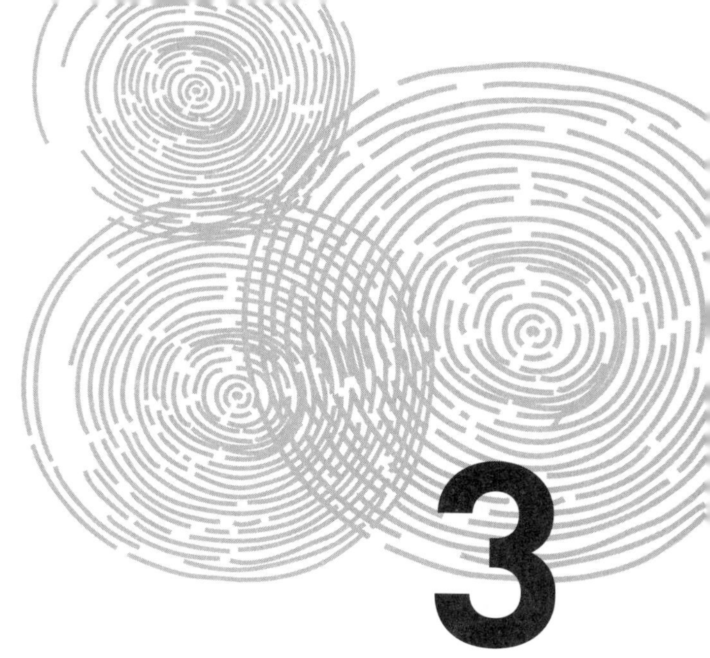

3

Basics about the Curriculum

Throughout our lives, but especially during adolescence ... less and less attention is given to what is coming from inside. We often need instruction on developing a healthy dialogue with our physical being.

—Andrea Olsen

Traditionally, the term *curriculum* implies a set of materials to be presented in a linear, step-by-step fashion, based on specific content to be cognitively understood and retained. The focus is generally on the learning of new material, with the teacher deemed the expert who will teach it—and then judge the level of success achieved by each student, often through some outside measure such as written testing. In contrast, this curriculum encourages experiential and personal research, with students making discoveries along the way while simultaneously being involved in evaluating their own progress. This method of body education brings students into dialogue with their inner and outer experience, giving them increased knowledge and self-awareness. A primary goal—and benefit—is a *shift in consciousness* toward self-care. The avenue is *movement,* which, along with cognitive study of anatomy, gives students practical knowledge of their own moving bodies, with the teacher as a guide and witness.

As a first step in this approach, as you read this book let yourself become curious about the miracle of the human body, engaging in your own personal research and allowing yourself to adopt a "beginner's mind." For readers who may be new to somatics, you might first explore each of the activities in parts III and IV on your own to gain your own experiential knowing—guiding your own embodiment process and contributing to your ability to potentially facilitate this process for others as well. This can take some time, in our otherwise busy lives, so consider how to make this a reality, perhaps setting aside a consistent time and place each week to begin this process. You may also want to establish your own journal writing to go along with this inner work. Although the activities are primarily designed to be facilitated with groups, some of the content can also be adapted for work with individual students or clients, and as such many of the activities can also be done on your own.

Curriculum Design and Structure of the Book

Each chapter of the curriculum in parts III and IV includes basic relevant anatomy information. Although many teachers may already be familiar with the anatomical information presented in each chapter, I include it where appropriate to facilitate the teaching of the material; this information provides content for your students. The curriculum relies on a very basic level of anatomy that teens can easily experience and practice fully embodying. Later, more complex anatomy and physiology may be added as appropriate to the context of the particular class and group. Simple approaches can help make somatic movement education real, inviting, accessible, and applicable for a range of children, teens, and adults.

In class, rather than introducing the anatomy material in a didactic manner, I incorporate it into relevant activities as well as in response to students' questions and interests. Sample methods for guiding movement activities and integrating specific information in this way appear throughout the book in the form of what I call "explorations," the primary content of this curriculum.

Explorations: Combination of Movement Activities and Discussion

"Explorations" are a blend of movement activities and discussions that comprise the core of the curriculum. This dual movement/discussion approach allows students to first learn through their own physical experience, compare their experience with that of others, and then share what they have learned. Students learn from one another as they begin to recognize the similarities and the differences in their experiences. Discussions either follow the activities or are incorporated into the activities themselves. For instance, in learning about joints, students locate and move their joints to discover the movement potential at each joint; in a discussion of breathing they place their hands on their own rib cage to feel its movement in inhaling and exhaling. They then describe the movements in their journals, and later share their experiences as a group.

Discussions that follow an activity also help students to integrate what they *already know* about the topic being studied with what they may have discovered through the class explorations. For example, in a related study of breathing, students are guided to rest, notice their breathing, and reflect upon and visualize the process of breathing. They then get in partners or small groups to discuss the mechanics and purposes of breathing and to make a list of what they know and/or discovered about their breathing. Discussions such as these give students a chance to recognize and share what they know, as well as give the facilitator a sense of the overall level of knowledge and experience in the class. Basically, it is important not to overload students with more facts than they will be able to integrate through their own physical class experience, while still presenting enough information for them to gain a fuller understanding of the topic being explored. This approach prioritizes the goal of embodiment, while also expanding upon students' cognitive knowledge.

Explorations include three main sections:

1. **Purpose:** summary of the specific educational goals of the activity.
2. **Activity:** guided instructions to read to the group or to be used as a sample of how to facilitate the activity.
3. **Discussion:** post-activity group conversations with sample questions to help initiate student discussion; teachers can alter or expand on these as appropriate.

I've included time estimates for each exploration for planning purposes. Each exploration includes one or more means of processing students' experience, such as drawing, writing in journals, or engaging in the final discussion in partners and/or in a full group. Some explorations also include a "Variations" section (with alternative methods of presenting the activity or related activities).

Lastly, a "Tips for Teachers" section gives additional suggestions related to the activity. Tips may include further suggestions for facilitating the activity, "Home Practices" (further related activities students can do outside of class), and/or "Related Projects" (further related research that students can undertake individually or as a group as an extension of the class content). Each of these supplementary topics is intended to help facilitators be successful and able to adapt the content to the specific teaching situation.

Each chapter includes a sampling of some of the initial exploration activities that I would include as part of that unit or topic area. In this sense, this book is designed to give readers a practical and conceptual overview of my approach to an embodied anatomy curriculum designed for teens. The explorations themselves are not *lesson plans* per se; rather, in each class you would choose specific explorations to be interwoven with related movement activities through what I call a "movement matrix."

This movement matrix allows you to build upon previous lessons, helping students review and integrate previous material, while introducing a next layer of material. These movement activities also provide a predictable format in each class that serves to bring cohesiveness to the overall curriculum.

Movement Matrix: Creating a Cohesive Context for the Class

The movement matrix allows you to integrate one or two explorations per class, and can be explained using a simple ABA format, with the following elements:

> **A) Movement:** an opening circle using body scanning or other body mindfulness activities, followed by more full-bodied movement throughout the room, and then
>
> **B) Explorations:** introducing a particular topic through specific explorations (such as in the explorations called Body Listening, How Do We Breathe, or Arm Circles for example), often initially done lying down with eyes closed
>
> **A) Movement:** a final body check-in, such as body scanning again, followed by guided movement to integrate the experience, and then coming back together for a group discussion (often included in the description of each exploration).

Using a movement matrix provides some essential predictability to the class content—since students generally don't know what to expect! As the curriculum progresses, this format of beginning the class by first standing in a circle for body scanning, and then moving—shaking out the joints, walking through the room, using imagery, noticing changes in the body, and so on—followed by a period of time lying down, can become familiar to students. It can also be used to review previous topics and integrate the next topics being explored. In a sense, then, this order of activities becomes the overall "score" for the class, a term used in improvisational dance or theater that indicates a set sequence that leaves room for creative variation each time. Having such a score enables you to layer the content, repeating some material while integrating new content. (This will be discussed further on pages 66–68 in the section on pedagogy in chapter 4.) The movement matrix keeps *movement* primary in the curriculum and, along with the discussion sections, provides a means for students to practice and integrate their psychophysical learning.

Having students begin and end in a circle is noticeably different than the structure of many traditional movement classes, such as yoga or some forms of dance, in which students tend to be placed in lines facing the teacher. The circle formation works much better for this type of class, as it allows for you to be on the same level as students—standing or sitting in a circle along with them—as well as for students themselves to each take an equal place in the group. Having students begin and end in a circle also creates a further sense of predictability and cohesiveness to the class.

Student-Centered and Project-Based Learning

In engaging students in this material, the curriculum needs to remain responsive to students' interests. In educational jargon this model of learning is sometimes referred to as "student-centered" or "emergent learning," with curriculum designed in this manner called "emergent curriculum." In an emergent curriculum, the teacher is seen as a "facilitator" who guides the students' own inquiry designed around a particular interest that has "emerged" from the group, rather than a topic proposed or determined by the teacher as in the more traditional model. The emergent learning process envisions students as curious learners who are actively seeking knowledge and then builds upon their interests.[1]

Although this program is not an emergent curriculum per se, in that the specific progression of body-mind topics is primarily predesigned, it is still geared toward *emergent learning* in several important ways. While I have organized the topics in this book in a progressive order, teachers can cover topics in a somewhat fluid way in response to students' interests. For example, you may be focused on a general study of joints when you discover that a few students have had knee injuries, and the group then becomes more curious about this particular area of the body. The curriculum model as designed allows for three ways to respond to such emerging interests: in-class activities, home practices, and related projects. If students want to learn more about the knee, for instance, you might incorporate further body-based exploration of the anatomy of the knee, with a corresponding focus on ways to care for your knees as a next class activity. As a home practice, students can color an additional anatomy coloring plate on the knee at home, and as a related project students might prepare a presentation on care of the knees for parents or others in the school.

In another example, perhaps you are focused on body alignment and students get interested in the role of the media in dictating their emotional responses related to various postures. In this case, you can use the exploration called "What's My Line?" that explores cultural perceptions of body image as a next class activity, even if you had expected to cover this later on. As a home practice, students can create a collage of media images related to posture, and then present their artwork for their parents or the school as a group project.

In designing individual or group projects, depending upon your teaching context, each student can choose one topic to explore further as an independent study, or the class can design a final group project by mid-way in the class. Whether done as part of or outside of the class, these projects allow students to follow their interests during the course.

These three aspects of the class pedagogy—in-class activities, home practices, and related projects—help students to feel a sense of agency, with ample opportunities to pursue their own curiosities, keeping learning fun and engaging. While it may not be necessary or practical to include all of these aspects with any one group, I provide examples of them throughout the book in the event they will be useful to you in some contexts. In this way, the curriculum can become a guidebook within which to improvise and respond to your group as needed.

Pathways to Teaching Somatic Movement Education (SME)

While you can apply the somatic movement education practices presented here in a variety of educational settings, the best context for offering the activities will vary considerably. You will need to consider many factors, such as the size of the group, other subjects being offered, the school or program schedule, as well as the expertise of the current faculty, school culture, and financial resources. As mentioned in the Introduction, I have taught this material in a wide array of circumstances and educational contexts, such as ranging from a semester course for academic credit at the high school level, to a PE unit in middle school, to a class for dancers at a local studio, to a college-level anatomy course. Depending upon your own situation, background, and interests, you can formulate a course context and structure that best suits the needs of the school or group with whom you are working.

In some sense, implementing a program in somatic movement education in schools may be best suited in situations in which a broader philosophical movement is already underway in the school district or individual school, such as through student-centered and project-based learning, smaller class sizes, and outdoor education programs. If your school has already implemented such innovations, or is offering social and emotional learning programs or perhaps is moving toward introducing yoga, aikido, or mindfulness practices, for instance, then key decision-makers may also be amenable to considering somatic movement education. In such cases, you might incorporate some of the simpler activities into a specific educational forum, such as in a mindfulness class, PE class, health class, advisory group, or an outdoor education program.

Another avenue would be to offer this material as an independent course, in which case the activities are taught cumulatively over time and covered in much greater depth. This is ideal, so that the teaching can be built upon progressively to support depth of learning and embodiment. In any case, each of these contexts will also likely require a different level of expertise by the teacher.

Teacher Qualifications

Because this curriculum is based in experiential learning, it is essential that you have your *own experience* with each of the activities before leading them with a group. This ensures that you are offering an embodied experience to your students—one that comes from your own *soma,* or lived experience. What can be taught from one's own physical, subjective experience will be more meaningful to teacher and students alike. We can only begin from where we are. In fact, regardless of their level of skill, many teachers who attend my trainings find that they really just need the time for *themselves,* and are less interested in the pedagogy at first. We each deal with so many responsibilities, it can be a relief to just take the time to focus within, move, and become more self-aware. Arriving first, we can then begin to focus on our students. Give yourself the time you need to feel ready to teach this material, as an extensive period of time may be needed to fully integrate these somatic practices.

To teach them also requires an ongoing involvement to sustain and grow your inner resources. Many somatic practices also require guidance by a practitioner to provide an "outside eye," along with skillful physical touch and movement facilitation, to help you learn and integrate new movement patterns. You may also find you need some support in processing any emotional responses. Therefore, while some learning can be done on your own, to reach a level of proficiency to teach this material to others will likely also necessitate seeking out your own training in somatics if that is not currently part of your background.

Embodied anatomy and somatic education are the primary trainings recommended. Some readers may already have an extensive somatics background. Other educators may have some previous experience upon which to build, such as in teaching dance, theater, physical education, yoga, or other movement forms; in this case you may have some minimal anatomy background, along with previous experience applying it to teaching movement. Many of the activities require some basic knowledge of anatomy, kinesiology, and physiology. While basic anatomy concepts are included in each chapter as a reference, you will want to be sure you are comfortable enough in your understanding of and experience with each topic that you can easily present the material. Other trainings in areas such as dance and movement education, mindfulness, cooperative learning, group dynamics, conflict resolution, restorative justice practices, and social and emotional learning can all support a more in-depth teaching of the material. Facilitators should also have previous experience teaching adolescents, preferably having worked with them in specific related areas, such as in teaching movement practices and in other areas like wellness, mindfulness, or social and emotional learning.

As you will see, some activities can be more easily taught by teachers with minimal anatomy and movement background, while other aspects require more in-depth anatomy background and further experience with somatic movement practices. If you are new to somatic practices and have no anatomy background, you can explore basic lessons by first engaging in the activity on your own or in a group with other educators, before leading it with students. Others may already have previous experience with leading some version of activities like body scanning, such as those teaching mindfulness in schools, and can presumably lead the versions presented in this book as well. With an addition of some anatomy study, such educators will likely feel comfortable teaching many of the basic activities presented in Level I, particularly chapters 7–9.

In facilitating movement repatterning and other activities that require a more in-depth anatomy and physiology background, such as those presented in chapters 10, 11, and 12 in Level I and chapters 13–16 in Level II, you would benefit from having further experience in somatics. This ensures the type of skills needed to accurately assess student responsiveness and progress throughout the curriculum. Certain movement assessment skills, like observing specific areas of the body in which movement is being initiated, detecting movement that is disorganized versus integrated, and determining an appropriate movement intervention if a student is having difficulty, are not possible to teach through the written word alone. Therefore, although I have provided some general "Tips for Teachers," which include tips on facilitating the activities, I haven't attempted to detail the full extent of the various methods of assessment to use when engaging students in each exploration.

As a general rule of thumb, if you aren't sure how to teach or assess a particular activity, you can seek out some further training to be sure that 1) you have experienced the activity or something similar *yourself* so you can bring your own embodied understanding to your teaching and 2) you have had a chance to ask questions about how to assess student participation related to the stated goals of the activity. This will ensure a level of confidence in working with your group and building upon your own level of skill. For further professional development in somatic movement education, you can refer to the ISMETA website for a more extensive listing of programs. For those interested in further training related to the curriculum in this book, my Embodiment in Education programs include short introductory classes for people at all levels of experience, as well as new more extensive teacher certification programs.

Finally, educators at any level of experience can benefit from reading and considering the pedagogy material presented in chapter 4. In some sense, I view this as the "gold" of this book—gleaned over thirty years of teaching—since it provides an understanding of the *essentials* that need to be in place for a curriculum such as this to be effective. My hope in presenting this material is two-fold. First, that those new to the field can gain insight into the type of multidimensional learning environment that somatic education provides, and second, that those educators with previous extensive somatic training who work with adolescents—or may become interested in working with them—can reference my pedagogy principles as a springboard to create further curricula for youth, based on the particular somatic disciplines in their *own* backgrounds. This is fertile ground, and given the wide range of creative resources available, this model can also serve as a framework for others to build upon.

Class Size, Schedule, and Space Considerations

When engaging students in this material, it is best if the class size is small, up to ten to fifteen students if possible, though I have also taught larger groups of twenty or so as well. An initial class series also needs to be long enough to allow students adequate time to practice and integrate new skills. For example, a class might be scheduled to meet for 45 minutes to an hour and a half or even two hours, depending upon the age group, meeting two or three times a week for three to four months. In this sense an ideal setup is that somatic movement education programs are sustained over time for at least several months, and offered throughout the school year at various grade levels. It's also best to evaluate the success of a particular somatic movement education program after a longer trial run such as I suggest here.

One of the next common issues to arise in teaching a movement-based program such as this, particularly in schools, is the question: Where will we offer it? Space is of a premium, and many schools have either classrooms lined with rows of desks, or a huge gymnasium—neither of which are ideal settings for this work. As many of these somatic activities encourage students to focus on their internal experience, they are less dependent upon the external environment, and therefore teachers can adapt the material to a variety of settings. That being said, I can offer some particulars to be aware of when creating the ideal environment for teaching the somatic practices in this curriculum.

Ideally, the space for these classes should be warm, have adequate lighting, and preferably have a clean, wooden, or otherwise uncarpeted floor. It is also best if the room can be private and quiet and conducive to still, inner focused attention, as well as to allow for students to be moving and expressing through sound without disturbing other groups in adjacent rooms. In a school setting, such a space will likely be the gym or multipurpose room, or possibly a dance or yoga studio space. A room without mirrors is also preferable, since mirrors often bring attention to the external image and thus may detract from a focus on the internal feeling and experience of movement. Some activities are also expressly designed to be done outdoors, although they can also be modified to an indoor setting if necessary.

In some situations it may be challenging to provide an appropriate space—you may not have a spacious, quiet room available, a safe outdoor environment, or the ability to offer smaller class sizes. In this case, you can adapt the material to your own situation, doing your best to work within the limitations you have, as well as to advocate for more supportive circumstances when necessary.

What Grades Should Participate?

This curriculum is designed primarily for high school students, ages fourteen through eighteen, with some activities suitable for younger middle school teens, as well as for young adults. In general I have found that some of the simpler activities in the Embodiment Basics—Level I chapters are suitable for teens of all ages (beginning in middle school, seventh and eighth grades, ages twelve and thirteen), while the activities in the Embodiment Fundamentals—Level II chapters work best with older teens (such as those in high school, ninth to twelfth grades, ages fourteen to eighteen).

When teens reach their final two years of high school, they are often the most motivated to gain the kind of self-understanding and related self-care skills addressed in much of this curriculum, as many of them face the looming transition of leaving home and entering the workforce or a college community. This period of their junior and senior years may be the ideal time for introducing these more complex topics in which teenagers can actively apply the learning from the previous Embodiment Basics activities. Older students also generally have an increased level of maturity—with an increased ability to introspect—to deal with the more complex personal and social issues that may arise in dealing with the body, such as examining the impact of cultural perceptions on their movement and their lives.

Teachers may also use some of the basic activities with preteens, depending upon the maturity level of any particular group. Many of these activities would need to be adapted significantly for working with younger elementary school–aged children, however, who need much simpler approaches; while it is never too early to learn about our bodies, these activities are not designed for that age group.

Further, although this book is focused on adolescents, from my experience teaching at both secondary and college levels, I have found little difference between high school seniors and their freshman and sophomore counterparts in college. I don't say this to imply they are somehow immature for their age; rather I mean that many young college-aged students seem to still be dealing with similar developmental challenges as adolescents. Recently, research in neuroscience and adolescent psychology has concurred, demonstrating that not only has puberty started to blossom much earlier for today's youth, but adolescence also *lasts* much longer—with some researchers suggesting this phase to last a full fifteen years, from age ten to twenty-five.[2] This attests to the increasing need to help our teens and young adults alike—whose challenging adolescent years are not necessarily over when they reach college or the workforce.

In this book, therefore, while the material is primarily geared toward teens in high school, much of my commentary throughout can equally apply to college-aged students. As such, along with anecdotes about the younger students, I've also included some stories about my older students aged nineteen to twenty-five and included some of their journal entries as well, to provide readers with a range of responses to the curricular material.

Lastly, in teaching this material with various age groups, ultimately *you* will be the expert on what is appropriate to offer to your particular group as you get to know them and pay attention to their responses in the moment. This is important to remember. Although we can postulate about young people's potential based on relevant scientific data about adolescent development, brain function, and the like—individuals themselves nevertheless vary in maturity, social-emotional skill sets, physical development, family and cultural upbringing, and so many other factors, which only you will be in a position to appropriately assess.

Introducing the Curriculum to Students

Teachers in regular academic courses whose basic content is familiar to students often take the first class meeting to explain the syllabus and scope of the class (e.g., in English class, teachers will say the class will cover short stories from the twenty-first century) and the types of activities that will be included (e.g., essays, discussions, oral presentations). In the context of a summer camp there may be a day of icebreakers and introductions to set the stage for the program. Somatic movement educators will need to do the same, and possibly dedicate parts of multiple class meetings to helping students get to know each other and understand "what this class is about," as the content may be less familiar. The sections that follow provide preliminary details for introducing the curriculum to students—such as suggestions for setting up the first few classes and establishing ground rules—along with practical basics of implementing the curriculum and preparing supplies. These essential details will help you in the planning stages as you consider the scope of the class, as well as to prepare an appropriate starting point and set the trajectory for success. This includes being clear in your intentions and thorough in your preparations, allowing you to be more present in the moment and teach with confidence.

Preliminaries: Initial Movement Assessment and Student Questionnaires

There are several methods you can use to introduce the curriculum to students, assess their needs, and set the stage for a successful program. While you may find alternate methods that work best for you, there are some general guidelines of methods that have proven most effective for me. You may want to start first with a few common icebreaker games to help students get to know each other. For example, I might go around the circle and invite students to each say their name, along with doing a simple movement. Then we all repeat the student's movement, while repeating the name, as we go around the circle one by one as a way to welcome each person into the group. Such activities help students get to know each other through movement in the first few classes and establish a common movement practice from the start.

Then, when beginning to work with a new group, I employ two methods of evaluating the needs of a group: a movement assessment and a written questionnaire. During the first few classes, I observe the movement of individuals in the class and of the group as a whole. In the first class, I talk to students briefly about the material we will be covering. Then I begin to engage them in the curriculum. I get them moving, laughing, playing. I ask them to be still and concentrate through imagery and visualizations. Finally, I ask them to talk about their experiences in the class that day. After a few days, my observations help me to get a sense of the group. I notice each person's physical vitality, movement preferences, predilection for movement or stillness, ability to concentrate, and way of sharing their experiences in a group. I also notice the particular dynamics between individuals in the group and of the group as a whole.

After the first class, I give students a written questionnaire. Students are asked about their initial level of interest in the class, as well as to rate a list of potential topics in order of their interest in each topic. These include topics such as stress reduction, increased concentration, developing greater flexibility, injury prevention, and learning anatomy. They are asked what physical activities they most enjoy and what injuries they have had, if any. This questionnaire tells me how the student feels about being in the class, as well as their particular interests and expectations. In addition, the questionnaire lets me know the interests of each particular group. These two methods provide me with both my intuitive responses to students' needs and the students' verbal and written responses. This information is essential to help me choose appropriate material and approaches.

Questioning students about their personal concerns also involves them immediately and engages their interest. In the next class, I present the group with an overview of the questionnaire results, giving us a chance to discuss and agree upon the goals for the course. In most cases, at least some students will have marked each of the potential goals listed on the questionnaire as a top priority, and while as a facilitator I can be quite certain that this will be the case, asking them first makes all the difference in gaining their interest in participating![3]

Some students may have studied some anatomy and physiology in previous classes. As they will discover, however, it takes time to physically explore and integrate that knowledge in the body so that it becomes a sensory resource to draw upon. While discussing this briefly can be helpful at the start, the experiences that teens *themselves* have with the activities will be their best teacher in helping them understand the difference between cognitive knowledge and somatic learning. Also, some students with very little "knowledge" of the body may learn kinesthetically quite easily, while other students who "know" all about it may or may not find this learning easily accessible. This will become evident with time, and you can support student learning in all of these cases.

Class Guidelines: Participation and Class Atmosphere

In the beginning of the course I encourage students to agree to participate 100 percent in each activity. As I explain, this is essential since they *can't judge an activity's effectiveness if they do not really try to do it!* "Try first, judge later" is a good motto in this case. This is an important concept to introduce explicitly, as otherwise students may infer that your request is merely a ploy to discipline them. Then, I remind them that the one exception to the 100 percent agreement is that they should first take responsibility for their own well-being. This means that if they have an injury, or know that they should not be doing a particular movement, like running or twisting, they should stop and not do that particular movement or activity. While I may already be aware of certain students' injuries from the initial questionnaire, I also ask that students let me know at the start of class if something new has emerged that they will need to be mindful of during the class that day. This might include emotional as well as physical issues that they feel may impact their participation.

After having discussed the questionnaires and set a trajectory for the course, you can work with the students to establish some further guidelines for class participation. I sometimes draw on a cooperative learning model,[4] using a group process in which students establish respectful behavior and communication guidelines necessary to create a safe space and that they then agree to uphold. Basic ground rules may include agreeing not to put someone down or make fun of them, neither verbally nor through body language, allowing another student to finish speaking without interrupting, and other positive guidelines. You can facilitate this conversation and add your own suggestions as well. Often we write these on a chart that can be later referred to, or on a sheet that each student can sign. For older students, often just having an open conversation about this together can feel sufficient, so see what works best for your group context. In some situations, students will have already done a similar process in another part of the school's program that you can draw on and then add any other relevant boundaries needed in this particular context. In yet other situations, there may already be enough of a conscious community established that an in-depth conversation is not as necessary.

You can also let students know they can observe a specific activity they don't want to engage in, or offer them the option of an "observation day," to allow for instances when they simply don't feel like participating. Girls may use this option on days they are menstruating and feel particularly achy and uncomfortable, for instance, or it may be used by a student with a particular injury or emotional upset, who may prefer to just observe. Sometimes a student will request an observation day, and then decide partway through the class that they prefer to participate. Or they may say they don't want to do a certain activity, and then decide to jump in anyway. Just being given flexibility often helps teenagers feel more comfortable, and ultimately results in more consistent and authentic participation. Students who choose to observe a class can also write their observations and submit it to you at the end of class. This helps them to hone their skill with perceiving movement and to recognize their judgments as their own, while giving you a chance to dialogue with them about their comments later on. You might also ask a student who is observing for their comments during the class, so they can offer their insights to the group as a means to still participate at some level.

The balance of structure and spontaneity, of laughter and quiet concentration, is also an important aspect of engaging students in this work. Humor can help pave the way to openness, and there are many ways to bring in play and spontaneity. You can draw from more ordinary, commonplace movements—like a suggestion to give someone a "high five" as you walk past each other. In other cases it can be fun to do something completely out of the ordinary, like slowing down a movement to the point of moving in slow motion, or suddenly moving very fast. This is especially fun to do with sports activities—drawing on something familiar that teens may have already seen or experienced—like pretending to be dribbling and shooting a basketball in regular speed, then in slow motion. Using references to sports may also help teen boys to feel more comfortable, as they often associate sports as culturally appropriate for them.

In any case, a certain element of surprise, used at the right moment, can be refreshing and uplifting; it can also bring a balance to the otherwise quiet and internal focus of many of the activities.

Student Dress for Class, Personal Supplies, and Preparing the Space

It's best if students wear loose, comfortable clothing and have bare feet or socks only. While some students may prefer to keep their socks on, bare feet are preferable, both to increase proprioceptive sensation to the feet and because socks can be slippery during the more active, locomotor movements like walking or running. You can negotiate this as you see fit, and as appropriate to each activity. Also ask those students who need shoes because of physical injuries to wear dance shoes, sneakers, or other shoes that have not been worn outdoors, because the floor needs to be kept clean and prepared for the possibility of lying down.

When working on the floor, students may want to use a towel or item of clothing to support any areas of discomfort, such as the head or the sacrum. If available, exercise and yoga mats may also be helpful, but in general, I prefer not to use yoga mats—given students' association of them with an actual practice of yoga—or to introduce them later in the course once our routine has been established. It is also helpful to have cushions or pillows for sitting on the floor during discussions.

School Supplies and Supplemental Materials

There are a variety of supplies and associated ancillary activities that I recommend to augment the curriculum—both in and out of class. Adopting them will be dependent on variables like time, budgets, and school homework policies. The resources described here are ones that I've found most helpful in developing a creative, dynamic learning environment; they also help to effectively integrate the various academic, kinesthetic, and socio-emotional aspects of the course.

PROPS AND SUPPLIES

Various props and supplies can be integrated into the curriculum during different activities—such as using physioballs, parachutes, skeletal models, organ models, Thera-Bands, and balloons—to better represent the anatomy material as well as to engage students in lively activities. At the very least, it is extremely helpful to have a skeletal model, either small or life-size, to work with during the class. One word of caution: some teen groups may at first find working with certain of these props to be "childish"; for example, using a parachute may remind them of games they played in elementary school, while other groups will welcome such creative opportunities. You will be the best judge of when and how to incorporate each of these elements to adapt to the sensitivities of your group.

ANATOMY COLORING PLATES

Corresponding anatomy coloring plates from Will Kapit and Lawrence M. Elson's *The Anatomy Coloring Book* are helpful supplements to the exploration topics. Coloring in the plates reinforces students' understanding of the visual size, shape, and location of aspects of the body, which is important to support the process of accurately visualizing the body. Students generally enjoy this activity, and though each plate takes some time, they find that it helps them to engage in the material, visualize their bodies, and discover further questions they may have. They can color the plates in class or at home, either on their own or as a group. One group of college students, for instance, reported that they regularly all went to the beach or park together in the afternoon before our evening class to color the plates, turning what could seem like an arduous task into a more relaxed group learning process. Another group of teens used to meet at one of their homes and complete the plates while listening to music.

On a practical note, you will also need to plan some time to introduce students to the book and how to color the plates, as explained in *The Anatomy Coloring Book* itself. Students can also draw the various anatomical structures, such as a vertebra or other bones, to get the feel of the shape and location, either by tracing specific anatomy plates, or by referring to the plates or to another anatomy book and drawing freehand.

BODY JOURNALS

Throughout the class, students can keep a body journal to respond to class activities or to specific topics. Examples for journal entry topics, to be done in class or at home, are offered throughout the book. Some journal entries draw on the practice of "free-association" writing, in which you follow a stream-of-consciousness process to respond to a particular prompt or topic, such as writing about a body part (such as "my feet," "my bones," or "my hands,") or a physiological process (such as "my breathing"). Such prompts may invite prose, poetry, a list of thoughts, and drawings. Other journal entries may be approached in a more open-ended manner, such as asking students to take a few moments to write about their experiences in the class that day.

Journal entries can be shared in class, either in partners, small groups, or as a full group. Some journal entries can also be handed in to you. In any case, students should be told up front if particular journal entries will be shared publicly or not, and should always be given an option regarding the material from their journals that they wish to share with others in class or will submit to you, versus material they wish to keep private. If you will be collecting journal entries to read, you might ask students to review their entries at home and select two or three of them to be handed in. Arrange this in whatever way will work best for your situation.

You can also discuss the issue of confidentiality, and decide together about how you will handle that as a group. You will also need to disclose any obligations you may be under to report sensitive topics a student may choose to share with you, either verbally or when handing in journal entries. All of these preliminary steps prepare the way for students to feel comfortable with the body journals and to use the process most productively.

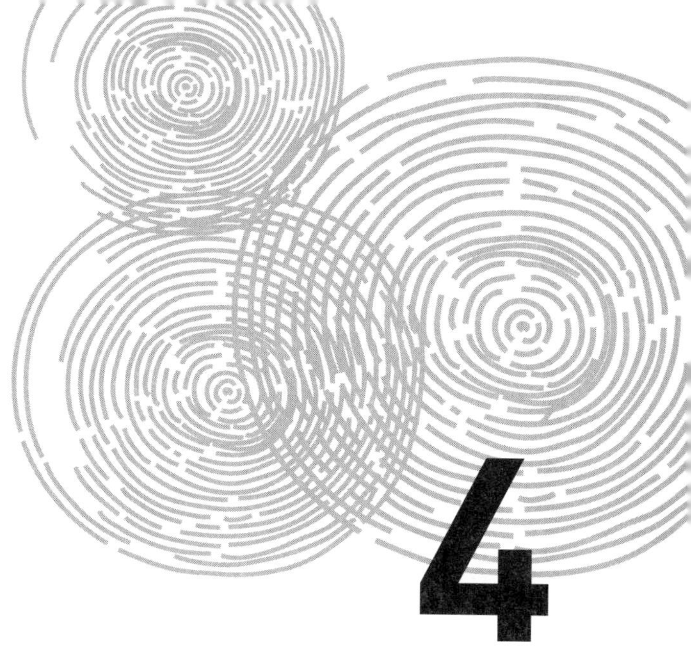

4

Eight Key Pedagogy Principles for Teaching SME with Teens

The study of the human body involves both mystery and fact: there is much known and equally as much that is left unknown. This paradox suggests that we need to value both the information and the questions about what it means to be human.

—Andrea Olsen

In learning about the body, there needs to be time for discovery. Especially in adolescence, students engage when they see themselves as an integral part of the learning process. Teachers become *facilitators,* whose objective is to set up a learning environment with activities appropriate to the specific group with which they are working. The teacher becomes the guide in beginning to engage students in a living understanding of the knowledge and mystery of what it means to be human.

When I was writing this book, I asked my sixteen-year-old niece if she might be interested in taking such a class at school—in which she learned about her body, her movement, and how her body, mind, and emotions might all relate. Her eyes lit up, and she nodded enthusiastically. "Yeah!" she said eagerly. But in the next moment she froze, and a very worried look came over her face. Then she quickly added, "Well, *actually,* it would depend on who was teaching it." Through this wise response, she had stumbled upon the key to opening adolescents up to their inner world: the container for the experience must be perceived as safe and well facilitated. After all, who wants to be in a group of peers and be asked to move and be vulnerable with a teacher who is, for example, overpowering or prone to ridiculing students? I can only imagine the memories of past experiences that flowed through my niece in that moment, of teachers whom she would *not* want teaching her in a class about her body!

Yet this issue is just as much about the personality of the particular teacher as it is about the class atmosphere created through the pedagogy with which the content is being offered. While we can't dictate personality, we can be mindful of our teaching methods to ensure the quality of our students' experience. Through teaching this material over many years, I have discovered that there are several core pedagogical elements that need to be in place to create the kind of trustworthy and caring container necessary for such a curriculum as this one to be effective with teens; without any *one* of them, the learning experience is often severely undermined. Although many of these elements overlap, I've distilled them into eight key pedagogy principles that, if enacted in each class and in the curriculum as a whole, provide a solid foundation for engaging teens in somatic movement education. (See appendix A on page 323 for a summary of these eight points.) While many of the principles are covered in greater detail in subsequent chapters—particularly those that deal more specifically with anatomy/physiology—this chapter provides a brief overview of each principle as it relates to the teaching of the material.

Include Subjective Experience

1. Provide a Balance of Objective Information and Subjective Experience

> **Core Principle:** To facilitate a somatic experience requires an approach to anatomy and movement that is inclusive of both objective information and subjective experience.

While information can be learned, true knowledge comes from one's own lived experience. To offer knowledge, then, we must offer experience. By focusing on students' own sensations and perceptions, we include their subjective experiences in the learning process. This is the *soma,* the body experience from within—the lived experience. All explorations are designed to initiate experiential activities that are grounded in applicable anatomy and that draw on students' own subjective body knowledge.

For such a method to be effective, students need time to process their psychophysical responses. This can take many forms, from drawing to journaling to discussing their experiences with a peer or with the full group. Thus, all explorations include some method of processing. This is explained further in the second pedagogy principle.

Use a Student-Driven Curriculum

2. Employ a Student-Driven Curriculum with the Teacher as a Guide

Core Principle: Start with what students already know, and build on their interests from there.

When you follow your interests, you feel engaged in the learning process. When you are given a chance to *discover what you already know* and *share that knowledge collectively,* you gain confidence from progressing from where you actually are, rather than measuring yourself against some outside standard of what you believe you should already know. As students share their perceptions, they also build community and create a supportive learning environment. These activities are designed to first provide experience and then elicit student input on the topic. A final step—one that has traditionally been seen as the main role of a teacher—would be to provide information *beyond what students already know.* This method prioritizes student-centered, embodied learning.

For instance, when students study breathing, they are first guided in an experiential exercise in which they close their eyes and feel the process of breathing in their own bodies. Next they reflect on the physical structures (anatomy) and processes (physiology) of the act of breathing: How do you breathe? What is happening in your body? What do you feel as you breathe? What is the purpose of breathing? After this internal investigation, students gather in small groups to discuss their experiences and create a list of what they experience and know about breathing. Finally, the groups come together to collectively "harvest" both their cognitive and their bodily knowledge as they share their discoveries.

From there, the facilitator can provide anatomical facts as questions emerge—provided no one else in the group is able to answer them. Common questions include the following: What are the lungs made of? How many are there? Is the diaphragm part of the lungs, or is it a muscle? How do the ribs move? Such questions can be followed up with further discussion, examination of the anatomy drawings or models, and related experiential activities. Other questions might relate to more emotional concerns, like examining why we hold our breath when we get upset. These more psychophysical aspects are also explored in other breathing activities in the curriculum.

Balance Sensory and Motor Learning

3. Provide a Balance of Sensory and Motor Experience in Each Class

> **Core Principle:** Create a balance of activities that provide both quiet inner sensing and active physical movement to keep each class engaging.

If you are always on the go, you end up feeling exhausted and needing a rest. But if you rest for too long, you often end up feeling tired, lethargic, or groggy. You may even just feel bored! It is the balance of rest and activity—or inner and outer focus—that is truly healthy and revitalizing. What we really crave is balance.

Providing a balance of sensory and motor activities within the curriculum can help teens stay engaged. Too much inner sensing—especially for active teens—can be difficult and overwhelming for a variety of reasons. When practiced in stillness, such as lying down, such sensing within may at first feel scary or disorienting to them. Because so little is happening on a physical (external) level, sometimes students are not sure what to do, since they are not used to paying attention at such a subtle level. Other times, by slowing down and focusing within, difficult emotions or areas of body discomfort or pain may rise to the surface of awareness. In any of these cases, stillness may be experienced as uncomfortable, or even repressive.

Yet to give students an underlying foundation of kinesthetic understanding from which to move, much of the experiential learning in this curriculum does focus on inner sensing. Such sensory activities stimulate the parasympathetic nervous system (related to inner sensing with an internal orientation toward the self), while motor activities stimulate the sympathetic nervous system (related to action with an outer orientation toward the environment). To provide a balance, then, you can plan your classes to include both active movement and stationary inner sensing.

For instance, I sometimes begin by asking students to walk through the room, first noticing the objects in the room, then one other, then the spaces between them as they walk. This generates playful group interaction with more of an external focus. As they continue to move through the room, I might ask them to pause, close their eyes, and bring their awareness to the weight on their feet. Then I might ask them to open their eyes and continue walking, maintaining awareness of the weight through their feet while noticing others in the room. (See photos on page 129 and the exploration

Walking on page 300.) When facilitated in this way, this activity encourages integration of external and internal awareness and helps students learn to shift their perceptions consciously from one to the other; this ultimately helps them learn to maintain mindful kinesthetic awareness of their physical sensations *while* moving.

Leading such an activity at the beginning of class also encourages full body movement within a group interaction—motor activities that stimulate the sympathetic nervous system. This provides teens with the "bridge" they need to slowly transition to a more inner-directed, parasympathetic state, which will be required for later inner-focused activities done lying down. Although for many adults such an internal focus can often be experienced as restful right away, active children and teens often find it easier to attend to their internal sensations in stillness after spending some time moving first. These initial movement activities help students experience a sense of play and external engagement that pave the way for the more internal sensing to be restful and enjoyable.

After some time, students begin to settle into a restful state more easily. Eventually, they enjoy the more active activities and the more still, inner-directed activities equally. To get to that point, however, the facilitator needs to attend closely to the level of group engagement in order to provide an appropriate balance of sensory and motor activity in each class on a given day.

While the inner sensing used in the curriculum is essential for reorganizing our nervous system, our process of thinking, and thus our movement, in order to act efficiently it is also essential that we can let go of this mental focus on our sensory awareness. As Bonnie Bainbridge Cohen says,

> It is different if you sense something, than if you feel it, than if you simply do it.... One of the things that I think is essential with sensing is that we reach a point where we become conscious and then we let it go, so that the sensing itself is not a motivation; that our motivation is action, based on perception.[1]

In addition to providing a balance for the more inner-directed activities, active movement activities encourage students to explore without consciously focusing on their movement—they move for the pure fun of moving.

When used at the end of class, these motor activities also help students integrate any physical changes that may have occurred during the class. In this final stage, body awareness becomes integrated into movement, so that awareness underlies action—without the need for a continued "mindful" attentiveness. Otherwise, it is like going to the DMV, getting your license, and then staying there. These somatic activities are meant to enhance your movement and your life, not merely to be a relaxing break in an otherwise hectic lifestyle.

Both improvisational "scores" (e.g., the walking activity) and specific, structured movement phrases (those from yoga, aikido, or dance, for instance) can serve as appropriate movement activities for this purpose. I often teach the Sun Salutation—a popular yoga phrase described in the curriculum—for this purpose as well.

At times, you may sense that your group needs a "party day"—with active movement throughout—or a complete "rest day" of calming, inner-focused activities. In these cases, it is best to follow the needs of the moment. In general, however, the balance of sensory and motor activities will be an important element to consider in each class to keep the learning engaging.

Teach about Proprioception

4. Teach about Proprioception and Orientation—and Allow for Some Measure of Discomfort or Disorientation

Core Principle: Teach about proprioception (our "self-receiver cells") and its relationship to learning new skills and movement patterns. This helps students develop patience with the process of kinesthetic learning, often new to them, which may include initial periods of disorientation as they "unlearn" old patterns in order to learn new ones.

Embodiment practices that rely on kinesthetic awareness can feel foreign at first, and students are quick to realize that this class experience is quite unfamiliar. Some students may find they enjoy the activities right away, as a tenth-grade girl named Giuliana noted in her journal after her first class:

> *My time today was really interesting. I felt very relaxed and at ease. It was very different than anything I have done before. It really made me think about my body in depth. It was eye-opening. It made me think about the way my body works, and why I feel certain ways at certain times. I enjoyed the experience.*

An eighth grader named Cameron wrote: "I had a very blissful experience. I felt relaxed and comfortable with the people around me. It was nice moving and learning more about human anatomy." And eighteen-year-old Cally noted after her first class: "Mindfulness, relaxation, body anatomy. Comfort with making sound and movement. Most of it was fun and relaxing and calming. Pushing my comfort zone."

Other students respond with less enthusiasm about having their "comfort zone pushed," and sometimes students' journal responses reflect an initial trepidation at the start of the class, only to have them recognize its value later on. Sentiments such as "At first the things we did seemed funny" or "I thought what we did was really strange" change as time goes by, as in this telling entry by Bryan, an eleventh grader, after his six-week gym unit:

> *This class surprised me, I wasn't sure about it at first. But after awhile, I started to realize how much tension I had in my body. Over time from doing Constructive Rest I got more relaxed while doing it and also after doing it. I also discovered that if I relax before a game my performance is 100 percent better. It helps me to center myself and get ready to play, and I concentrate better in the game.*

Maintaining this larger perspective, knowing that some measure of discomfort may occur—and will likely pass—you can help your students understand the process they are going through by teaching them directly about proprioception and kinesthetic sense using specific experiential activities (see chapter 10). As readers will discover in greater detail later in the book, proprioceptors are nerve cells in the muscles and joints that provide the body awareness necessary to feel our position in space and to learn new movement patterns. Combined with the sensory receptors called interoceptors that are located in our internal organs, proprioceptors contribute to our kinesthetic sense, or our awareness of our body when in motion.

Before we can learn a new movement pattern, however, we must first *unlearn an old one*—a process that may leave us feeling disoriented since we are no longer relying on the previously established proprioceptive pathways in our nervous system, and yet have not yet formed new pathways to help us reorient. Knowing this, a facilitator needs to be prepared to allow for *disorientation* and the resulting "discharge" that may occur—yawning, laughing, making jokes—as students attempt to get comfortable in a new situation, understanding this as a precursor to "reorientation" and new learning. While this may be true in any new situation, it is particularly evident in somatic learning. Teaching students about proprioception will provide them with a cognitive framework for realizing the necessity of some measure of newness in their experience—which may translate to them as strange or weird—in order to develop new proprioceptive and interoceptive sensations and thereby expand their movement potential, allowing them to be more patient with the process. This will also help the group to become more understanding of themselves—or others who may be navigating this sometimes awkward but necessary transitional stage—as they pass from discomfort to comfort with the material.

Later on, as they become more experienced with these types of somatic activities, students tend to take greater responsibility for their responses and come to enjoy this process of moving, repatterning their movement, and learning about themselves. This phenomenon has also been noted by other somatic movement educators when working with college-aged students.[2] As students come to understand any awkwardness and resistance they may have, and can discuss this openly as it *relates to the anatomy/physiology of kinesthetic learning,* you can reach a common ground that allows you all to feel more comfortable.

Further, as is true for those of us who have been a teen or known a teen—that is, all of us—remember that many young people are quite uncomfortable with their bodies. They also may be struggling to adapt to myriad body changes, such as boys who have grown facial hair before or after many of their friends, or girls who are ahead or behind their peers in developing breasts or beginning their menstruation. Even beyond the complex issues of body image and self-esteem, some teens have unfortunately come to simply fear their own bodies. These classes can support students to overcome some of their initial fears and awkwardness with their bodies, as reflected in this final journal entry by Jeanne, a tenth-grade girl, after her four-month course:

> *I started out feeling very self-conscious in this class. I think I was afraid of my body. But being aware of what's in my body and how I move makes me more at ease. Having the knowledge about my body allows me to be a little more confident.*

Other students remark on how little they know about their bodies. And while many teens are quite curious and enthusiastic to learn more, others express an initial hesitancy or squeamishness about it. This has been true for students at all levels of experience, from middle school to high school to college. Our bodies have on some level become foreign to us.

As an educator, the more you reflect on and come to understand the many complex challenges—as well as the gifts—that you are presenting by offering embodiment practices, the better your chances are of successfully negotiating the potential difficulties inherent in introducing teens and young adults to this type of kinesthetic learning process. Teaching about proprioception, interoception, and kinesthetic awareness can significantly ease the way.

Use a Layered Learning Approach

5. Use a Layered Learning Approach in the Progression of Curricular Material

> **Core Principle:** Teach using a layered learning approach to help students to experience some level of proficiency and ease without being overly challenged. This also allows you to add new material that builds on previous experience to keep students engaged.

You can help facilitate students' comfort level in the class by keeping a balance of old and new material—that is, reviewing activities from previous classes while integrating new movement activities. As dance and movement educators know, this type of layered approach ensures some level of familiarity with the material while challenging students with new approaches. This method also respects the process of psychophysical learning—appreciating the need for new proprioceptive stimulation yet understanding students' desire for some measure of comfort within which new body learning can occur. Through this type of layered learning, students can experience some level of proficiency and ease without being overly challenged.

For instance, when introducing students to rolling down the spine—bending forward from the waist to release one's upper-body weight toward the floor—you can guide them to relax their chin down toward their chest and then release their upper-body weight toward the floor. After studying the spine and learning that it is composed of vertebrae and intervertebral discs, students learn to roll down by first releasing the weight of the head forward and then progressively releasing each vertebrae, while allowing for the spaces between the vertebrae—the discs—to expand with the weight of gravity. They can also feel the buoyancy of these spaces as they roll back up the spine. In a subsequent class, students can learn another layer: the names and number of the specific vertebrae—the seven cervical, twelve thoracic, and five lumbar—and you can then guide them to articulate each section while naming them specifically, such as counting C1–C7 for the cervical, T1–T12 for the thoracic, and so forth. This approach serves as a cognitive review of the information learned while progressively inviting more nuanced and articulate movement in each class. The activities become familiar without being merely repetitive, as the new information and challenges keep students engaged.

This type of training is often referred to as "scaffolding," and is considered an important aspect of adolescent education.[3] In his book *Age of Opportunity: Lessons from the New Science of Adolescents,* Laurence Steinberg advocates for this approach as a primary means to effectively teach adolescents: "The training needs to be *scaffolded.* By this I mean that the activities should be demanding, but not so demanding that they overwhelm the adolescent's current capabilities.... An effective school-based intervention should be calibrated to fall into the 'zone,' so that it's challenging but not so difficult as to frustrate or discourage the child. Once the child has mastered a particular task, the degree of difficulty should be increased, but just slightly."[4] Examples of ways to layer, or scaffold, activities over time are included throughout the book.

Another way to layer in small bits of experiential learning is to teach a few students and then have them teach other students in the class. For example, when your students are writing in their journals or coloring anatomy plates during class, you can teach a related simple activity to the first few students to finish, like feeling how the leg (femur) rotates in the hip socket (acetabulum). Each student can then teach one other student who has finished. Once everyone has experienced the new activity, when you can come back together as a group, you can make any necessary additional suggestions or adjustments as you observe them in the activity, or answer any further questions that may have arisen. When teens teach each other, they gain ownership of the material. They also discover their questions, since if we don't really understand something for ourselves, it's hard to teach someone else! This also helps to build a strong sense of community among teens, as will be discussed further in the next principle.

Create a Safe Container and Sense of Community

6. Create a Safe Container and Build a Sense of Community

> **Core Principle:** We learn best when we are respected and approached with love and compassion. Create a community of mutual respect and kindness as a foundation for growth and learning.

Creating a safe container for teaching somatic work for teens is no small task. Going within and focusing on your body—even for adults—can be wonderful one day and fraught with challenges the next. The previous pedagogy principles have already included information relevant to creating a safe container for students (such as layering the curriculum to keep activities within a reasonable comfort zone) and to building a sense of community (such as by creating a context for students to openly share their discoveries through discussion). Safety and community are intricately connected, since building a sense of community builds trust among the group members, which in turn helps create a safe container for somatic work. And of course movement itself can help build community. Moving together is a powerful bonding experience that can reinforce a sense of warmth and belonging.

Several interrelated important factors contribute to the creation of a strong and appropriate container in which to safely engage teens in somatic work.

COMPASSION, KINDNESS, AND EMPATHY

Recent research in psychology and neuroscience has clearly demonstrated what we all know intuitively: we learn best in an atmosphere of care and compassion. Compassion is about relationships, both intrapersonal and interpersonal. To create a compassionate environment, there are three levels to be considered: self-compassion, the relationship between ourselves and our students, and the relationships between the students themselves.

First, how can we achieve the necessary level of compassion and empathy toward our students? One supportive attitude is to maintain the basic premise that individuals are wise, whole, and resourceful while remembering that they are also experts on their own subjective experience. Simultaneously, you can perceive that each individual is also growing and learning—evolving over time—and is likely to have areas of both strengths and weaknesses, leading to both successes and individual challenges. Maintaining this perspective helps to draw out the best in others while giving you a measure of patience with the more challenging moments when individuals are not acting out of their highest natures. It's also important to remember that the same is true for yourself: provide an equal measure of compassion for your own growth and learning. Then, as you aspire to facilitate this material to the best of your ability with each group, be open to self-evaluation and critique as well.

How can we help develop a safe, compassionate, and kind community among teen peers? First, we can help teens develop compassion and kindness toward *themselves.* Recent research on compassion such as that by Kristin Neff has shown that self-compassion leads to increased self-care, the benefits of which are many, including lowered anxiety and depression, increased creativity, and better overall health.[5] Many of the explorations support students in gaining self-compassion and self-care, as they give them a tool set for integrating body and mind, and teach them to move and engage in life with greater ease. As students feel more confident and comfortable in themselves, they often become less judgmental of—and less reactive toward—others as well.

We can also help students begin to recognize their basic commonalities as human beings—such as that we all have a skeletal system—which evokes empathy and kindness toward oneself and others. Studies have demonstrated that when individuals recognize a common trait with another person, their empathetic response—often measured as the level of kindness extended toward that individual—increases.[6] This perceived similarity elicits our natural capacity for concern for others, while our refusal to recognize such similarities can result in reactions that are contrary to our empathetic natures, leading to all manner of negative behaviors toward others—from stereotyping to objectification and dehumanization to demonization.[7] When teens develop an embodied understanding of their similarities, it affects many layers of related social issues that stem from an inability to embrace the "other" as similar to oneself.

To create a truly compassionate—and safe—environment for all, we also need to allow for differences. Several pedagogy methods in the curriculum are designed to address the creation of such an inclusive atmosphere. For example, in facilitating the discussion sections, we can include a variety of individuals' experiences, so that students come to see that it is safe to express dissent. Imagine, for example, that others are saying they felt relaxed and refreshed after an activity, while you found the same experience to be uncomfortable. Or you were left feeling tenser than before, rather than more relaxed. Now what would you do? As a teen looking to fit in with your peers, likely you remain silent. Yet in somatic work, noticing tightness in our body or feelings of discomfort, boredom, or sadness, or even feeling grossed out may be part of the experience at times and are just as important measures of the experience as positive responses, like feeling relaxed and open. Of course, this can also play out in the opposite way: many individuals have expressed feeling discomfort or dissatisfaction of some sort, while the student who enjoyed the activity is afraid to speak out.

One way to ensure space for all experiences, which I learned from Bonnie Bainbridge Cohen, is to ask the following question after some students have shared: *"Did anyone have a different experience?"* This way we *invite* difference rather than just tolerate it. Students also come to see that you are open and respectful of various experiences, ideas, and opinions—helping them gain the courage to share in the group, even if their experience differs from that of their peers. You can also speak about this directly. This permission invites them to be more authentic.

Remember that this also invites individuals to express reluctance, resistance, apathy, and other emotions that may normally be deemed disrespectful to express to a teacher. Yet opening the discussion to *all* experiences is essential if teens are to feel truly safe. While many teachers may feel comfortable with this level of discussion, others may not have as much experience facilitating this type of dialogue; therefore I've included some examples throughout the book of how to facilitate potentially difficult conversations that may arise from such open invitations. Additional training in areas such as conflict resolution and community mediation may help you feel more confident and open when dealing with a wide range of diverse expressions. Without this training or at least a certain comfort level and proficiency in dealing with conflict, this type of class can easily deteriorate into a power struggle between teacher and students: not a healthy atmosphere in which to invite inner work. When well-facilitated, open, inclusive dialogue allows students to voice and sort out their own perspectives, as well as to respect differences among them.

ORDER AND DISCIPLINE / STRUCTURE AND SPONTANEITY

In addition to a compassionate atmosphere, students also need a certain element of order and discipline to stay focused on the task at hand, as well as to feel safe. Adolescent developmental research has shown that teens do best when given both firm discipline and warm understanding.[8] Steinberg advocates this concisely: "Be warm. Be firm. And be supportive."[9] To facilitate the focused environment needed for somatic work, it is important to establish *clear directions and boundaries* in all activities. (This is especially important with those that may involve touch; see chapter 6, "Touch and Other Touchy Subjects," for more discussion.) It is also important to keep a balance of *structure and spontaneity* appropriate to the comfort level of the group. This helps keep the learning fun.

In this regard, some of the curriculum relies on structured improvisations, or "scores"—a game with rules: the rules and goals are defined, but the method of accomplishing the goals is discovered by the participants. In working with adolescents, a clear set of rules helps them feel safe and builds a measure of trust between you and the group. If the score is too free-form, open-ended, and improvisatory, teens immediately feel threatened—not knowing how to measure if they are "doing it right," or even why they are engaging in the activity at all. They also often experience the context as being too childish if there is too much freedom, since they have come to associate unstructured free play with elementary school, which by middle and high school is generally experienced as definitively beneath them. Over time, as students become more familiar with the structure of the class and the type of somatic awareness practices involved, it becomes easier to introduce some more free-form exploration as well.

On the other hand, if the structure is too rigid and repetitive, teens will likely either space out or rebel. When we take a *psychophysical* perspective on such behavior—rather than immediately labeling it a behavioral problem—we can begin to recognize it as a likely sign of an imbalance in the learning environment and make necessary adjustments. (This topic will be discussed further in the next chapter; see the section on Perceiving and Describing the "Mind of the Room" on page 85.) In any case, finding an appropriate balance of structure and spontaneity is an important aspect of creating a safe container for teens to engage in these embodiment activities.

RESPECT THE NEED FOR MOVEMENT

As educators, we have been conditioned to associate stillness with attention: if our students are still, we know they are paying attention. We may also feel some measure of confidence from feeling we are in control by assuming we have gained their attention. Yet in many cases, this could not be less true! To be able to pay attention—especially when the task at hand is a cognitive one, such as sitting in a group discussion—you may actually need to change your physical position once in a while to maintain your focus. While we often assume this to be true for students diagnosed with learning disabilities or ADHD, it may also be true for *all* students, as well as for many of us as adults. In fact, research into the benefits of movement—and the detriments of sitting—has led to an influx of technological innovations for introducing movement into the classroom, ranging from standing desks to balance balls to pedal desks.

In facilitating these classes—particularly the discussion sections—students should be encouraged to check in with themselves regularly about what they need, and should be free to change their position as needed, such as getting a physioball to sit on or grabbing a chair if sitting on the floor is uncomfortable. When teaching from a somatic perspective, we don't want a chaotic, "anything goes" environment, but we do want students to feel free to move when needed. This more permissive approach may also necessitate a new measure for *you* as to what it means for students to pay attention respectfully, since movement in a classroom is often seen as acting out—even if no other disrespectful behavior is being exhibited. Here again, striking a balance of respectful listening while slightly expanding the idea of what that might mean can provide an atmosphere more conducive to somatic learning. Students need to be free to move, but not to the point that it becomes overly disruptive for you or others in the class. This balance can be negotiated by the group or can be discussed outside of class with a particular student if necessary.

TEACH WITH LOVE

Many educators have advocated for the importance of a loving relationship as a basis of learning. This is especially true in our work with teens, who often feel harshly disciplined by exasperated adults. Research in neuroscience has shown that secure and loving caretaking relationships form the foundation for emotion-regulation skills among adolescents,[10] while mindfulness educators drawing on this research have noted that when children are cared for with a measure of predictable sensitivity, their tolerance for discomfort increases.[11] Providing a loving educational context becomes especially important in somatic work, which inevitably requires a certain level of discomfort in order to invite new learning via movement. A loving environment allows adolescents to gradually trust that their feelings will not overwhelm them and to develop further self-care skills. This capacity continues to develop as a progressive stage of self-regulation in adolescence.[12]

Teaching with love goes beyond merely holding love and compassion in our hearts for our students. We demonstrate our caring for students as human beings by *valuing their opinions and experiences as part of the educational process.* In this way, we let students know that it's OK to be themselves. A college student of mine expressed this beautifully in one of her journals:

> *I often wonder why it is that when we fall in love or are finally accepted by someone is when we can settle into ourselves. With love, the weight of life is seemingly lifted from our shoulders.*

Including students' own experiences also shows them that we are looking beyond their outer appearances and social status to get to know them as individuals. We also encourage them to do the same as they view one another; these somatic practices encourage students to look deeper than what kind of cell phone they have, the clothes they wear, or the color of their skin. Bringing loving attention to students' inner experience as part of the educational process can equip them with a level of self-esteem conducive to entering into new learning challenges. Teaching with love, we are best setting our students up to learn.

Provide Time for Integration

7. Provide Time for Integration of New Material / Experiences

> **Core Principle:** Include a motor activity at the end, such as walking, to help integrate the more inner-directed parasympathetic activities often explored in somatic exercises and to help students reorient as they prepare to move on to whatever activity follows your class or session. Leave time for a final discussion section as a further way to help students integrate their experiences that day.

While in certain instances it may be fine to end a class with a quiet, inner-focused activity, in many cases students will be entering a very stimulating environment after your class—the lunchroom, the hallway, the city streets, the subway—and may benefit from a transition period to adjust to the outside world. At the very least, it is generally best to end with a brief eyes-open activity, which allows for a transition back to a more outer-oriented perception. To allow time for that, in planning your session you will need to finish any eyes-closed individual or partner work at least five to ten minutes before the actual end of class. Many movement activities or games can be used for this closing piece—walking through the room, doing "the wave" (or passing a similar gesture around a circle), or clapping out a particular rhythm pattern. These activities can be initiated either by you or by the students themselves.

You may also find that the group does best with a more specific and established closing ritual, such as the ringing of a bell or students clapping together three times in a circle. This chosen activity may be used as an opening ritual as well, so that there is consistency in how you begin and end. Opening and closing rituals contribute to establishing a clear and predictable container for the class.

Leaving some time before the end of a session also allows time for the class to regroup and for you to ask for any comments or questions that may need to be addressed before students leave for the day. Stay aware of and monitor the amount of processing time that may be needed to provide adequate closure to each class. In fact, it is more important to allow time for such processing if necessary than it is to adhere to a certain goal of covering particular material on any given day. While with experience we can often predict how much time we may need for an activity, each group and each day is different. When facilitating somatic work, it is especially important to remain flexible to keep the priority on adequately meeting the needs of the moment.

This may include recognizing when it is best not to speak at all, and letting students have time to process and physically integrate the material on their own. In such cases, you may find it best to start with an opening circle check-in at the next class, to see if there is anything left from the last class that needs to be discussed, once students have had some time and distance from the experience.

Teach from Embodied Knowledge

8. Teach from What You Know and Have Experienced in Your Own Body; Trust Yourself While Acknowledging That You Are a Student in This Process as Well

> **Core Principle:** Remember that you are teaching by transmission through your own movement, as well as by the structured activities you are offering. Be willing to demonstrate that you are both a student and a teacher in this process.

In teaching embodiment practices, your physical presence will speak louder than your words. Your own embodied experience—past and present—is central to your ability to facilitate the material. This makes sense on a practical level, but it also makes sense on a psychophysical level. In teaching mindfulness practices, for instance, you likely know that if you want students to meditate but you are in a nervous state yourself, chances are good that things will not go very well. Why is this?

EMBODIMENT AND MOVEMENT TRANSMISSION

We help to initiate certain states in others through our own movement and presence. For instance, a meditative state when embodied brings about a sense of rest and calm, associated with the parasympathetic nervous system. Your *own physical presence* is actively transmitted to your students through cellular resonance, which in this example inspires a calmer state in them as well. In somatic movement practices, we aspire to embody *all* aspects of our body systems and their correlating states of mind. The more comfortable you are with expressing a wide range of movement, the more you can guide your students to find their own expression. To help others, we must first do the work ourselves.

BEING BOTH TEACHER AND STUDENT

Regardless of the extent of our previous experience, we are all still students in the process of embodiment and in learning about our bodies—because the *mystery* of the human body and human consciousness is just so great. Don't be afraid to let your students know that you are also engaged with them in the learning process. Sometimes this means discussing your particular background and skill set up front, so that students understand the context of your knowledge. Otherwise, since the class material relates to the body, students will often assume that you know everything about it.

In my class, I often briefly discuss my previous dance and somatics experience, while letting students know that I don't have a particular medical background. I learned to do this over time, since students would inevitably ask me about myriad medical conditions. In discussing the heart and circulatory system, for example, they might ask me how open-heart surgery is done; or in a discussion after a certain breathing activity, they might want to know more about treatments for asthma. If they are asking out of curiosity, it is fine to simply say "I don't know" or direct them toward more independent research; or if they are inquiring due to a specific medical condition they themselves may have, you can direct them to talk with their parents and to seek out an appropriate health care professional. In any case, speaking at the outset about the limitations of your experience helps the class stay focused on the learning at hand while still inviting students' curiosity.

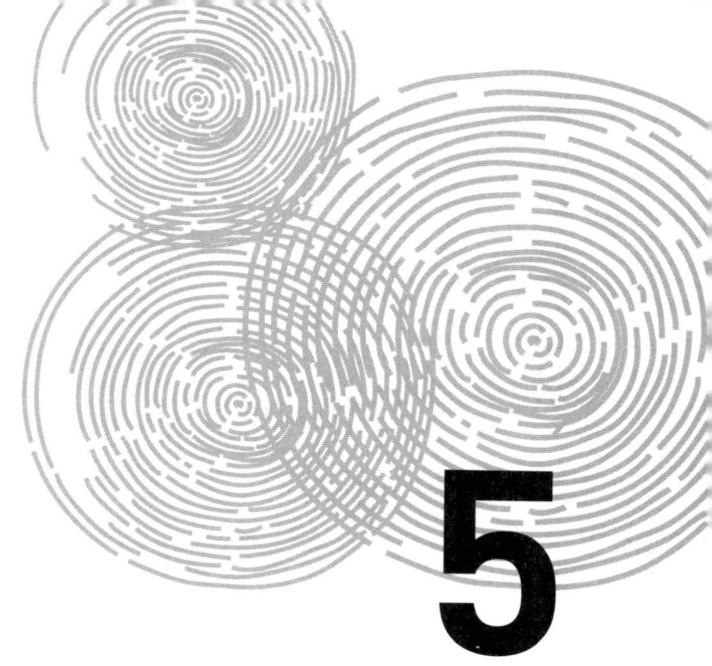

5

The Language of Embodiment

The point of doing these exercises is to create a way of moving and being that opens perception, so habitual ways of operating are discovered and replaced with awareness. It is in this place of awareness that innovation can be born and the inquiry into what it means to be alive, in a human body, gets interesting.

—Caryn McHose and Kevin Frank

Movement itself is a language. As somatic movement educators we help people to develop and build upon that language in physical and nonverbal ways. The essence of embodiment occurs at primarily a cellular level. The verbal language we use is not unrelated to the physical activities we teach and encourage, however, since our language perpetuates certain perspectives. When used with care and intention, language can skillfully guide individuals more accurately and deeply into their experience. In teaching somatic work, we need to be particularly mindful of the words we choose and the *responses* that our words elicit: are they helping or hindering the students' learning process? Are they inviting awareness?

Being mindful of and consistent in your language also develops a shared vocabulary for speaking about the body and movement that can be used throughout this cumulative curriculum. This enables all students to gain ownership over the terms used in the classroom, and have language to describe their experiences. Here are just a few of the most important concerns, particularly when working with teens, which relate to both how we speak to students in the classroom in general, and how we use language related specifically to anatomy and physiology.

Inviting Student Participation

Positive vs. Negative Directives

In teaching from a somatic perspective, keep directives positive. For example, rather than saying, "Don't do x, y, and z," you can focus on what you are encouraging students to do, by saying something like "I invite you to ..." do such and such. Such a phrase is more encouraging, as well as much simpler for students to understand and process. I once saw an amusing animated film that illustrated this psychological effect. It portrayed two children who had climbed up very high in a tree in the yard. Their parents stood at the base of the tree wondering what to do to help their child get down safely, when a big gust of wind came by and started to sway the tree. One parent called out, "Hold on tightly" to their child, while a parent of the other child shouted, "Don't fall!" The first child held on, and then slowly started climbing down the tree to safety, while the other one became startled and promptly fell out of the tree. The moral of the story was that the child who was told not to fall had to first *imagine themselves falling,* and then *physically inhibit that response,* while the other child was free to follow the directive offered. In this sense, positive directives can be more easily followed.

So for example, rather than "Don't lift your shoulders as you reach your arms up," you can say, "As you reach your arms up, allow your shoulders to soften and relax," or even pose this as a question, such as, "As you reach your arms up, can you allow your shoulders to relax?" Another even more open-ended version, which invites further somatic inquiry, would be to merely suggest: "As you reach your arms up, notice what happens in your shoulders." Or ask, "As you reach your arms up, what happens in your shoulders?" Rather than serving as an elicitation for mere obedience, each of these methods is an invitation that provides an opportunity for *increased awareness.* These distinctions are subtle but important, in that the former runs the risk of perpetuating an automatic habitual response, while the latter invites an inquiry process.

Ask before Telling

Remember to ask before telling by allowing *curiosity,* rather than *assumption,* to guide you. This process respects students' own perspectives and experiences, rather than overlaying your own opinions as a means to judge and evaluate. For instance, when looking at a student's drawing, you might first ask a few questions before offering your own observations. Or if a student is having a certain response to a movement activity, such as keeping their eyes open when you have suggested multiple times that they try the activity with eyes closed, you can ask why they might prefer to keep their eyes opened—which inevitably gives you more information to work with in any case. While some behavioral issues or obvious disruptions to the class will of course require further intervention to sort out, beginning with curiosity is never a bad idea!

To do this takes a certain amount of mindfulness on our part, however, along with a willingness to inquire into why we might hold certain tendencies ourselves. By approaching *ourselves* with curiosity as well, we are more likely to have the resources to allow space for our students' perspectives.

Activity vs. Exercise

Although physical activity can be approached in many ways, the term *exercise* has come to be associated with the physical fitness model. We exercise for a purpose: to become fit, to trim down, to lift up, or perhaps to fit in. The focus is generally on *accomplishing* the movement, rather than on *how* we are doing it. In somatic practices, you pay attention to the internal experience of the movement as well—how we may feel and what we perceive—instead of merely measuring whether or not we have been successful or unsuccessful in completing some task. Of course, we can approach any form of exercise with more or less somatic awareness. And although there are distinct purposes and benefits to many types of physical movement, it is important to discern the difference in approach if somatic education is to be understood on its own terms.

In this book, therefore, I use the term *activity* rather than the term *exercise* when referencing a specific movement practice done in the curriculum. (As described previously in chapter 3, when a specific movement activity is presented with a defined purpose and a related concluding discussion, I refer to it in its totality as an "exploration.") In your own communication, I would suggest discussing "activities" in the class rather than referring to the content as "exercises."

You All vs. You Guys

Although the colloquial expression "you guys" has become so deeply engrained in American culture that it would seem like splitting hairs to discuss it, it's worth examining its usage and considering the message we are sending by using it to address our students. With the English language's lack of a plural form of *you, you guys* has been widely used as a gender-neutral term. Of course that is not the case, as the term *boy, man,* or *guy* is used for a male, with its equivalent in the word *woman, girl,* or *gal* used for a female. Just imagine if we were to reverse this usage, for instance, and casually refer to a roomful of boys and girls, or men and women, as "you gals" rather than "you guys." How do you think that would go over? In consideration of eliminating any unnecessary division and exclusion of any one or more genders, in any case you can consider using "you" or "you all," when referring to your group, and get rid of the need to reference gender at all.

Using Embodied Language

My Body vs. the Body

In the language in this book, I use—and recommend—a very specific use of possessive pronouns. When referring to general anatomy and physiology, such as in a discussion, I use the term "*the* body," such as referring to the bones, the breath, or the organs. When referring to students' own bodies, such as in the activities themselves, I use the subjective possessive: "*your* arm" instead of "*the* arm," for example, or "your body" instead of "the body" or even "it." This is again a subtle but important distinction.

Imagine, for instance, being asked in a yoga class to "reach the arms up," rather than to "reach your arms up." While not true for everyone, many people find that use of the subjective pronoun invites more personal engagement, while the use of the word *the* promotes a more mechanical use of your body. I have found evidence to attest to this when working with adults in my private practice as a somatic movement educator, and those who refer to their own bodies with terms such as "the body" or "the leg" often are quite unconscious of doing so. In some cases, they may also later discover elements of trauma in their own body history, with such terms used as a means of subtly distancing themselves from their subjective and sensory experience. As they become more comfortable with their bodies, such people often spontaneously begin to refer to themselves with more subjective terms: *my body, my breath, my legs.*

Paying attention to the language our students use gives us clues and information about their experience, while choosing our language thoughtfully can invite them into a more personal relationship with their movement.

Colloquial Terms vs. Anatomical Terms

In referring to the body, it can be helpful to begin with common terms that students will be most familiar with, such as the spine, neck, head, hips, torso, and shoulders. As the course progresses and students learn more anatomical terms, you can begin to weave them in. For instance, as students study the skeletal system and learn locations and names of specific bones, the neck can be referred to as "the cervical vertebrae," moving the leg becomes "moving the femur in the acetabulum of the pelvis," and so forth.

This use of body-based language can also extend to movement references, such as using terms like core and peripheral movement (referring to whether a movement is initiated in the axial skeleton, the core, or the appendicular skeleton, the periphery), or to proximal versus distal initiation (referring to movement of the limbs, with proximal being the joint closest to the axial skeleton and distal being the joint furthest away). In this way, you begin to use anatomical language to support both more specific understanding of the body and more nuanced movement choices.

Anatomically Accurate Movement Directives and Invitations

In inviting movement it is important to use anatomically accurate prompts, yet many times our colloquial language falls short of the reality of our bodies! Take for example the common saying, heard in schools, yoga studios, and meditation halls alike, to "Straighten your spine" or to "Sit up straight." While this directive does get people to *change something,* it also often invites greater tension as you attempt to push or pull yourself into what looks like a straighter alignment. Rather, I find it more helpful to suggest, "Lengthen your spine," which invites a more internal adjustment, while respecting the anatomy of the spine—which is naturally *curved* rather than straight.

This is just one example, and throughout this book I include further discussion regarding how to use language to assist in creating an accurate perception of one's body and invite more ease of movement.

Words of Perception: Feel, Visualize, Imagine

To effect change in the body, you can bring your attention to your body in a variety of ways. One way is to bring your attention to your physical sensations, such that you *feel* your feet on the ground for instance. With increased awareness, you might also notice if your weight is shifted more forward on your toes or backward on your heels, for example. If you are asking students to bring their attention to their sensations, then, you might use words like "feel" or "notice."

Using general directives like "Feel your body" or "Notice any changes" can be helpful phrases to use when you want students to learn from their own experience in a more open-ended way. Used at the end of a particular movement activity, for instance, this give students an opportunity to discover any changes that emerge most prominently in their own awareness.

On the other hand, more specific directives can be used when you want to invite students to pay attention to a particular aspect or area of their bodies, such as "Notice if you feel your weight more on one foot or the other." These more specific instructions make it easier for students to learn how to notice *sensation*—helping them know where to specifically put their attention—especially as they are getting introduced to this process. Keeping this in mind, you can use a mix of both general and specific language in your instructions depending upon the goal of the activity, as modeled throughout the curriculum section of the book.

In much of this somatic work, we also use a process of visualization to bring awareness to particular aspects of our bodies that we can't see visually, such as visualizing the organs within our bodies, the bones of the rib cage, or the movement of the blood moving throughout our veins and arteries. This process supports learning about your body, as well as distinguishing between body systems for the purpose of both shifting your felt sense and increasing the articulation of your movement. In other instances, you might combine visualization with imagery, such as imagining that your feet are growing roots down into the earth. Much of the work in Ideokinesis, as described earlier, is based on such use of imagery to effect change in the body.

In fact, muscles respond better to *imagery* than to directives, since muscles function in groups rather than in isolation, as noted by Andrea Olsen in her book *BodyStories:*

> [T]he body is unable to respond to a directive to "release the sternocleidomastoid muscle" of the neck; instead, either a functional directive [used when lying down] such as relax the head to the side, or a visualization or image of relaxing your neck into a pillow, will affect the release of that muscle in particular, accompanied by all of the muscle groups involved in head support.[1]

This is an extremely important concept to understand, and also helps to explain why much of this curriculum is based on the bones and the use of imagery, rather than extensive study of the muscles as in some other physical training approaches, such as sports training. Although we often think of the muscles as directing our actions, it is actually often more effective to clarify the bone support and use imagery, than it is to simply train the muscles.[2]

Individuals will vary in the way that certain images affect them, depending on their own associations and background of course, so you can experiment with what works best for you and the group with whom you are working. Suggestions for using visualizations and imagery are mentioned throughout the curriculum.

Specialized Terminology

There are a few key terms and concepts that will be used throughout the book that may not be familiar to you, even if you are versed in traditional anatomy, kinesiology, and physiology. Understanding these concepts will help you to recognize the deeper psychophysical learning inherent in these activities, as will be introduced here briefly and expanded upon later in the curriculum section of the book.

The "Mind" of the Body Systems

According to the principles of Body-Mind Centering (described previously in chapter 2), expression of a certain body system activates a certain state of mind, just as entering a certain state of mind will activate that body system. For instance, moving from the bones may initiate a state of clarity and directness, while moving from the muscles may initiate a state of resistance or vitality. On a basic level, you can perhaps understand this in this way. Imagine if you are feeling very tense and anxious. Often your movement will be more constricted and have a tense "muscular" quality as well. Our language reflects this intuitive understanding, such as when we are told to "muscle-up" or to "just muscle through it," suggesting we should push through our resistance. On the other hand, engaging our muscles can be empowering, as reflected in expressions like "put more muscle into it," meaning to take control and act. In this sense, an emphasis on moving from the muscles can express a range of states, from tension and resistance to vitality and power. As Body-Mind Centering teacher Linda Hartley notes, "any movement will express a particular quality of attention, perceptual process, energy, and direction of focus ... which relates to the 'mind' of that particular movement."[3] Each system expresses a different quality: in BMC you learn to make contact with and embody different systems and initiate movement from them so that each of their qualities becomes available as a means of expression.[4]

We can also learn to perceive certain states in others, both by observing them moving and by being in their presence, as my teacher Bonnie Bainbridge Cohen describes in this now-famous quote from a 1984 interview:

> I see the body as being like the sand. It's difficult to study the wind, but if you watch the way sand patterns form and disappear and reemerge, then you can follow the pattern of the wind, or in this case, the mind.[5]

Becoming familiar with this way of perceiving—viewing movement as an expression of a certain state of mind or *being*—you become more skilled at understanding your own movement and the movement of those around you. You can also then understand movement as a powerful intervention to help yourself or others, as changing your movement can also initiate a change in your state of being.

Why is this important to understand? Each of us has developed certain tendencies in our own expression that have essentially become our way of being in the world: body systems we tend to express are in the forefront, while the systems that we tend not to express remain largely in the background or the unconscious, serving as support. Although these tendencies give us our individuality and are not necessarily wrong or bad, if we are always expressing in one way, that system becomes overworked and fatigued, while the supporting system becomes underdeveloped and weak. To quote Bainbridge Cohen again: "What we are strong in we do all the time, so that we over-fatigue that system. In doing this kind of work we don't all end up being equal in every system, we end being … more fully ourselves."[6]

By getting to know our tendencies and becoming comfortable with expressing more of ourselves, we bring a much-needed balance to our nervous system and our entire body-mind to help us in our self-care in practical ways in our daily life. For example, someone who is more inwardly directed all the time might find that going out hiking with friends or joining a basketball or soccer team will bring them out in the world and make them more balanced.

We might also then make the opposite observation, in that if you are always on the go and outwardly focused—as is true for our often overscheduled teens—you might need more inner-directed activities, such as meditation and body awareness practices, to bring a balance to your hectic lifestyle. As students learn to observe their own perceptive state, they can also learn how to shift activities to bring a balance and renewed focus as needed. On an individual level, this might translate into a student who can tell that she is feeling tired from extended computer time and gets up for a bit, or notices when an interactive learning activity is becoming overstimulating and takes a break to go be alone before "acting out" to get away. Conversely, this can be a student busy studying alone who goes out for a walk, or chats with a friend for a few minutes, before resuming his homework. Rather than becoming drained, depleted, and overtired, with self-awareness, students can apply self-regulating skills to remain engaged. This kind of inner awareness leads to an increasing independence as they learn to maintain their balance in myriad ways.

I worked with one college group who was still learning about this in an anatomy for dancers course I taught. As the class lasted two-and-a-half hours, we often took a break midway through the session. During these times, I noticed that nearly all of the students were on their cell phones for most of the twenty minutes. I also noticed that they became increasingly tired and "spaced out" during the second half of the class, regardless of the activities we engaged in. One day at the break, I reminded them to consider how they were using their break time, related to the topic of balancing the nervous system that we were exploring that week. "Don't check your cell phone, check yourself!" I advised. This must have hit home, as they burst into laughter at this thought. Yet as the course progressed, I saw that they began to use that time differently, and we all soon noticed that the quality of our time together in the second part of our class also markedly improved. As we learned, increased individual self-awareness contributes to the whole as well—as balanced, energized individuals lead to a more creative and productive learning environment for all. These skills also become lifelong awareness tools that can help to build resilience and vitality—both personally and collectively. This empowers students to become more consciously involved in their own health and growth process.

Introducing students to the concept of engaging in recuperative activities, as well as giving them experiences that encourage a wider range of expression—and vocabulary to name these states—helps them expand their comfort zone and gain new self-care skills. Engaging in a wider range of body-mind expression also enhances students' resilience, opening them up to learn, change, and adapt more readily. Through this process, they gain an understanding of these more psychophysical processes referenced in the concept of the "mind" of the body systems to draw upon as needed.

Perceiving and Describing the "Mind of the Room"

Just as moving with an emphasis on any one body system is understood to evoke a certain quality of "mind" or state of presence, a group of individuals can also be expressing a collective "mind" through their presence and physical expression, which can change from moment to moment. Bonnie Bainbridge Cohen refers to the quality of presence expressed by a group at any one time as "the mind of the room." Perceiving this state is not a cognitive measuring tool that emerges from what you think about; rather you sense the "mind of the room" through your own physical presence and the presence of others in the room. For example, the mind of the room of a group of people who had just been meditating would be very different than that of a group that was engaging in aerobics or kick-boxing. Likely, if you walked in the room you would experience the mood and the quality of presence of the individuals to be quite different! Perceiving this difference requires an open attentiveness and expansive state of awareness to sense the whole.

Learning to perceive the "mind of the room" is an essential skill for the facilitator of somatic movement activities—and for any teacher or group leader—that can be cultivated through our attention. In this curriculum, you will have many opportunities to use this open awareness to sense the "mind of the room" as you present various experiences, and begin to "read" the group. You may already be doing this. After students engage in an inner-focused activity, for example, you may sense that this has created a calm in the group that can then easily lead into a next quiet activity (such as sitting with a partner to talk about the experience). Or, conversely, you may notice that students now look rather "spacey" and groggy from so much inner focus, and then choose to add an active movement game, such as passing a ball around or clapping together in a certain rhythm, to help them reorient and bring a balance to the more inner-directed activity.

After some time, you can also talk with your students about these various "facilitation choices" you have been making, as a means to help them discover why you initiate certain activities related to the body systems. Once understood, this type of perceptual awareness and self-regulation can also be initiated and applied by the group itself. Over the course of working together, I have experienced students becoming so aware of the perceptive state of the group that they begin to notice the "mind of the room" independently and make suggestions to help the group to stay engaged. For instance, after sitting for some time during a discussion one student may suggest: "Let's get up and do that clapping rhythm game, it's getting kind of 'sleepy' in here!" Or another student may notice that the group is not really paying attention any longer as there is too much activity going on, and suggest we take a five-minute break to lie down or write in their journals. This knowledge base of *experiential knowing* helps to transfer the authority from the teacher to the group, as they begin to monitor their own interest level and discover what they need as a group to stay involved and to use their time productively.

By reading the mind of the room you can also perceive if certain states you are aspiring to teach are being physically *actualized* or not by your students. In some cases, you may see that the material has become embodied, even if students may not have noticed this themselves yet. This can mean that the learning has occurred in their bodies at a cellular level, but has not yet been registered in the higher processes of the nervous system such that they "know what they know." Bonnie Bainbridge Cohen expresses it this way:

> One of the main characteristics of my teaching is that I tend to teach both to the unconscious and the conscious in the student. For example, when I present an exploration in class, as soon as I feel 'the mind of the room' resonate with the consciousness or mind state central to that exploration, I'll move on to another exploration. The moving on might be premature for people in the class who did not recognize *consciously* that they were in that state or exactly what that mind state was. They knew something had happened but had no idea what that was.[7]

By teaching in this way, we are teaching to the *body experience first,* and secondarily to the conscious awareness or ability to verbally articulate that experience.[8] This type of body learning may be very different than what we are used to expecting as educators, when we generally assess only what is understood cognitively as a measure of growth and learning.

For instance, there is a difference between the kind of cognitive learning this curriculum offers, such as that students learn the names of their bones, or learn to acknowledge "the body as a dynamic ecosystem rather than an object"—measuring *concepts* that can be understood. Other learning experiences relate more directly to specific measures of body knowledge, some of which can be achieved with or without cognitive recognition, such as learning to shift your point of movement initiation, or to shift from shallow breathing to fuller breathing, for example. Eventually, students often come to understand such newfound body knowledge more consciously as well, and as somatic educators we value both methods of learning. You can similarly aspire to teach in a way that encourages both cognitive and physical body knowledge appropriate to the level and goals of the group of students in any given situation. Ways to create this balance will be addressed further throughout the book.

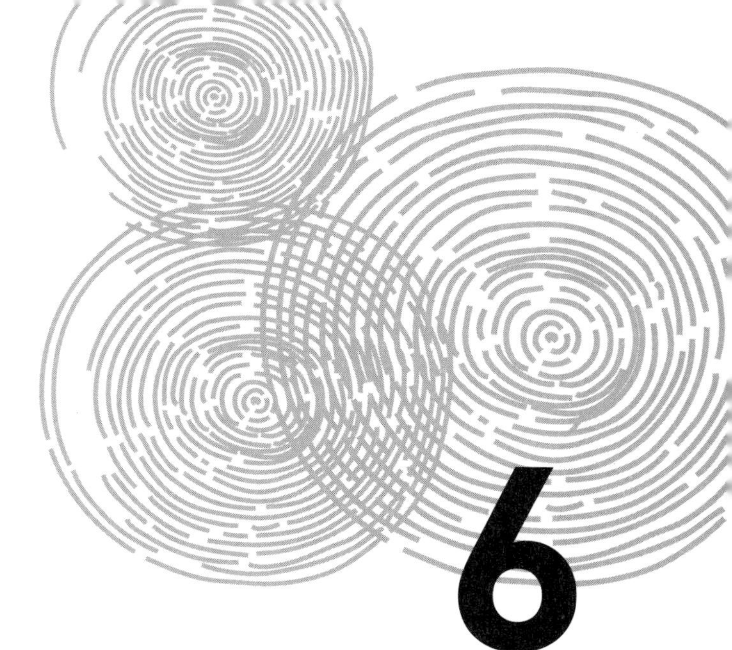

6

Touch and Other Touchy Subjects

Touch is the other side of movement. Movement is the other side of touch. They are the shadow of each other.

—Bonnie Bainbridge Cohen

Many of us have become quite devoid of the sensual—movement and touch—in our hectic lives. Yet our senses of touch and movement are developing in sync from early in the womb, as the developing fetus learns about itself and its surroundings through cellular awareness. The individual cells interact with the fluid around them, while the body relates with the lining of the womb, first through movement of the mother and then through our own self-initiated movement. This dance between movement and touch establishes a fundamental basis of self-knowledge—one that can continue to develop through our lifetimes.

Through both movement and touch, as children and adults we can experience new modes of relating to the world within and without. Just as we move from the direct knowing of the cell to the complex sensitivity of the nervous system, we also develop through our ability to differentiate self from other.[1] Given appropriate support and time to integrate new perceptions, both touch and movement can each provide distinct, direct means of introducing new proprioceptive feedback, eliciting fresh awareness that expands our perceptual base. In an educational model of teaching to the whole person, movement and touch are essential domains to draw upon to develop sensory vitality and enhance our well-being.

In his book *Touched by the Goddess,* Deane Juhan advocates for the need to provide students with a safe and nurturing environment that includes healthy, respectful, and nonsexual touch to support their development. To substantiate this claim, Juhan cites several scientific studies, such as one done in the early 1900s investigating the cause of death in orphanages, which was discovered to be the result of understaffing that led to a lack of affectionate touch being given to each infant—effectively proving that no infant can survive without tactile stimulation. Other studies he cites, done with monkeys in the 1950s, showed that infants preferred touch even over food, suggesting that touch itself is an essential food, without which development was shown to be severely limited both physically and emotionally. As Juhan notes, "Much of what passes for learning disabilities or poor school systems may to a significant degree be the result of these kinds of depressed physical and mental performances.... Appropriate, affectionate, nourishing touch is one of the main missing ingredients in our social fabric."[2]

Contemporary scientific research concurs. Studies on the effects of touch include a plethora of physiological benefits, from decreased heart rate, blood pressure, and cortisol rates, to enhanced immune functions and increased levels of oxytocin.[3] These benefits are particularly efficacious for teens. For example, one study conducted with adolescents in forty-nine cultures showed a direct correlation between violent behaviors and a lack of nurturing touch, while demonstrating that touch-based therapies brought about decreases in depression, anxiety, and violent behavior.[4] Clearly touch is a primary human need.

Despite the proven necessity of touch to human survival and well-being, our contemporary society maintains a complex, often fearful relationship with touch, especially in relation to education. Touch has all but been eliminated in our schools, burdened as they are by an unfortunate legacy of abuse of power in the dynamic between adults and children. As educators, we have to ask ourselves difficult questions: What happens to children when no distinction is made between friendly and harmful touching? And yet, could it be that learning to touch each other in healing, positive ways is indispensable to integrated learning for the individual and to productive change in society as a whole?[5] Insomuch as healthy touch helps to establish a sense of well-being and belonging, it may indeed be a key factor. And after essential survival strategies are established, the next level of human need may be the need to belong, experienced even more acutely during adolescence.[6] To establish a healthy context for the educational use of touch with teens, we can begin to engage students in curricula that provides more positive touch-based interactions that enhance, rather than undermine, a sense of respect, community, and belonging.

Somatic movement educators, along with other health practitioners or certain dance and movement educators, are some of the few professionals who may have developed touch-based skills and can hope to successfully introduce them to a next generation through curriculums like this one. With care and attention, we can begin to include movement and touch within specific guidelines appropriate to an educational setting. This next section will discuss some of the areas to be considered in designing an educational context to teach what I will refer to here as "intentional touch," meaning touch that is included with a specific purpose, intent, and educational goal.

Working with Intentional Touch in Education

To engage students in somatic movement education practices in general, or in this curriculum specifically, it is not necessary to include activities in which students touch each other. Methods of self-touch, along with movement activities, can be helpful in and of themselves in eliciting new proprioceptive feedback that heightens body awareness. That being said, when approached responsibly and with care, partner touch activities can be a vital and engaging part of the curriculum as well. If you are going to include touch activities of any kind, there are a several important things to keep in mind related to offering touch-based activities in schools or other youth programs. This is necessary both to ensure the well-being of the students participating in the curriculum as well as to address potential concerns that may be voiced by parents, administrators, and students themselves.

First, if touch-based activities will be a significant part of the curriculum, you will want to be sure that there is adequate support within the school or program—among teachers, parents, and administrators—for including touch in the class. This begins by clarifying the purpose and scope of the activities ahead of time (related to self-touch or partner touch) with all those involved in the decision-making process; you may also want to share some relevant articles or sections of this book in support of your work. In getting parents on board, some schools decide to send an information sheet home to parents before the start of the class, or they may just have more informal group and individual discussions. In college contexts, I and other colleagues I know of have often included a description of the type of touch activities involved directly in the syllabus. In any case, you can decide what works best based on the context and sensitivities of your situation.

In working with the students themselves, it is important to help students develop basic self-touch skills and establish a basic comfort level with touch. To that end, I have several recommendations for how to successfully—and responsibly—introduce touch in the class. Then, after students are familiar with self-touch activities, if you do want to include partner touch activities as well, such as several in this curriculum, there are some additional considerations and guidelines presented here. The following four key pedagogy guidelines should be helpful in setting the stage to include touch responsibly in all of these cases.

Four Basic Guidelines for Teaching Intentional Touch

1. Begin with Self-Touch

Core Principle: Introduce self-touch activities first, so students can become familiar with basics of touch for body-awareness and learn self-care skills.

Beginning with self-touch activities gives students a chance to become comfortable with touch, as well as to learn specific types of touch that activate proprioceptive awareness. Once familiar, such self-touch activities—like tracing the bones of the feet, for instance, as included in this curriculum—give students easy and effective self-care tools to do on their own. Self-touch is also an essential aspect of experiential anatomy in that you can discover distinctions in form and function in your own body through touch and movement, rather than merely looking at plastic models or drawings.

2. Give Specific Guidelines in Each Touch-based Activity

Core principle: Use clear guidelines and be specific as to the goal and type of touch to be used.

In introducing touch activities, using clear guidelines can help students learn about and distinguish between various types of touch, such as types of pressure (hard, light, and so forth), or touch that is initiated from a particular body system (such as bone touch versus a more muscular touch). These types of touch will be explored further in various explorations in the curriculum. It is also important to be specific as to the goal of the touch, and how that relates to the type of touch being used. This sets the stage for *intentional touch*, that which has a stated purpose and method.

For example, in the exploration called Bone Tracing—The Feet, students touch their own feet to feel the many distinct bones of the foot. This activity also helps them learn to use touch to distinguish between the bones and the other soft tissues, like the muscles and ligaments, and creates space between the bones as the muscles relax. In this case, you would tell students directly: 1) the purpose of the activity ("This exercise will help you to feel the many bones of your foot by tracing each one"); 2) the type of touch to use ("Use a directed bone touch, so you are touching the bones rather than pressing on the soft tissues like the muscles and ligaments"); and 3) why that type of touch is being used ("This helps you to locate each of the bones of the feet and make space between the bones to help your muscles relax.") Being clear in your directions will help students to feel more comfortable, in both self-touch and in partner activities, as they have a clear context and purpose for the activity.

3. Working with Partners: Set an Educational Context for Touch-Based Activities

Core Principle: Be clear to set an educational context, rather than a therapeutic one, especially when working with touch as a group or with a partner.

Although engaging in somatic practices can clearly be therapeutic, this curriculum is meant to establish an educational context for students, rather than to provide individual or group therapy or to diagnose or fix specific physical problems. Even so, as students begin to work in partners with touch they often have many preconceived ideas and cultural assumptions about the relationship between the person touching and the person being touched. Many are familiar with massage or bodywork, for instance, in which case the one touching is the "practitioner" and the one being touched is the "client." The stereotypical assumption is that you are coming to the practitioner for help, and that this professional knows more about your body and your needs than you do. This relationship between "toucher" and "touched" in this case is related to a certain perception of a therapeutic context of touch. Therefore, when setting up a partner touch activity, it is important to bring awareness to these assumptions by explicitly discussing them, and then to create an alternate context for the touch experiences to be explored in the curriculum that is educational, rather than therapeutic, in nature.

In the context of this curriculum, rather than "practitioner" and "client", both people are seen as "learners"—students in the process of understanding more through the inclusion of touch. For instance, in studying about the spine, one student sits behind the other and traces the curves of the spine of his or her partner, feeling the curves with a flat palm and pressing gently along the spine while moving the hand down, starting at the neck and moving down along the surface of the back. In this case, the person touching is getting a chance to see and feel the variations in the curves of the spine: some areas, like the cervical and the lumbar spine "curve in" or curve anteriorly, while other areas like the thoracic spine feel like they "bulge out" or curve posteriorly. Simultaneously, by receiving touch along the spine the person being touched is able to learn about the curves of his or her spine as well, through the sensation of the touch that brings greater proprioceptive awareness of that area. Discussing these two aspects of learning reframes the touch activity—from a primarily therapeutic context to a more educational one—and puts both students on equal ground as participants in the experience.

Another important aspect to shifting toward a more educational context is to explicitly invite verbal feedback from each partner, particularly from the one who is receiving touch. Again, this is necessary because in the stereotypical therapeutic context, such as the massage session discussed previously, it is assumed that you would generally not speak during the time you are being touched. This can create an implied "passive" role for the person being touched, such that they feel they can only speak up in an extreme case, like if something really hurts or is very uncomfortable. To help counteract this unconscious tendency and provide a sense of agency for the person being touched, you need to discuss this tendency, and then explicitly give permission for each person to talk during the process as needed, as discussed more specifically below.

4. Working with Partners: Establishing a Protocol of Consent and Communication

> **Core Principle:** Set the stage for touch-based activities done in partnership by creating a system of establishing consent and appropriate communication between individuals, while keeping the main focus on sensory experience.

In all touch-based activities, you should establish a protocol of consent—but keep it simple. Once students each know that a specific activity will include touch and have seen it demonstrated and agreed to participate, having students ask one another if they are ready to be touched, or having the students agree as to when they are ready to begin the activity, is still important. You can derive a formula that works best for you for this process, such as having a student simply ask the partner, "OK, can we begin this now?" or "Are you ready?" with the other person responding, "Yes, you can start now," or simply "Yes." Such detailed communication establishes trust and safety. You might think of this in terms of how copilots navigate a flight, for instance. Before the flight starts, one of the two pilots is designated the captain, whose job is to fly the aircraft, and the second pilot is the assistant, whose job is to communicate with ground control and assist them in flying the plane. Sometimes the captain needs to transfer the control to the assistant, however, and so to be sure this is clear and there is no miscommunication as to who is flying the plane, the captain might say "You now have control" and the assistant pilot would respond "I now have control" to indicate that the flying roles have switched. As strange and detailed as this may sound, this protocol is always followed during a flight to ensure the safety of all involved. Similarly, establishing a common language and system for speaking during touch activities makes the situation more predictable, and ultimately, more respectful as well.

You can also give a few examples of what can be said during the activity, such as that the person being touched might ask for touch to be slower or to be done with more or less pressure, or might ask the person touching to wait a minute or to simply stop. You can even have students practice saying some of these phrases, if that does not feel too contrived for your situation. The person touching can also be reminded that they can speak to ask questions, or check in with their partner as well. This often helps them to feel free to do their best, asking questions when needed, since they may feel insecure about their abilities in this new role.

All that being said, once a protocol of consent and communication has been established it is equally essential to remind students that the touch activity is primarily meant as a means to learn through the physical experience, and that keeping a focus on the sensations and perceptions of one's body is important—so they should still try to keep their talking to a minimum. This is important to emphasize so the activity stays focused and is not overcome by needless chatting.

At the same time, keep in mind that sometimes if students are feeling particularly self-conscious with the process, like the first time that they work with touch in partners, they may use chatting as one way to feel more comfortable and ease into the experience. If I sense this is the case, I generally let it go on. Later on, it is not uncommon that students develop greater ease and concentration such that this is no longer an issue.

Finally, you will also want to be sure you have a student's consent to touch them as well, whether demonstrating before or assisting during an activity, by asking them directly. Simple, direct language is helpful, such as asking, "Would you like me to assist you with that by touching your arm?"; you can also offer help by saying something like, "I can help you feel where that vertebra is through touch if you like." Other times you might say something more general, like if you are going around the room to assist during an activity, in which case you might suggest that those who would like you to come help them through touch can raise their hand, put their palms up, or some other sign that you can establish together. All of these protocols help in establishing a safe context for touch in which students can feel free to choose touch or not in the moment.

Other Touchy Subjects: Teen Stress, Trauma, and Sexuality

In advocating for a body-based curriculum for adolescents, along with the issue of touch there are sure to be some other *touchy* subjects to address. By this I mean that they are complex and sensitive, particularly in the context of working with adolescents.

Each of these areas I'll discuss here—stress and trauma, sex and sexuality—could obviously encompass books in and of themselves. While beyond the scope of this book to cover each topic in great depth, it's important to bring awareness to them and provide some overall discussion and guidance.

Teens, Stress, and Trauma

Among other things, somatic movement practices can help us to become aware of various levels of tension and stress as it manifests in our body. When approached slowly and gradually, this process of self-awareness can lead to decreased tension and increased acts of self-care. As such, it can be both freeing and empowering. Yet no matter how careful we are to craft a safe and inspiring context for somatic movement education, it's important to be aware that many people have deeper levels of stress from intense life experiences. When working with teens, this can encompass instances beyond their control, such as past physical accidents, illnesses, physical or sexual abuse, or a history of mental health issues, including self-harm and eating disorders. Primarily, this curriculum is intended for a general population and would need to be adapted quite significantly for work with teens who are known to have more extreme psychophysical needs. Yet as we invite groups of teens into somatic practices, there will inevitably be students who need more support and/or interventions than can be realistically provided in a group context. In many cases you will know who those teens are and be able to identify them ahead of time. In other instances you may be entering into unknown territory, and discover such students along the way.

When engaging students in somatic movement education it helps to have a basic understanding of possible responses that indicate distress or trauma, along with a few basic interventions. If you can recognize specific behaviors that touch, movement, and learning about the body may trigger, you'll be able to identify particular individuals who may need extra support in approaching this material. You can also become aware of when you may need professional support to assess whether the curriculum is appropriate at all or is contraindicated, either for a particular student or a particular group, or when you may need to refer a particular teen to an outside professional. Although some educators may already have experience in this realm, I've included some preliminary guidelines for those who are not as familiar with such signs and interventions.

To begin with, when delving into body awareness activities, body memory and related emotions may arise that can feel overwhelming or confusing at times. In such cases it is not uncommon for individuals to either "freak out" or "shut down," colloquial terms for two clinically defined trauma responses, which we can understand as instincts of self-protection. An initial reaction can be the "fight or flight" response, an activation of the sympathetic nervous system (SNS) that results in a variety of physical symptoms—increased heart rate, sweating, dilated pupils, and a dry mouth—often referred to as hyperarousal. As you likely know from your own experience, this may also be expressed emotionally in varying levels of frustration, anxiety, and anger. Conversely, another reaction may be a state of disassociation or emotional repression, often referred to as a freeze pattern, in which an individual feels unable to respond effectively, or even to respond at all. This may be expressed more subtly as emotional withdrawal, apathy, or dullness, or more dramatically as actually experiencing some level of physical paralysis.

If you feel that a student or group of students is having a more extreme response to an activity that may indicate it is too overwhelming for them, the simplest intervention is to switch gears. In somatic work this can perhaps feel counterintuitive, as a student may be involved in a quiet, still activity, which we might otherwise assume would be calming and restful. Yet if a student is overwhelmed from inner sensory work, it is usually best to get them up and moving. In a group context, you can draw on several modes of active movement described in this curriculum, such as having students walk through the room, or initiating a playful rhythm activity, for example. After a lot of inner sensing work, as another mode of intervention you can end the class by discussing some unrelated, more mundane topic. This helps bring their awareness back to the present moment and engage in light, lively conversation before heading to the next class or activity. In somatic work refocusing on the outer—rather than the inner—environment in cases of psychophysical overwhelm can be key to regaining emotional stability. This is not to say that we want to encourage students to ignore or override their feelings, but just that it is best to first help them to stabilize emotionally when the context is not immediately conducive to further processing of their psychophysical needs.

Another extreme reaction to overstimulation of the sensory-motor system can be a state of physical shock, in which the body temperature drops, the heartbeat speeds up, and one may experience fatigue or dizziness. In this case, you want to help the individual to be quiet, restful, and warm, such as covering them with a blanket or coat, while the body has a chance to recuperate and regain its homeostasis. While these instances of extreme body reaction in class are quite rare, you should become familiar with these basics as a precautionary measure, and consult other specialists as necessary. There are also specialized fields of somatics, such as somatic psychology, or particular related somatic methods, like Somatic Experiencing® and other disciplines, which deal more directly with trauma responses; you may also want to seek out further professional development in these areas. Ultimately you will know your population best to determine the level of experience you need, but generally I have found that in most cases the pedagogy already in place in this curriculum effectively serves to build an accessible bridge to somatic practices that is both safe and engaging for teens.

Sex and Sexuality

Clearly teenagers need support in becoming comfortable with their own bodies, which includes their sexuality. This introductory level curriculum explores the body systems in general with a focus on movement education and overall well-being, and is not meant to serve as sex education. In further curriculum development any one system—such as the reproductive system—could be chosen as an area of more detailed study should you want to include it in more depth,[7] a study which could also include related issues like sexual preference and gender identity. Though the topic of sexuality doesn't need to be avoided in the classroom context of this curriculum, it doesn't need to be expressly invited either.

I remember an amusing story told by a student of the Zen Buddhist monk named Shunryu Suzuki who, as a young aspiring monk, had asked him the question: What is sex? To which Suzuki replied simply, "Once you say sex, everything is sex."[8] And while this may just inherently be the case with some adolescents no matter what you do or don't say, given their infamously raging hormones, I find that introducing the topic of sexuality—with teens who may already be a bit apprehensive about dealing with their bodies—just makes them more uncomfortable. Instead, you can be clear with students about the intent and content of the curriculum without mentioning what is not covered, and then stand ready to sensitively incorporate whatever topics should emerge in the course of your work together. This may or may not include discussions of sexuality, related to anatomy, gender, sexual abuse, or any other more personal perspectives and psychophysical concerns. You will also need to access your *own* comfort level in dealing with topics related to sexuality, and consider how you might prefer to handle various topics if they come up in certain contexts.

For example, the topic of sex and sexuality often naturally emerges in certain sections of the curriculum, such as when looking at the structure and functions of the pelvis, and in that context can be appropriate to address. I find it best to allow students themselves to bring this up, however, which gives them more of a sense of agency. For example, I recall a moving journal entry by one of my students written the week we studied the pelvis. She shared that as we approached the skeleton to go over the bones of the pelvis, she noticed that she had become really anxious. Then, as we began to name the specific bones and discuss the various functions of the pelvis, she felt so relieved that we were dealing with this part of the skeleton as we had with all the other parts, and was glad to learn about this part of her body in a factual way. She went on to write that she hadn't realized how much anxiety she had about her pelvis, which evoked all sorts of issues about her sexuality, digestive functions, and more, and shared that she had spent the next night coloring her anatomy plate on the pelvis and writing more in her journal about these complex issues.

While in the next classes we did also discuss some of these related topics, like sexuality and eating disorders, beginning with the concrete anatomy of the bones had given her a safe avenue to open—on her own—to her more subjective experience. Other students may find it easier to approach these topics initially in small group discussions in class with their peers first, before addressing them in a larger group conversation. This type of experiential curriculum—that deals directly with the body—opens up a frank discussion and helps students to develop a healthier body image, self-respect, and clear and strong physical boundaries. These experiences can also positively impact their relationship with sexuality.

Students can also take on related research projects if they like—such as learning about differences in the skeletal system of males and females, researching hormonal changes of adolescence, or examining issues of gender identity, for example—as an ancillary part of the class or as a group project done in class. This type of emergent learning can reinforce their autonomy while deepening the learning process for the group, and even the larger community if they later share their discoveries in discussions and school-wide presentations.

Finally, the issue of whether or not the curriculum directly deals with sex and sexuality can be important to bring up with parents and administrators, who might have questions about the scope of the class content. This helps the community at large to feel comfortable and welcoming of the class, as well as helping you to incorporate any concerns or suggestions they might have into how you structure the material. These discussions can also lead to collaborative curriculum design, such as coordinating lesson plans with others, like the biology or health teachers, or with planning for particular guest speakers on relevant topics that may be needed to support or augment the curriculum. In any case, be sure to take the time to clarify the goals and scope of the course with the school community.

PART III

A CURRICULUM IN SME: EMBODIED ANATOMY FOR TEENS

Embodiment Basics—Level I

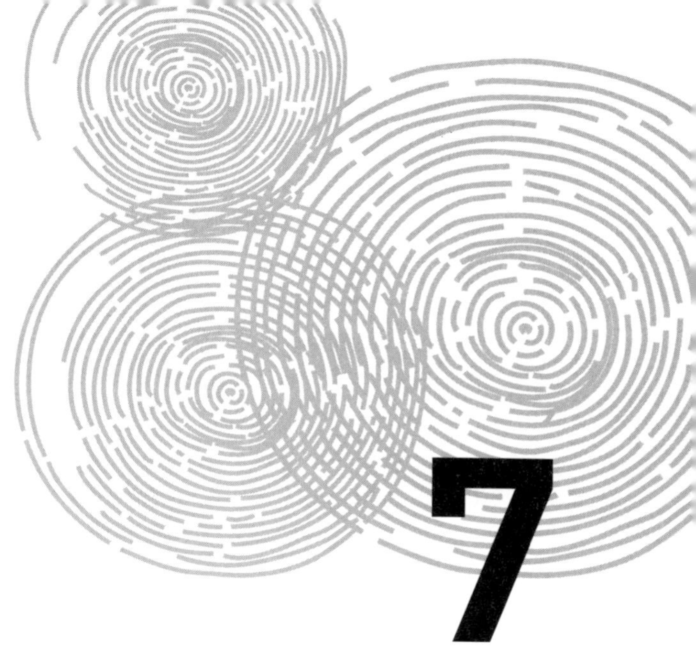

7

Body Listening

Just as you are sitting, reading this, take a deep breath … in … and out. Feel the weight of your body sitting. Notice the position of your back, your shoulders, your neck, your head. Now take another breath … in … and out. Notice your feet—are they touching the floor? If so, notice the weight of your feet on the floor. Notice your legs. How are they placed? Bring your awareness to their position. Don't try to change your position; just notice. Breathe in again, and as you exhale, allow your weight to be supported by the earth. Rest here for a moment.

This is the thirty seconds it takes to become present and begin to focus within, first on a body level: to shift your awareness to your physical sensations, to "re-member" body and mind, to integrate sensation and thought. In addition to relaxing, you may have noticed tensions or discomfort of which you were previously unaware. In fact, you may have felt an impulse to change your position, to readjust in a way that might alleviate any strain you were experiencing. Our bodies speak to us when we pay attention.

Most often, however, we are just not listening. For instance, when we are sitting at the computer for hours, we may not notice our increasingly slouched position, which then causes tension in our neck and shoulders. Or forging ahead on a project, we may forget to eat when we are hungry and only later quickly grab something on the run, which then leads to indigestion. Or while obsessively exercising to attain a better physique, we may not notice our need to rest, which creates a state of exhaustion. Throughout the day we often slip into *override mode* to push through our many obligations, rather than paying much attention to our bodies. Teens experience this as well, with their many obligations and often overscheduled lives.

Ramifications of inattentiveness to our bodies' signals can range from minor bodily discomforts and illnesses to the kind of stressful lifestyle that leads to more serious health issues. Teens may also often experience a corresponding sense of "dis-ease" within themselves—a nagging feeling of being self-conscious or generally uncomfortable in their own skin. When teens begin to pay attention at a body level, they develop an increased level of self-understanding and self-care. With such heightened sensitivity, they gain the skills to manage their health and well-being—releasing built-up tensions, developing greater embodied presence, and ultimately becoming freer and more at ease.

What Is Body Listening?

Body listening is a term I use to refer to a means of actively turning our focus inward to the sensations of our body—to first become aware of what we are sensing.[1] Only then can you begin to have a relationship to those sensations. Through body listening, we become aware of our body in a nonjudgmental way as we learn to listen rather than direct, to experience as well as to achieve, as we observe both our inner and outer posture. The outer posture refers to specifics of our body, such as the position of our spine, the weight on our feet, or the degree of tension in our shoulders. The inner posture refers to the way we direct our thoughts and the related state of our internal emotions. To balance body and mind, the ability to notice thoughts and emotions objectively and to quiet the mind is as important as developing body awareness. Awareness of the inner and outer posture is an essential component of effecting change in our body-mind relationship.

As a starting point, this curriculum begins by helping teens cultivate the essential skills of *mindful awareness* and *nonjudgmental observation* through body listening. Body listening allows us to take the time to arrive in the present moment. This essential body listening practice has many practical physiological benefits, which students also learn about through these activities, adding to their motivation to use it in their own daily lives. As the curriculum progresses, they also learn about the anatomy and physiology of their own bodies through movement, helping them develop an inner *body mindfulness—being while doing*. This supports them in recognizing physical tensions and self-defeating movement patterns and psychophysical attitudes. Other activities help them discover new, healthier patterns and perceptions. The focus is not so much on teaching specific movement, but on facilitating a process in which students' own movement will be teaching them about themselves. They gain access to their own body's innate intelligence to integrate body and mind, to gain ease of movement, and to develop greater health and vitality.

Two Approaches to Body Listening: Body Scanning and the Constructive Rest Position

The explorations related to body listening begin with *body scanning,* a term that is used in many awareness practices, such as Vipassana meditation, as well as in many somatic education disciplines. Body scanning is a method of paying attention to sensations and changes in your body. When standing, for example, we might notice the weight on our feet or the length of our spine. Students first practice body scanning while standing, and then lying down in the Constructive Rest Position. In this position, you lie on your back (supine) with the knees bent and feet on the floor, generally with your eyes closed. The Constructive Rest Position (also referred to simply as Constructive Rest or CRP) is described by Mabel Elsworth Todd in her book *The Thinking Body* as the position that uses the least amount of muscular activity to support the body in gravity *(Fig. 7.1)*.[2] Here the skeletal system and organs are supported by the floor, allowing the muscles of postural support to release.

When in Constructive Rest, as we focus our attention through body scanning we might bring our attention first to the weight of our feet touching the floor, then to the weight of our legs, then to each part of our body progressively up to our head. This step of bringing our attention to particular areas of our body also gives us a specific mental focus that helps to calm the mind as we settle into gravity. This allows our body to fully rest.

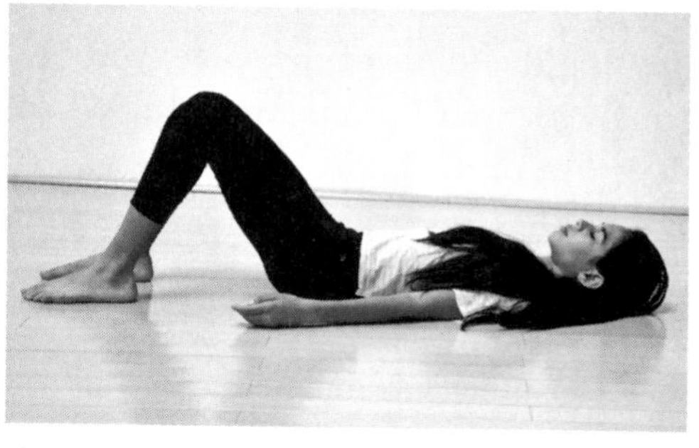

Fig. 7.1. Lying in the Constructive Rest Position requires the least amount of muscular engagement to support the body in gravity.

Sometimes when students first lie down in Constructive Rest, they may be nervous, fidgeting, or laughing, especially younger teens—which are often first steps to "settling in." They may also at first "peek" to see if their peers are actually doing it. Others immediately appreciate this chance to rest, and relax more readily. Others may find it initially uncomfortable to just lie still, or may notice particular areas of tension or pain that they find distracting. The room soon settles down as students begin to concentrate. Then after lying in Constructive Rest for even five to ten minutes, students generally find they feel more relaxed and refreshed, with renewed physical energy. There are several reasons for this.

Benefits of the Constructive Rest Position

Constructive Rest has concrete physiological benefits, especially when practiced daily over time. We often underestimate the importance of rest for physical and psychological health, and youth especially have such quick recuperative powers that they often consider rest as nonessential. Yet knowing how and when to rest is an important first step in developing body-mind awareness, as well as in gaining ease in our movement. When we accumulate muscular tension throughout the day, tightened muscles constrict the flow of blood in the muscles and other tissues. Muscular tension pulls the body out of alignment, creating imbalances in posture. Over time, the fascia layers, which encase muscles like moist plastic wrap, also begin to lose their viscosity and harden—further solidifying the resulting postural patterns that arose from the initial muscular tension. Lying in Constructive Rest allows these deep postural muscles to release and, practiced over time, helps to realign the body and gradually allows more blood flow.

The shift from upright weight-bearing to a supine position also allows for more space in our joints, as compression from gravity is lessened and joint spaces can expand. This is especially true for the joints between the vertebrae of the spine—the fibrocartilaginous intervertebral discs—that begin to decompress. Many students even discover that they feel taller after resting in this position! To help with this process of decompressing the joints of the spine, you keep the knees bent in this position rather than lying with your legs outstretched. When lying down in a more outstretched position, the curve of the lumbar spine increases, putting increased stress on the back muscles and the intrinsic muscles along the spine; in Constructive Rest with knees bent, the lumbar spine retains its natural curve and requires less muscular engagement.[3]

As students learn about and experience these many benefits of Constructive Rest, they are invited to practice it for ten minutes each night before going to bed. Just as flossing the teeth maintains healthy gums by eliminating a buildup of plaque, lying in Constructive Rest clears the daily tensions before they have a chance to accumulate and create embedded restriction within the body. After doing Constructive Rest for ten minutes each night for even a few weeks, many students experience improvements in various postural problems, such as lower back pain, shoulder tension, or knee strain. Rather than forcing themselves into a "better" position, this approach helps them regain their inherent body integrity, as the postural muscles used throughout the day relax and a more balanced alignment emerges. Student athletes and dancers have found Constructive Rest to be especially helpful, since they create new daily stresses from their workouts or technique classes, but rarely take the time to truly recuperate. Constructive Rest can become part of their daily hygiene routine and can be an enjoyable and recuperative addition to their busy lives.

Another advantage of practicing Constructive Rest is that it alters your physiology toward greater balance. With a hectic lifestyle, students are mainly encouraged to be active and attending to their outer environment—a sympathetic nervous system (SNS) response that over time can create mental exhaustion and a high level of bodily tension. In this hyper-aroused state their adrenal glands produce the stress hormone cortisol, which builds up in their bloodstream, contributing to this ongoing self-perpetuating stressful state. In contrast, Constructive Rest initiates relaxation and triggers a parasympathetic nervous system (PNS) response that releases serotonin into the bloodstream; this chemical works as a neurotransmitter to help maintain emotional balance. Many students find that using the body scanning exercise as a means to focus their attention helps them to feel restful in this position. Others find it helpful to use body scanning initially and then to simply focus on their breathing. They are guided in this restful position to clear and calm their mind so they can fully relax.

With the many responsibilities and emotional turmoil of adolescence, students find this to be a particularly useful skill to learn. Even after practicing Constructive Rest for the first time, students often remark on how much better they feel, as one high school junior named Cristiano noted in his journal after his first class:

> *Today's adventure felt really new and relaxing. I felt my mind go blank. I became much more aware and mindful. I currently feel less stressed, my body has let go of much of its tension, and my mind is more fixed on my body and mind.*

And here is another account from a tenth-grade girl named Giuliana:

> *I really liked doing movement that I typically don't do on a regular basis. That was fun. My favorite was the Constructive Rest position. It made me feel more grounded and solid afterward when I stood up and then did movement. I also liked it because it made me feel very peaceful and relaxed which is a great contrast to our busy everyday lives!*

After time in Constructive Rest during each class, students gradually feel more comfortable, achieve a deeper level of concentration, and become enthusiastic about practicing it on their own at home. Although it can be difficult to create a new habit, once they integrate Constructive Rest into their routine the results can be substantial, as another student noted in her weekly journal:

> *When I lie down in Constructive Rest on the floor before I sleep, it puts me back in balance. One of the benefits I have found is that it lets me find time to really focus on myself in my busy schedule! The combination of doing it with the body scanning helps me to find a calm mindset. I also notice that the days that I do it, I wake up feeling less tired than usual, and seem to have a lot less soreness in my back too.*

As teens discover, the benefits of this activity also increase over time, giving them an essential practice to feel calmer, refreshed, and energized.

The explorations that follow first introduce students to body scanning while standing, followed by body scanning when lying down in the Constructive Rest Position.

Exploration: Body Scanning

(10 minutes)

PURPOSE. To observe physical sensation and the state of your attention; to practice focusing your attention and calming your mind; to experience the changes in your body-mind from using such focused attention.

Activity

Begin with students standing in a circle.

- Close your eyes and take a minute to feel yourself standing. What do you notice as you stand? What draws your attention? *(Pause.)*
- Are you able to observe or are you thinking of other things? What do you notice about what you are thinking? Feeling? Take a few breaths, inhaling and exhaling deeply.
- Now notice your weight on your feet. Is your weight more on one foot than another? More on your toes or on your heels? Don't try to change your position. Just feel how you are standing.

This next directive can be said very slowly, allowing time between each body part before continuing to the next.

- Bring your awareness to your feet again ... then to your lower legs ... your knees ... your thighs ... up to your hips ... your torso ... your neck and head ... your shoulders and arms ... your hands and your fingers.
- Feel your whole body, standing on the earth. What do you notice?
- Take another deep breath, inhaling and exhaling fully.
- When you are ready, open your eyes and walk around the room. How do you feel as you walk? What do you notice in your body? What draws your attention?
- Now let's come back together to share our experiences. *(Students can share in partners or small groups, or proceed directly to the group discussion.)*

Discussion

- What did you experience? What did you notice as you were standing? Was it difficult to focus your attention? How were you feeling? What were some of the things that drew your attention? What did you experience in your body?

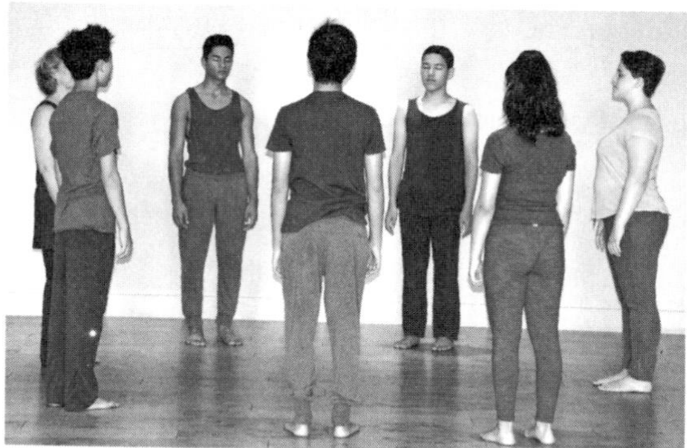

Fig. 7.2. Students practicing body scanning while standing with eyes closed.

Tips for Teachers

- Body scanning can be used before and after any other activity as a means of comparison to discover any changes that have occurred from having engaged in that activity. This is explained further in chapter 16, "A Somatic 'Warm-up'"; see the description of check-in activities on pages 291–293.

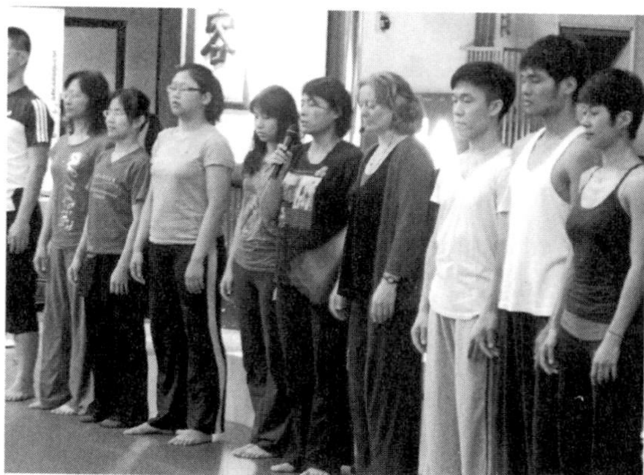

Fig. 7.3. Adult educators practicing body scanning: We teach best from our own experience. (Photo courtesy of the Somatic Education Society of Taiwan.)

Exploration: Body Listening and the Constructive Rest Position

(20–30 minutes)

PURPOSE. To observe physical sensation and the state of your attention; to begin to notice and respond to inner movement impulses through body listening; to practice focusing your attention and calming your mind; to release muscular holding patterns through relaxation; to initiate a parasympathetic nervous system state of rest; to observe the effects of Constructive Rest.

Activity

Begin with students standing in a circle; this activity begins by repeating the previous body scanning activity, a version of which is included in the following description.

- Close your eyes and take a minute to feel yourself standing. What do you notice as you stand? What draws your attention? *(Pause.)* Are you able to observe or are you thinking of other things? What do you notice about what you are thinking? Feeling? Take a few deep breaths. Inhale and exhale.
- Now take another deep breath in, and allow any sound or sigh to emerge as you exhale. *(Model this by doing it with them: inhale, and exhale with an audible sigh.)*
- Let's try this again: inhale, and exhale with any sound. *(Do this together again.)*
- Notice your weight on your feet. Is your weight more on one foot than another? More on your toes or on your heels? Feel free to change your position if you notice an impulse to move a bit forward or back, to one side or the other, to feel more balanced.
- Notice if you feel like moving in any other way now. Maybe your shoulders feel a bit tight and you just want to move them a bit, or your neck is bothering you and needs to move ... just see what you notice and allow yourself to respond in movement in any way that would feel good. Still keep your eyes closed. *(Pause to allow a minute or two for students to explore this.) (Fig. 7.4)*

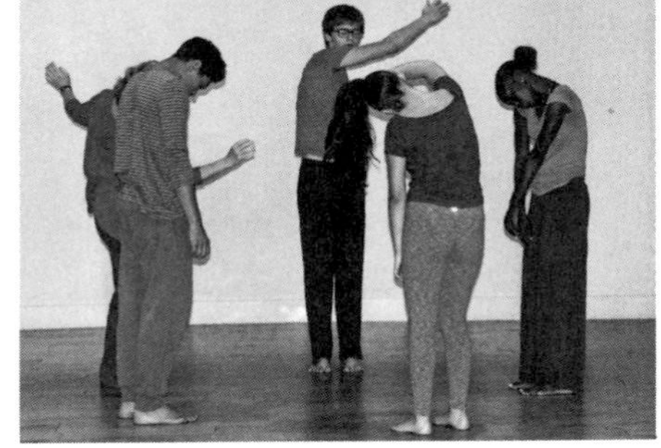

Fig. 7.4. After doing their body scans in stillness, students initiate their own movement as they begin to pay attention to what they need.

- Now begin to come back to stillness, and come back to standing in your center. What does it feel like to do that? What does "center" feel like? Feel the weight on your feet again, and notice any changes you feel in your body now. Take another deep breath in, and out. *(Fig. 7.5a.)*

- Begin to let your head relax forward toward your chest. Feel the weight of your head. Slowly begin to allow the weight of your head to pull you down toward the floor. *(Fig. 7.5b.)* Just go as far as you can, letting your shoulders relax as you roll down. Notice how this feels. Be sure to bend your knees if that feels more comfortable. *(Students will be bending over from the waist.)*
- Let your knees bend and as you come down to a squatting position, use your hands to balance. *(Fig. 7.5c.)* Then come down to sitting. Still with your eyes closed, use your hands on either side of your body to lower yourself down to the floor so you are lying on your back. Keep your feet on the floor so your knees are bent. Let your arms relax at your sides. *(This is Constructive Rest.) (Fig. 7.5d.)*

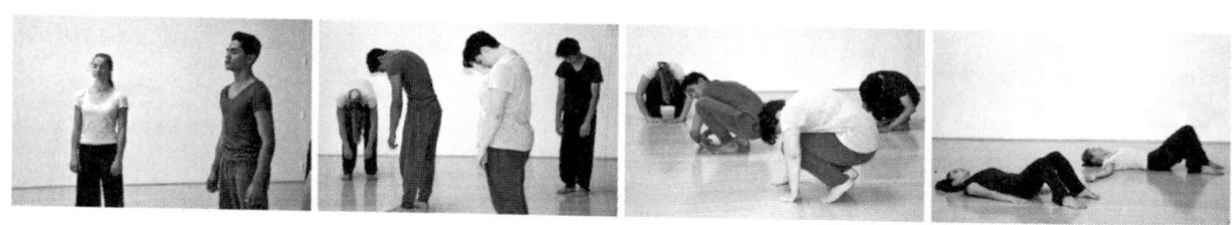

Fig. 7.5a, b, c, d. Rolling down the spine to lie down in Constructive Rest.

- Take a deep breath, in and out, allowing any sound or sigh to emerge again as you exhale. *(Do this with them again.)* See what you notice as you lie here.... What draws your attention? Is it easier for you to focus now than it was when you were standing? What parts of your body are you most aware of?
- Feel your weight on the floor. See if you can line up your feet with your ankles, your ankles with your knees, and your knees with your hip sockets. Let your weight be supported by the floor, by the earth.
- Now, as you did when standing, bring your awareness to your feet, feel their weight on the floor. Feel your feet being supported by the earth, and let them sink into the floor.
- Feel your lower legs and knees, with the weight of your lower legs flowing down through your ankles and into your feet. Then feel your upper thighs, with the weight of your upper legs flowing into your hip sockets and pelvis ... feel the weight of your pelvis and torso supported by the earth ... all the way up to your neck and head, as you feel them resting on the floor ... and now bring your awareness to your shoulders ... to your arms, hands, and fingers, as you feel them resting on the floor.
- Then feel your whole body relaxed on the earth. Breathe, and just allow yourself to rest here for some time. *(Pause for three to five minutes. During this time, be sure you are also sitting or standing in a way that you can be comfortable and relaxed.*

Focus on your own body and your breathing, as they are doing, while still keeping a sense of monitoring the group.)

- Take a few deep breaths again, inhale ... and exhale. Take another deep breath in, and allow any sound or sigh to emerge as you exhale. Now inhale, and exhale with any sound.
- When you are ready, let your knees fall to one side or the other, and feel the rotation in your spine created by this new position. Then roll gently onto that side. Use your arms to help push yourself back up to sitting, still with your eyes closed.
- Then, as you are ready, find your way slowly back up to standing, still keeping your eyes closed. You can roll back up your spine, like you did when rolling down, or just get up in any way you like. Once you are standing, take a deep breath, in and out. Take a minute to feel yourself standing and see what you notice.
- Feel yourself standing on the earth. How does this feel compared to when you began this exploration, that is, before lying down? Do you notice any changes in your body? Your breathing? Your weight through your feet? Your emotions? Just take a few moments to see what comes to your attention.
- Now repeat the body scanning on your own, starting with feeling the weight on your feet and bringing your awareness to each part of your body up to the top of your head.
- In a moment, I'm going to invite you to open your eyes. As you do, feel your vision meeting your eyes the way the earth meets your feet.
- Open your eyes slowly. Let your vision meet your eyes the way the earth is meeting your feet. *(Pause.)*
- Now, take a walk around the room. See how you feel, what you perceive, what draws your attention.

Students can then share their experiences in partners or small groups first, or proceed directly to the group discussion.

Variation

Students may do this variation lying in Constructive Rest at any point in the exploration to support further relaxation of the eyes and facial muscles:

Have students cup their eyes with the palms of their hands, with their fingertips resting on their foreheads, and take a few deep breaths. Generally this is enough time to rest the eyes and face, while holding this position for much longer may create tension in the shoulders. Mention this to students, and guide them to relax their arms back down when they feel ready to do so.

Discussion

- What did you experience? What did you notice as you were standing today? Was it difficult to focus your attention? How were you feeling? What did you notice when you were lying down? What were some of the things that drew your attention?
- When you stood up, what did you notice? Was your experience different from your experience the first time you stood? How? How did it feel to walk around after you had gotten up? Did you experience any changes in your body? What drew your attention?
- Was anyone uncomfortable? Did you enjoy this? Why or why not? Did anyone have a different experience they want to share?

Tips for Teachers

- If you find that some students have fallen asleep during this activity, don't despair. Rather, this provides a wonderful opportunity to discuss why this may be happening, related to our need for both active (SNS) engagement and restful (PNS) repose. You can talk about this as part of the discussion.
- When you first invite students to make sound, even with something as simple as sighing, be prepared for a variety of responses! Some students may like this. Other students may feel self-conscious, and either refuse your invitation or, alternatively, exaggerate the sound by exhaling very loudly. This is often done unconsciously to get a response of laughter from others in the group, breaking the tension they experience from your invitation to use the voice. After some time, students generally get over this initial discomfort and very willingly participate.
- If many students seem to find this uncomfortable, you can discuss this with them, either the first time you introduce sound or on a subsequent day, beginning with asking your students how they are feeling. As a culture, we have a limited range of vocal expression that is considered socially acceptable or "normal," especially in a school environment. You can help to normalize a wider range of expression by allowing students who were uncomfortable to express their feelings. You can also ask students who *liked* making sound why they enjoyed it or found it helpful. By including all perspectives equally and addressing the issue of cultural context, you also demonstrate to your students that you find it more important for them to learn from their *own authentic responses*, than to "get it right" or "follow the rules." Simultaneously, you show that you are willing to address their resistance or discomfort by hearing them out and discussing their perspectives. You can also talk directly about some of your reasons for including vocal expression in certain activities, such as that making sound encourages fuller breathing and may help them to release body tension.

- Making sound also serves to break the silence of the quiet atmosphere often associated with these more internal sensory activities, which can feel repressive to some students. Once it becomes familiar, vocal expression invites a sense of play and freedom that creates a more relaxed atmosphere.
- Discussing all of this also gives students a chance to become conscious of their preferences—while perhaps even expanding their comfort zone of expression—rather than merely acquiescing to any initial discomfort to allow them to feel more immediately at ease. That being said, you may also choose to hold off on introducing the use of the voice until a bit further in the course, once you feel that students are more accustomed to some of the activities.

HOME PRACTICES

- Invite students to practice body listening on their own, by lying in Constructive Rest on a hard surface, such as the floor, as a way to rest before going to bed at night; a minimum of ten minutes is optimal to let both the superficial and the deep postural muscles release. The benefits of this are explored further in chapter 13, "Structure and Posture," but can be introduced here by using the dental floss analogy (see variations listed below). They can also practice Constructive Rest for a few minutes in the morning. Bringing awareness to their morning routine by discussing it together can be especially helpful, as many teens begin their day on their devices, by reading their email or checking out social media. Practicing Constructive Rest instead can help them replace such tendencies with a healthier daily habit.
- Students can record their experiences with Constructive Rest in their body journals over the next few weeks.
- After they have become familiar with Constructive Rest, invite students to practice it somewhere in nature: their own backyard, a nearby park, or the beach. If you know this will prove difficult for many students to find a safe space, consider arranging a field trip where you can facilitate the activity and ensure a safe container for them. Resting in nature can be particularly calming and refreshing *(Fig. 7.6)*.

RELATED PROJECTS

- Students can design individual or group research projects based on their areas of interest, such as learning more about the nervous system or the function of neurotransmitters in the body, such as serotonin, which are released when resting.

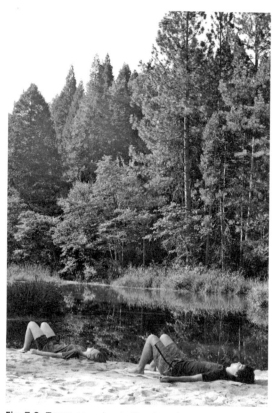

Fig. 7.6. Teens engaging in Constructive Rest in nature.

Variations: Further Discussion and Activity

As you continue working with your group, on subsequent days you can clarify specific aspects of the Constructive Rest Position, such as tracing alignment and weight support, learning how to get out of the position most easily, and understanding the benefits of Constructive Rest. Here are some brief examples of such discussions as further variations.

Alignment—Tracing Weight in Constructive Rest

The position you were lying in is called the Constructive Rest Position, or Constructive Rest. Why do you think it might be called that?

Explain the name by asking for a volunteer to lie in Constructive Rest. Trace the weight of the student's body to see how it is being supported: the weight of the lower legs falling into the ankles and feet; the weight of the thighs falling into the hips; the weight of the pelvis, torso, spine, neck, and head supported by the earth; the arms and shoulders supported by the earth. This demonstration explains why this position is considered to use the least amount of muscular effort to rest in gravity *(Fig. 7.7a).*

Compare this with how the weight is taken when lying down with the legs outstretched, in which case the lordosis of the lumbar spine increases, putting increased stress on the back muscles and the intrinsic muscles along the spine *(Fig. 7.7b)*. Have students lie down and try each of these variations to feel the difference. They can also explore this in partners, with one person lying down and the other one sitting to the side and placing one hand under the partner's lower back. With the legs extended there will be more space between the lower back and the floor; with the legs bent and the soles of the feet on the floor, the space will decrease and they can often then feel the weight of their partner's back on their hand. *(Fig. 7.7c, d.)*

You can also go over specifics of aligning the feet with the knees, and the knees with the hip sockets, as well as looking at the alignment of the spine. Some students may also need a book or small towel placed under the head to properly align the head and spine; demonstrate this as well.

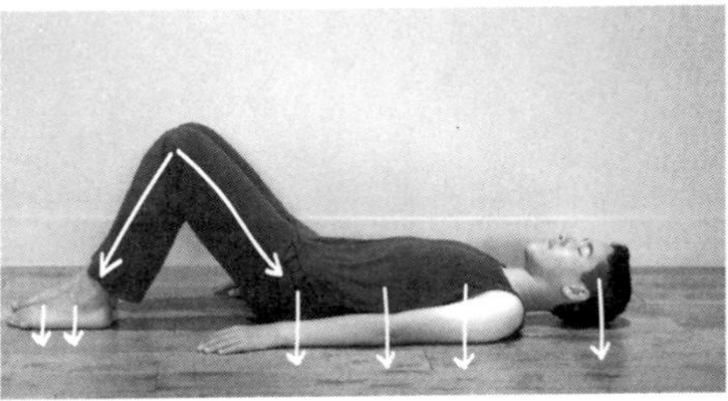

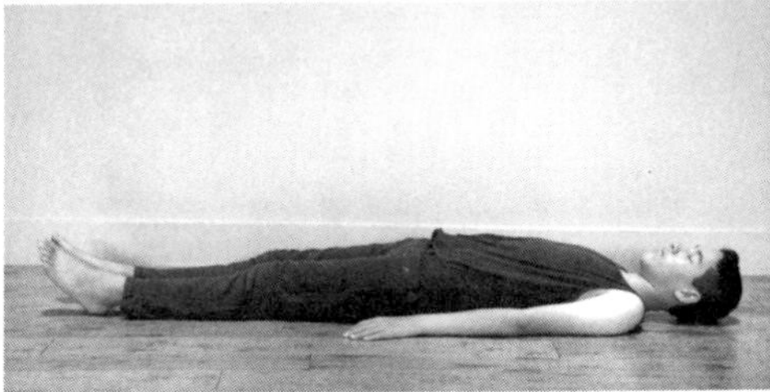

Fig. 7.7a, b. With feet on the floor more of the spine is supported; with the legs outstretched there is increased strain placed on the lower back.

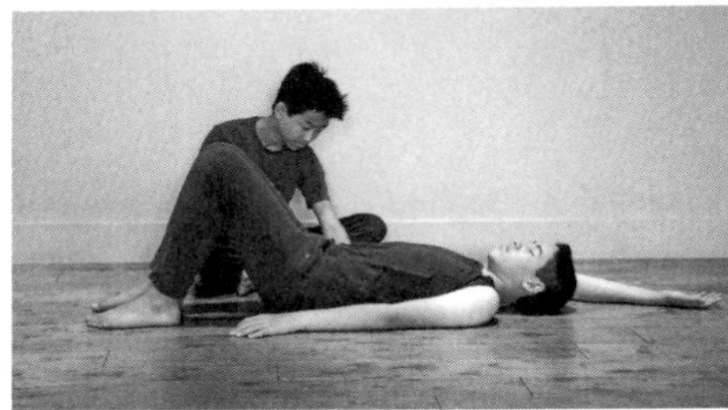

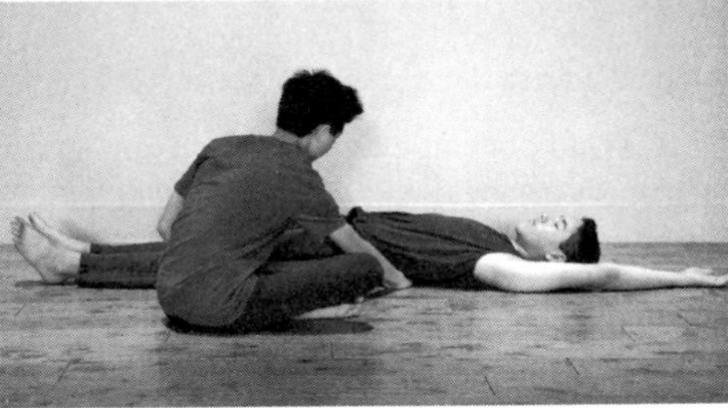

Fig. 7.7c, d. Working in partners, students can feel the variation in the curve of the lumbar spine in each position to help them understand the benefit of placing the feet on the floor, rather than lying with legs outstretched.

Transitions—Getting out of Constructive Rest

When getting out of this position, students will often roll up directly by tucking the chin and coming up to sitting as if doing a "sit-up." By sitting up in this way many of the benefits of resting are often undone, however, since you may reengage habitual patterns of tension in your shoulders, upper back and neck muscles. This uses much more muscular effort than when rolling to one side and using your hands and arms to support you.

You can help students understand the best way to get out of this position by having them try each method of getting up, and then discussing what they experienced. Then discuss the benefits of rolling to the side to sit up. Once they have *experienced* these two versions and compared them, they will generally choose the more easeful pattern.

Benefits—Constructive Rest as Dental Floss for the Body

The Constructive Rest Position is like the "dental floss for your body." Why might that be? Why do we use dental floss?

As students respond, continue to elicit their knowledge by asking them questions. You can then relate that to the purpose of Constructive Rest. For instance, plaque between the teeth not only harbors bacteria, but it also presses on the gums, restricting blood flow to the surrounding tissue—just as does tension in the muscles.

You can also ask students what other ways they may have to clear tension in their bodies. Examples might be physical activities, such as swimming or jogging, that actively get their blood flowing, or more passive means such as getting a massage. A subsequent discussion can include the distinction between the sympathetic and the parasympathetic nervous system, and the related benefits of deep relaxation, such as they may experience when practicing Constructive Rest on their own.

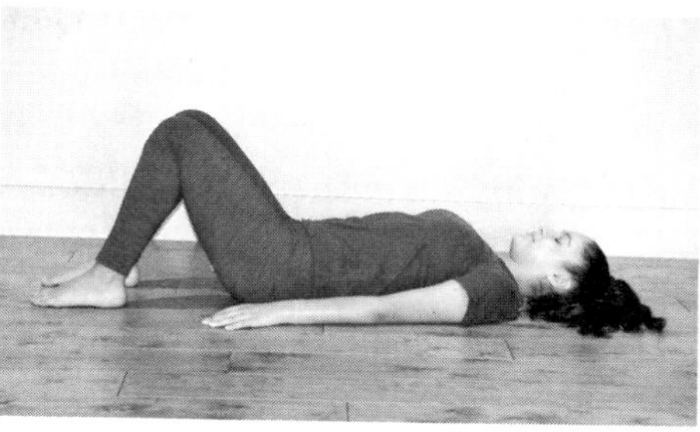

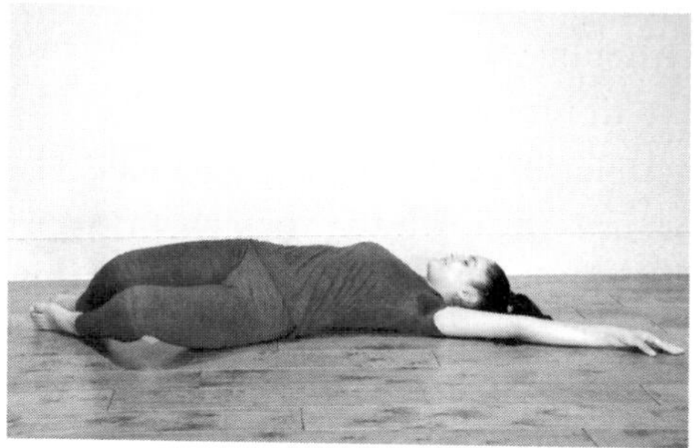

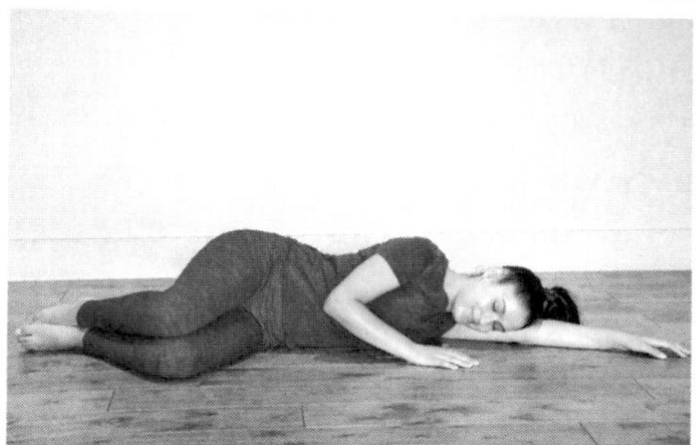

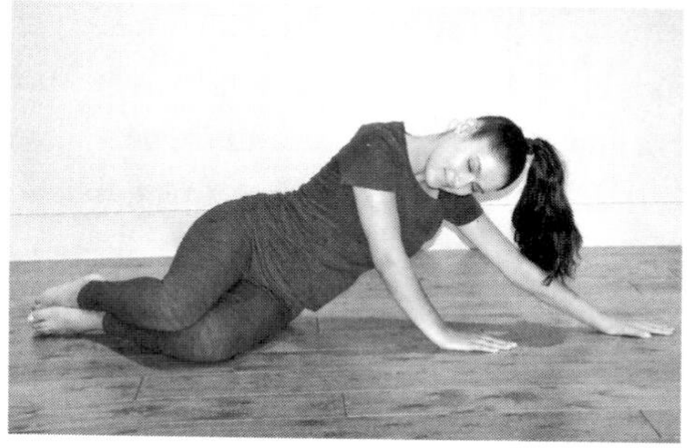

Fig. 7.8a, b, c, d. The best way to transition out of Constructive Rest (a) is to let the legs drop to one side (b), roll to the side (c), and then use the arms to push up to sitting (d).

Orienting to Both Weight and Space

After students have gained experience with orienting to gravity through the sensation of the weight of the body in Constructive Rest, they can begin to explore using imagery to enhance this feeling, as well as to orient to the space around them. Rather than using our minds to *observe* our bodies, as in the previous mindfulness activities, in this process we actively engage the mind to *initiate change* in our bodies through the use of imagery. As an example, while you are reading this, begin to imagine your head as a helium balloon floating up. Or you might try reaching upward through the top of your head, like you are reaching up toward the sky. As you do this, you'll likely feel a lengthening all along your spine. Orienting to space involves relating to the environment around you, as you just did by reaching through the top of your head to initiate movement in your spine. You might also feel your feet sinking in sand, or growing roots into the earth to experience your weight more fully.

Many somatic educators identify this skill of orienting to weight and space—and the ability to shift between the two, or even activate both at once—as fundamental to developing easier, more proficient movement. Somatic pioneer Hubert Godard refers to this as "tonic function," a model of orienting through weight and space in relation to how we prepare to move. Tonic function emphasizes using our perception to change our coordination to move more effectively and with less effort. Godard's students Caryn McHose and Kevin Frank use the term *gravity orientation* to refer to a similar process, one that serves to restore healthy movement.[4] There are several methods that can help students learn this fundamental skill, as we will see below.

Imagery

In this curriculum, I incorporate imagery in many of the movement matrix activities used throughout the class as a means to help students learn how to actively shift their orientation between weight and space, and then to activate them both simultaneously. According to the principles of Ideokinesis, when imagery is activated in *at least two directions*—such as feeling your feet sinking in sand while imagining your head floating upward like a helium balloon, as used in a next exploration—a *tensile dynamic* is created that activates the neuromuscular system. This ability to orient to weight and space at the same time—by using imagery to initiate both a downward and an upward force simultaneously, for example—activates further postural tone and gives both groundedness and buoyancy to our movement. The Shifting Perceptions exploration gives a good example of this.

This sense of "going down to go up" can be understood on many levels: picture a tree with shallow roots getting blown about in a windstorm or hurricane, versus one with deep roots extending down into the soil; the downward support of deep roots allows for the upward strength to resist the outside force of the wind. Or envision the height of the dancer who must first plié, or the basketball player in a leap who must first bend the knees, in preparation for extending upward; the deeper the bend, the higher the jump. As infants, yielding into gravity underlies our later abilities to push, reach, grasp, and pull—all movements that allow us to actively engage with our environment. Further, as you learn to yield your weight, you gain a corresponding sense of rest, safety, and security that creates a foundation for your movement out into the world. Primarily, yielding gives the deep support necessary for the ability to push up and away from the resistance of gravity.[5] In the Shifting Perceptions exploration, students explore imagery to effect change in their bodies—yielding downward and expanding upward—and then reflect on their experiences in the subsequent discussion.

Counterbalance

After this discussion, you can use a demonstration of the concept of counterbalance as a fun way to help students understand why they might have experienced actual *physical change* in their own bodies—simply by using imagery. In this demonstration, two people stand and face each other while holding hands, and then are asked to simultaneously lean backward. If only one person leans back, of course the other person will be pulled forward and both will fall. But if both people lean backward at the same time, a *counterbalance force* is created that prevents them both from falling. If they stand and face each other, place their palms together, and then lean forward, again a balance point is created between them that prevents them both from falling forward. Counterbalance creates a *third force,* which is the tensile energy between the two points. This activity demonstrates how counterbalance works in your body when using two contrasting images at once.

You can also use this counterbalance activity to help students become more grounded through their pelvis, legs, and feet. For instance, when leaning forward, if you are not releasing your full weight through your lower body, you will likely not be able to release your weight through your arms; rather you will be "holding" your body up and then need to actively push forward with your shoulders and arms to keep your balance. As you release your weight through your legs and feet your weight naturally releases forward toward your partner, and there is no need to strain in your upper body. When both people achieve this, a very easy and solid-feeling state of counterbalance is created. This activity becomes a fun process of discovery into how we each inhabit our bodies, as students begin to recognize the complexity of achieving such a simple movement task!

Experiencing a new groundedness in their physical bodies also helps students to feel more confident—particularly those who tend to be shy or insecure—as they not only *experience* this sense of rootedness, but are also *seen* and *experienced* as strong and rooted by their peers. Teens develop a sense of agency—developed from within—that helps them recognize that they can choose how they move and embody themselves.

Exploration: Shifting Perceptions—Imagery

(20 minutes; 30 minutes with variation)

PURPOSE. To activate imagery in your body related to weight and space; to activate postural tone and vibrancy in your body through imagery; to create groundedness through your lower body and lengthening through your spine; to create length through your neck and relax your shoulders (see variation); to discuss the use of imagery as it relates to movement repatterning and effecting change in the body.

Activity

Have the students stand in a circle or spread out throughout the room.

- Stand and take a moment to close your eyes and do a body scan. Just notice what you become aware of today.
- Imagine yourself standing in sand, letting your weight be taken through your feet into the earth. *(Fig. 7.9a.)*
- Begin to shift your weight slightly forward *(Fig. 7.9b)* and then back to center. Then shift your weight slightly back, and then once again back to center. Notice the weight shifting on your feet as you do this.

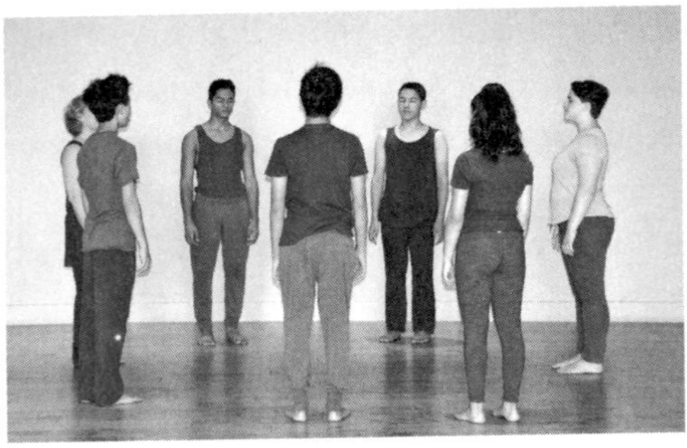

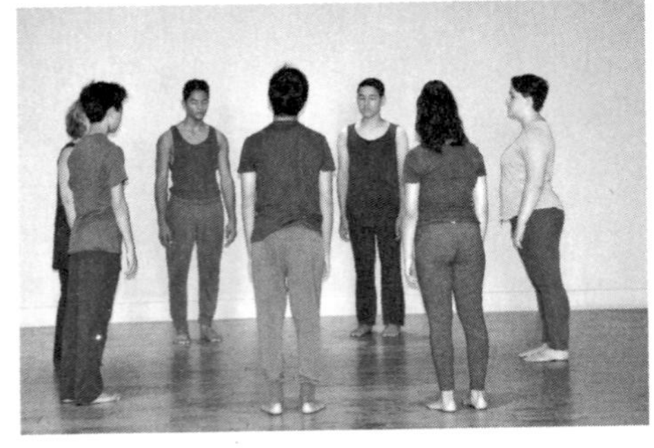

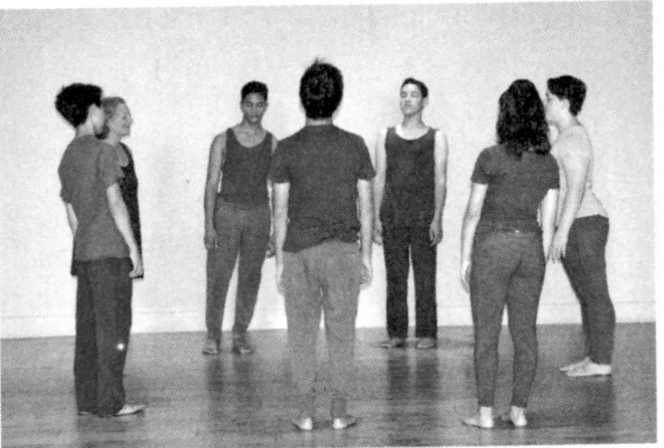

Fig. 7.9a, b, c. Students standing in "sand" (a), then leaning forward (b) and back, and then beginning to circle their weight on their feet, while still keeping the spine lengthened (c).

- Shift your weight again slightly forward. Now shift your weight slightly to the right, slightly back, and then slightly onto your left foot. Then again forward, to the right, to the back, to the left, until you are shifting your weight around in a small circle. Keep your spine lengthened rather than bending at the waist as you shift your weight through your feet. *(Fig. 7.9c.)*
- Imagine you are standing in soft, warm sand on the beach. Feel the sand shift as you move your weight around. Let your feet spread out in the sand.
- Change the direction of your circle whenever you like.
- Come back to center, and pause there a moment. Use a finger to tap the center of the top of your head, and then relax your arm back down. *(Fig. 7.10.)*
- Feel the spot you have tapped, and lengthen up from that spot, as if your head were floating upward like a helium balloon, up and up toward the ceiling or sky.
- See if you can keep this feeling of lifting, and relax your muscles. Perhaps you've lifted your shoulders along with the top of your head, or perhaps you've lifted your chin or tightened your knees ... Let all that release, and still feel the lift through your spine and up through the top of your head.

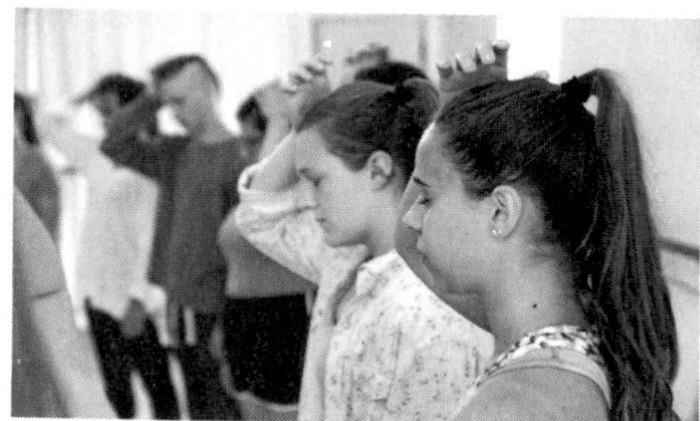

Fig. 7.10. Students tap the top of their head to increase their proprioceptive awareness at that spot. This helps them begin to initiate movement from the top of the head to lengthen the spine.

- Now imagine you have a colored crayon at that spot on your head. What color is it? Imagine it growing up and up and up, until it reaches the ceiling. Check to see that your muscles are still relaxed.
- Now "draw" a tiny circle on the ceiling, by allowing your weight to shift on your feet as you did before: forward, to the side, back, to the other side. Let the circle get just a little bit bigger. *(Watch to see that the head and spine stay aligned.)*
- As you draw your circle on the ceiling, bring your awareness to the weight shifting on your feet, from the front to the side to the back, other side, and front again, around in a circle. Can you still feel your feet in the sand? ...
- Let your circle get a little smaller ... and smaller again. Can you still be aware of the crayon on your head, or did you lose it as you were focusing on your feet? See if you can notice both at once, drawing the circle on the ceiling and feeling the weight shift in your feet.
- Let the circle continue to get smaller until you find yourself balanced in the very center.

- Open your eyes, letting your vision meet your eyes like the earth is meeting your feet. Walk around the room, keeping this awareness of the warm sand under your feet and your tall crayon. Can you feel your feet on the earth? Can you "see" the patterns that you are drawing on the ceiling as you walk throughout the room? You can nod hello to each other from the top of your crayon as you go. How is that the same as or different from nodding with your head as you usually do?

Variations

Done Standing: After you have done this exploration with the group, you can add in additional visualizations to this basic formula as you repeat it over time. This is another example of using visualizations and movement to help students establish a physical sense of both groundedness and upward expansion.

- Stand and take a moment to close your eyes and do a body scan. Just notice what you become aware of today.
- Imagine yourself standing in sand, letting your weight be taken through your feet into the earth.
- Now reach your arms up above your head, as if you're reaching starting with the soles of your feet. Can you feel your feet as you reach your arms up? *(Fig. 7.11.)* OK, then relax your arms back down.
- Let's do this again, reach your arms up, but this time reach as far up as you can, and let your shoulders come along so they are reaching up by your ears! *(Fig.7.12a.) (Demonstrate this by doing it along with them.)* Great, now, let your arms drop back down, but keep your shoulders where they are! *(Fig. 7.12b.) (Demonstrate.)* Now, let your shoulders drop back down too. *(Fig. 7.12c.)*
- Now lift your arms and shoulders up again. Now, instead of keeping your shoulders up, just let your arms and shoulders drop back down. *(Do this along with them.)*
- Once more, lift your arms and shoulders up as far as you can as you breathe in, and then hold for a moment, now this time as you exhale, let your arms and shoulders *float* back down slowly as you open your arms to the sides. *(Do this with them.)*
- Close your eyes, take a moment to do your body scan and see what you notice. Take a moment now to tap the top of your head, so you feel that spot at the center, and relax your arm back down.
- Now open your eyes and we'll do this one last time. Reach up with your arms and shoulders as you breathe in *(Fig. 7.12d)*, and now as you exhale, let your arms and shoulders float down, while your head floats up! *(Fig. 7.12e.)*
- Close your eyes now and try this again on your own, on your own timing, reaching up, and then letting your arms and shoulders float down while your head floats up.
- Then take a moment to do your body scan again, and when you are ready you can open your eyes and take a walk through the room.

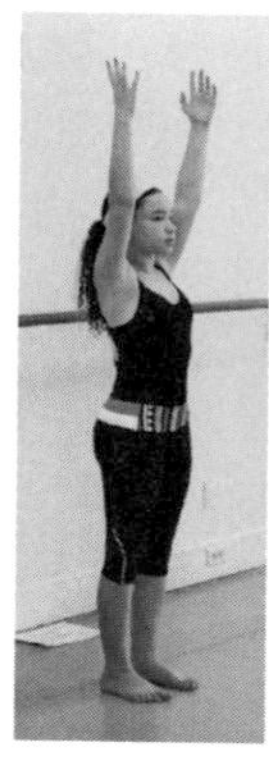

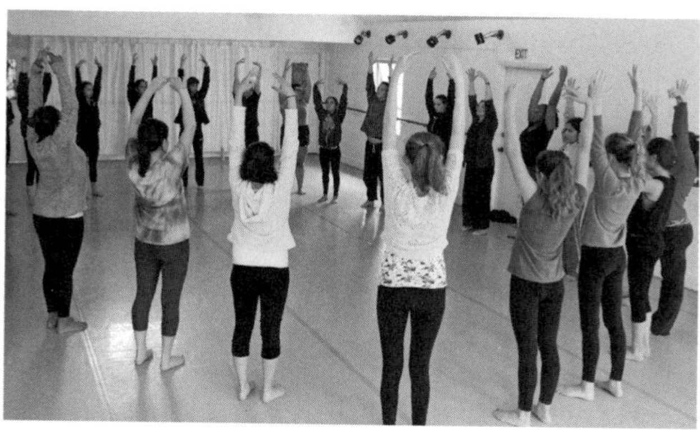

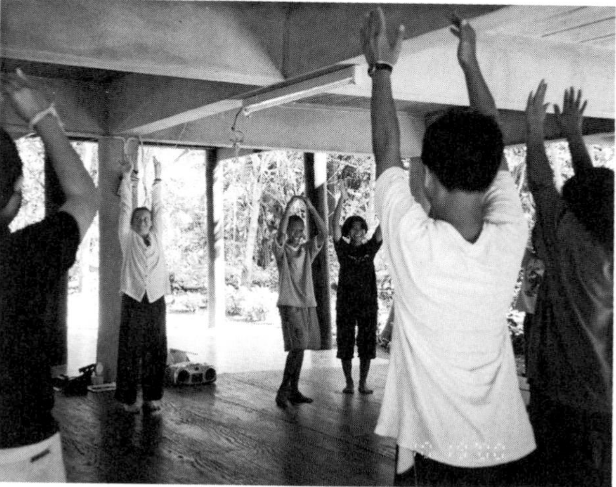

Fig. 7.11a, b, c. Students reaching their arms up "from the soles of the feet," so the movement travels through the whole body. (Photo c, teens in Thailand at Moo Baan Dek School.)

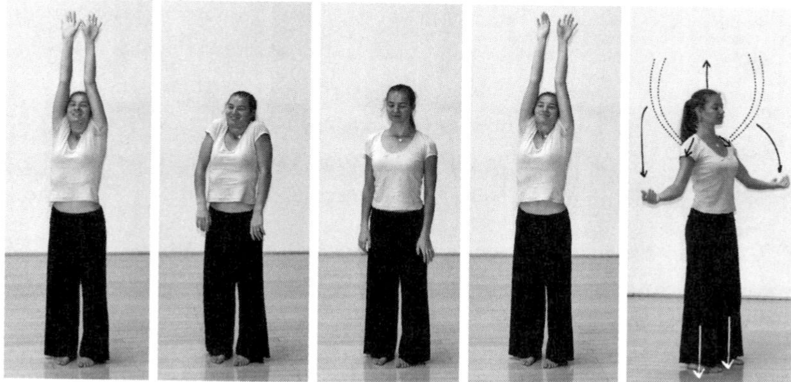

Fig. 7.12a, b, c, d, e. Variation of Shifting Perceptions—Imagery exploration. Using visualization and movement combined helps students to relax their shoulders, activate postural tone, and gain a sense of both groundedness and upward expansion.

Done in Constructive Rest: Another variation can be done while lying in Constructive Rest, using imagery to relax the muscles of the neck and head. Have students slowly roll their head to one side and then the other, noticing how that feels. Then they can repeat that using various images that you can suggest: rolling a water balloon or a sand bag side to side; resting their head on a pillow; or imagining the floor underneath their head tilting to one side and then the other, rolling their head as it lifts. Suggest several images, or offer one image, and experiment with others on subsequent days.

Discussion

- What did you notice in this activity? How did the imagery affect your body? Your movement? Could you stay focused on two images at once? What happened when you tried to do this? How did it feel to walk using these images? What did you experience? What did you learn? What questions do you have?
- Why do you think you experienced these changes?
- *(For variation done standing)* What did you notice from this activity? Could you feel your feet still while you lifted your arms? Did you notice any changes in your body?
- *(For variation in Constructive Rest with head)* What did you notice as you rolled your head? How did the image affect your movement? Which image did you prefer? Why do you think that was true? Did anyone have a different experience?

Tips For Teachers

- When using imagery to activate movement initiation, students may end up unconsciously creating additional tensions in their bodies, as was indicated in the exploration itself when students were asked to notice if they may have also lifted their shoulders while lifting through the top of the head. Being able to visually perceive these subtleties in your students' movement is a core skill that allows you to help them become more aware of the various shiftings in their bodies. Later in the curriculum when working in partners, students also gain experience with learning how to see changes in others' movement as well. This helps them gain compassion for each other and develop patience for the process that we all go through when learning something new.
- If some of the imagery used here seems to elicit a more general "stiffness" in your students, particularly in the spine, you can introduce the exploration called What is Balance? The Small Dance (see p. 234) to invite greater ease.

Exploration: Counterbalance

(20 minutes)

PURPOSE. To experience groundedness through your lower body; to experiment with finding your core support; to understand the concept of counterbalance and reflect on how that relates to the use of imagery as a method of body and movement repatterning.

Activity

This activity can begin with a demonstration, by having two students stand, face each other, and join hands to experience leaning forward or back, as described previously. There are a variety of ways to facilitate this demonstration; here is one example.

Have the students stand and face each other. Then ask them each to lean first forward, and then back of their center, to get a feeling for this. Then ask them to come back to center and place their palms together.

- ❍ Now slowly lean forward again, and let's see what happens. *(Pause while they do this, and wait while they find a balance point between them; prompt them to use their full forearms, not just their hands, to support the weight.) (Fig. 7.13a.)* Now come back to center.
- ❍ What would happen if only one person leaned forward now, and the other one didn't? What do you imagine? Let's try this. *(Have the students try this, carefully and being sure there is nothing behind each of them that they would bump into if they moved backward.)* What just happened?

Then you can have students come back to center, take a step back, and hold onto each other's wrists.

- ❍ Now when you are ready, slowly each of you can start to lean back. *(Pause while they do this, and wait while they find a balance point between them.) (Fig. 7.13b.)* Again come back to center, but keep holding onto each other's wrists for a moment.
- ❍ What would happen if one person leaned back now, and the other one didn't? *(Pause to let them answer, but don't have students demonstrate this version, as it is all too common that a student could fall backward onto the floor.)*
- ❍ What is this called when you find this point of balance between you?

After demonstrating and discussing this, students can try the counterbalance activity in partners. Facilitate this in a similar fashion as the demonstration, so students can practice both leaning forward and leaning back with their partners *(Fig. 7.14a, b).*

Discussion

- What did you experience from this activity? What was easiest to do? Hardest? What did you discover or learn? Did anyone have a different experience?

Discuss the relationship between counterbalance and using visualizations that activate movement in two or more directions.

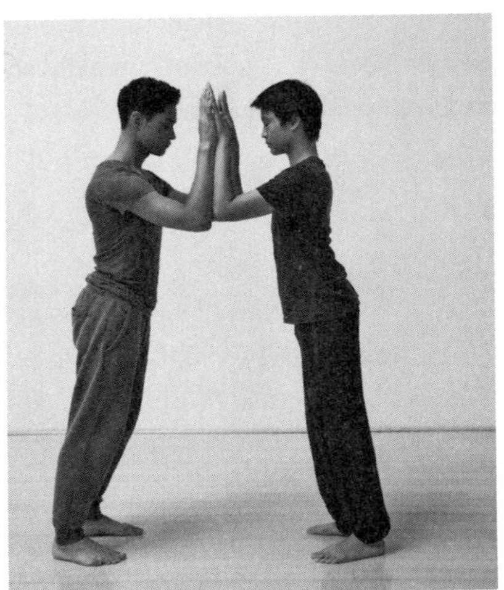

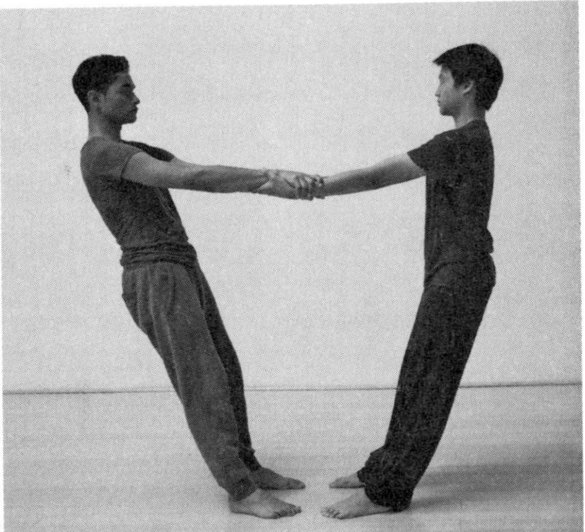

Fig. 7.13a, b. Teens demonstrating counterbalance, forward and back. This activity serves as metaphor to help them understand the dynamics involved in using imagery in two directions; it also helps them ground through the pelvis and legs.

Tips for Teachers

- When doing the counterbalance activity, it can be helpful if partners are somewhat the same height and weight if possible. If particular students are having difficulty either giving or receiving weight, you can begin by making suggestions as to what might help them based on your visual observations. Alternately, you can partner with that student yourself for a moment; this helps you to get more direct sensory feedback as to what may be happening, such as if they are holding tension in a particular area of the body, allowing you to introduce more direct sensory feedback through your own movement. This type of direct movement intervention is often much more helpful—and effective—than verbal explanation or suggestions alone.

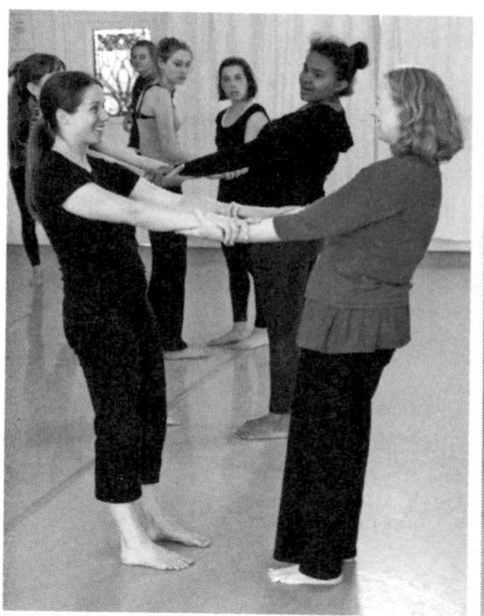
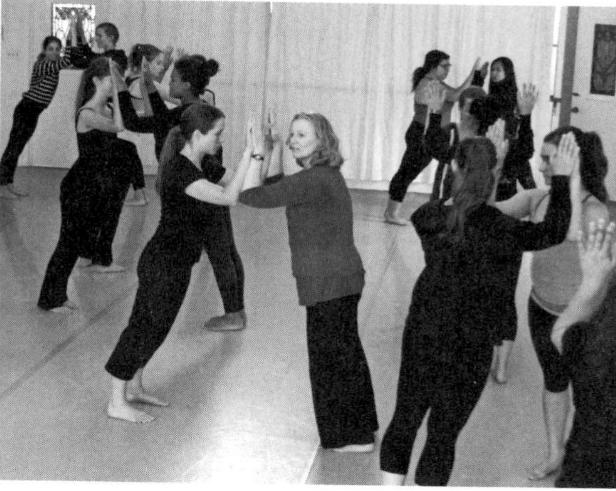

Fig. 7.14a, b. You can also demonstrate the counterbalance activity, and have students practice this in partners. (Author demonstrating counterbalance with dance educator Mo Miner, with students trying it as well.)

Using Body Scanning, the Constructive Rest Position, and Visualizations

As classes progress, students use body scanning and Constructive Rest to focus on sensing and visualizing various structures or processes of the body they are studying, such as the bones, muscles, organs, and breathing. These activities help them to discover what they know about their internal bodies, as well as to become aware of questions they may have. We'll use these foundational practices throughout the curriculum.

Using a Movement Matrix

As mentioned in the description of the movement matrix in chapter 3 (and explained further in chapter 4 on pedagogy), remember that although classes can do each of the explorations presented in this book separately, it is often best to begin and end each class with more active movement. A simple formula for the start of class can be to have students begin standing in a circle, closing their eyes to do their body scan, and then opening their eyes to walk throughout the room.

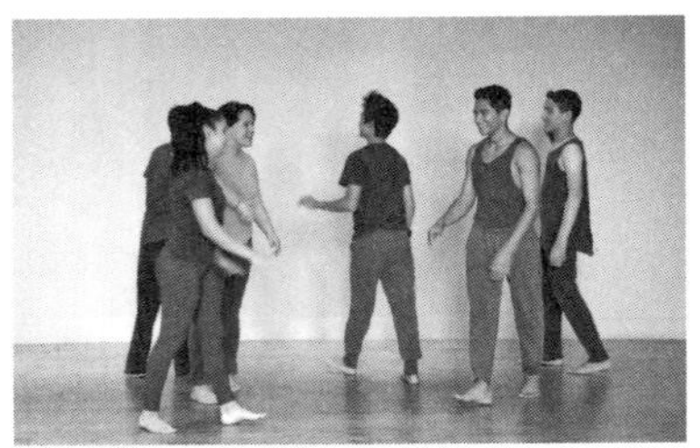

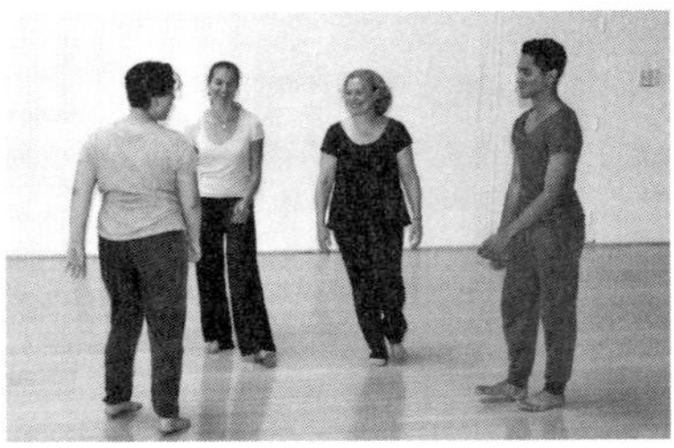

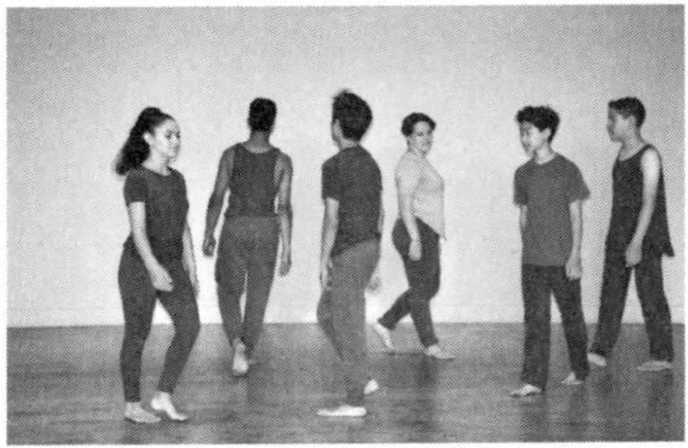

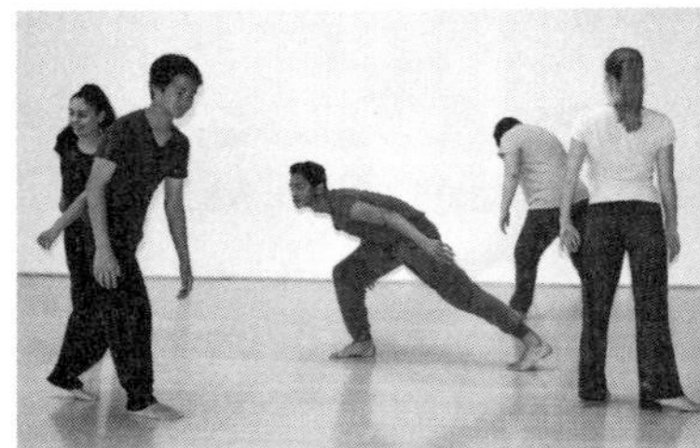

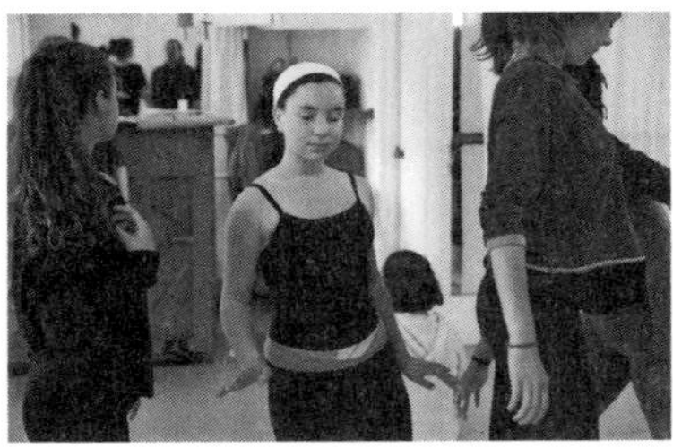

Fig. 7.15a, b, c, d, e. Students walking with a more external focus first (a); you can initially walk with them to get the energy going (b); then students transition to a more internal focus, feeling their feet as they walk (c), or pausing to close their eyes and do their body scan in whatever position they are in (d, e).

Here they can be guided in a progression from a more external focus, such as noticing each other as they walk by, to a more internal focus, like feeling their weight on their feet as they walk, or pausing to close their eyes and bring their awareness to whatever shape they are in in that moment, or shifting back and forth between an internal and external focus on their own *(Fig. 7.15a–e and Fig. 7.16).*

If your group is already comfortable with more improvisational modes of moving—such as in a dance class in which students have already been using improvisation—you may want to also introduce the Responsive Moving exploration (see chapter 16). This process, which allows students to move in a more self-directed way, can serve as another effective method of "body listening" that can be used as part of the movement time. For many teens, however, this free-form practice is better introduced much later in the curriculum, once there is less self-consciousness—and more body awareness and group cohesion—to support this more vulnerable process of eyes-closed, inner exploration through movement.

Finally, if you know a subsequent activity will include a long period of time in relative stillness, such as many of the explorations done in Constructive Rest, you might also add a faster and interactive aspect to the walking activity at the start of the class. This might include having students move quickly through the spaces between themselves, give each other a "high-five" as they pass by each other, or run and pretend to be dribbling and shooting a basketball as they move. All of these activities create a fun break from the more inner-directed focus, as well as providing a bridge to prepare students for a next, more inner-directed process.

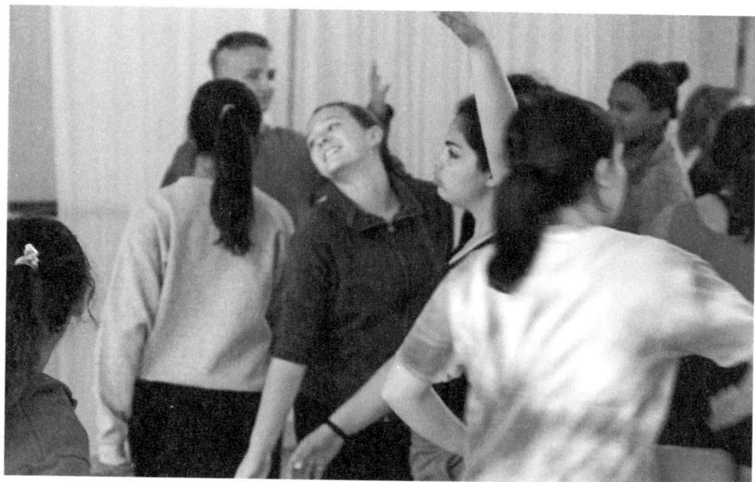

Fig.7.16. Students can 'shape' their way through the spaces, maintaining awareness of their bodies as they also notice each other, moving back and forth between an internal and external focus as needed.

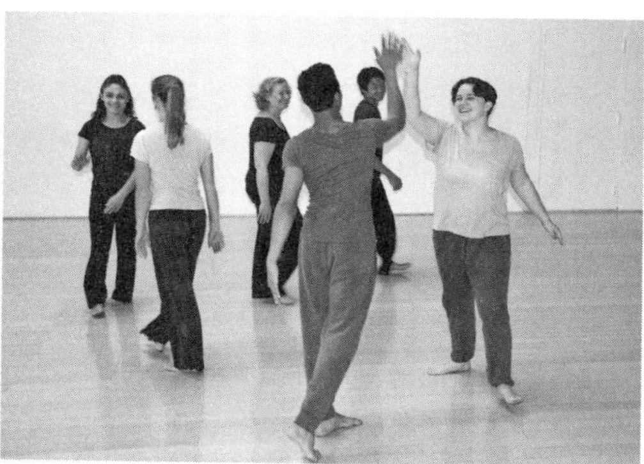

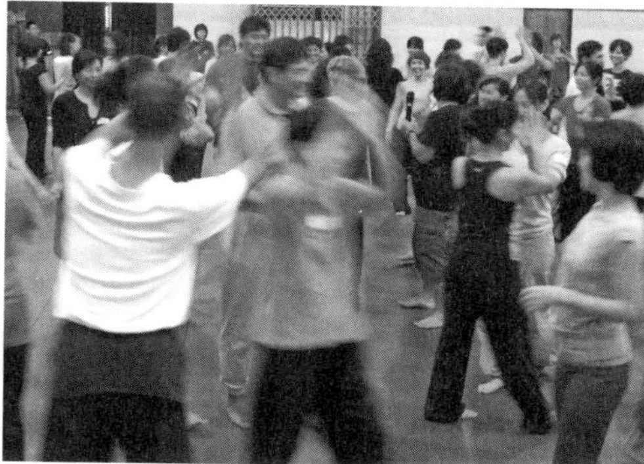

Fig. 7.17a, b. Giving a high-five as they pass by encourages lively interaction among teens and adults alike. (Photo b courtesy of Somatic Education Society of Taiwan.)

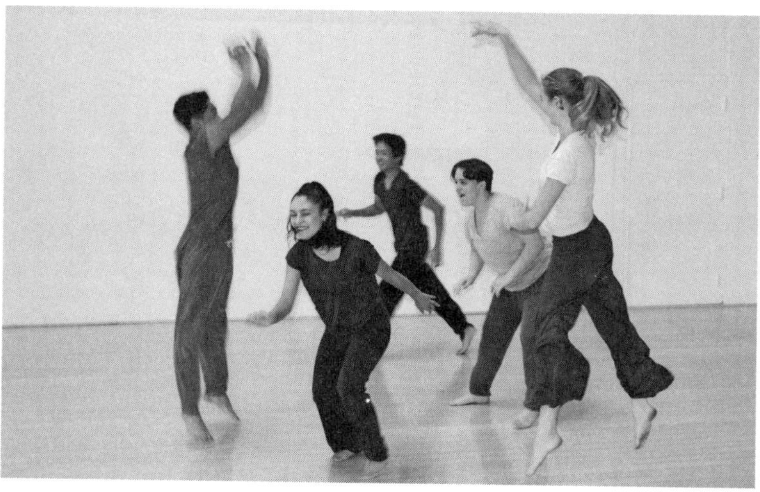

Fig. 7.18. High-energy movement, like pretending to be dribbling and shooting a basketball, can provide active teens with a bridge to the more inner-directed movement to follow.

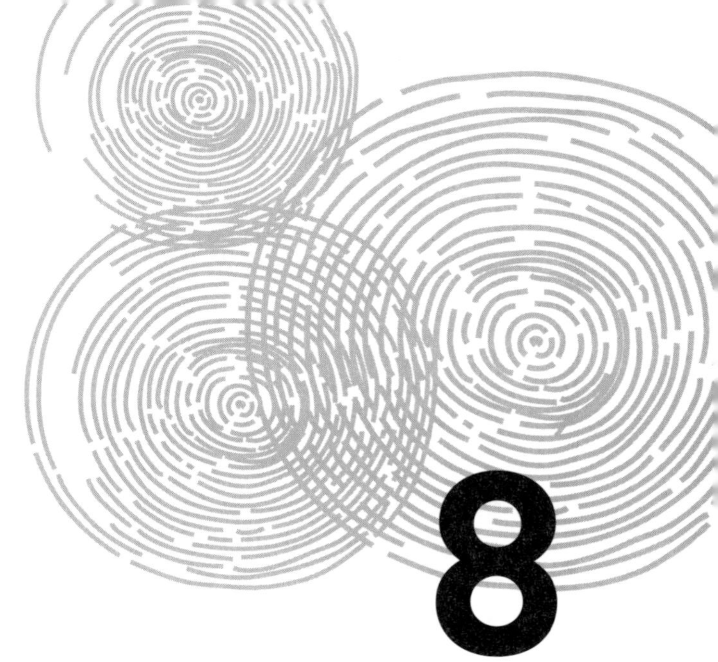

8

Body Systems

The mystery of the human body is apparent when we look inside our bodies at the myriad cells, tissues, and systems within. Yet how much do we know about this amazing complexity within our own bodies? How much did you know about your own body as a teenager? Learning about our body systems and their respective and interrelated functions is relevant to every human being. Through the explorations in this chapter, a holistic approach to physiology becomes a living topic of study for students.

Inside the Body

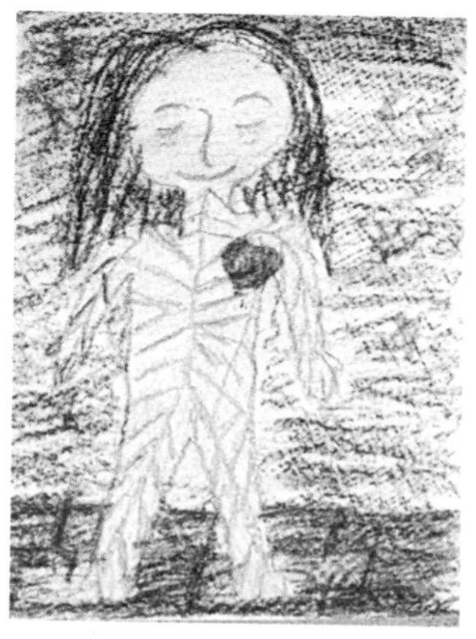

As a means to explore the body systems, students are first guided to imagine what is inside of them while lying in Constructive Rest, and then afterward are invited to draw their perceptions. After this activity, they look at each other's drawings and discuss the body systems together. They learn to identify the body systems individually, and see how they function interdependently. The Western scientific model divides the body into twelve distinct systems, with a system defined as a collection of organs and structures that share a common function. These are the skeletal, muscular, cardiovascular, lymphatic, nervous, endocrine, integumentary, respiratory, digestive, urinary, immune, and reproductive systems. The organs of a particular system share a common function but are located throughout the body. The cardiovascular or circulatory system, for example, includes the heart, blood, and the blood vessels of the veins, arteries and capillaries that extend throughout the body, and yet is considered one body system.

While many students can easily identify at least a few body systems, such as the skeletal, muscular, or cardiovascular system, others may mention less commonly known systems, such as the endocrine or lymphatic systems. It often turns out that these students have heard about them from a family member who was ill or is a health practitioner. Other students know intricate anatomical details about certain parts of the body, such as the knee or shoulder girdle, because they had an injury in that area and learned about it for themselves. As the group "pools" their knowledge, you can add any additional relevant information according to the students' questions and interests.

As students become aware of the many systems inside of them—working interdependently—they gain a fuller perception of their living bodies. Here is how one eighth grader put it in his journal:

> *Today we did another walking around the room exercise, but this time we had already taken a look inside at all the organs and stuff in there, and then drew them. Visualizing my bones, muscles, and other systems as part of my movement was a realization ... learning that not only my bones and muscles are moving as I walk around, but my respiratory and digestive systems are moving around too. Of course it's so obvious, but I just never thought about it or really felt it before!*

Just being asked about what they know about their bodies can be empowering for teens, as it allows them to focus on their bodies in a frank and practical way that they find both surprising and relieving. Their curiosity about aspects of their bodies—some of which may be repressed or overlooked—often emerges as the silence about the body is broken.

A group of young teens in Thailand, for instance, engaged in this activity in our first day of working together. Rather than doing individual drawings after the visualization activity, they instead worked in groups by tracing one person's body on a large piece of paper and then filling it in together with whatever they had perceived. The boys all gathered together, while the girls formed another group. The girls drew pretty clothes on their female figure, with a few outlines beneath for the heart, lungs, and some bones of the arms and legs. The boys' group, on the other hand, included all sorts of bones, organs, intestines, and blood vessels on their male figure—along with a marked big pile of poop at the bottom of the drawing.

When we gathered back together, after some general conversation facilitated by my Thai translator about what the students had experienced when visualizing their bodies, I began to comment on the drawings. When we got to the boys' group, they sat in stillness awaiting my response, glancing over at each other with mischievous looks in their eyes. Clearly they thought they were in trouble. The translator then relayed my words: rather than reprimanding them, I had discussed the different body systems they had represented in the drawing, including the digestive system that provides for both intake of food and output of wastes through the elimination of urine and feces, as they had accurately portrayed. I also mentioned that we don't often talk about these things, as many of them relate to body functions that happen in private, and while it is important to respect personal privacy and adhere to certain cultural norms, it is also necessary to understand and appreciate all the ways our miraculous bodies keep us alive and functioning. This response initially shocked them, but soon opened up a rich discussion, as the group came forth with a barrage of additional questions about the body over the course of the next few days. Looking within and drawing their perceptions is a potent first step in students' individual and collective learning about themselves and their bodies.

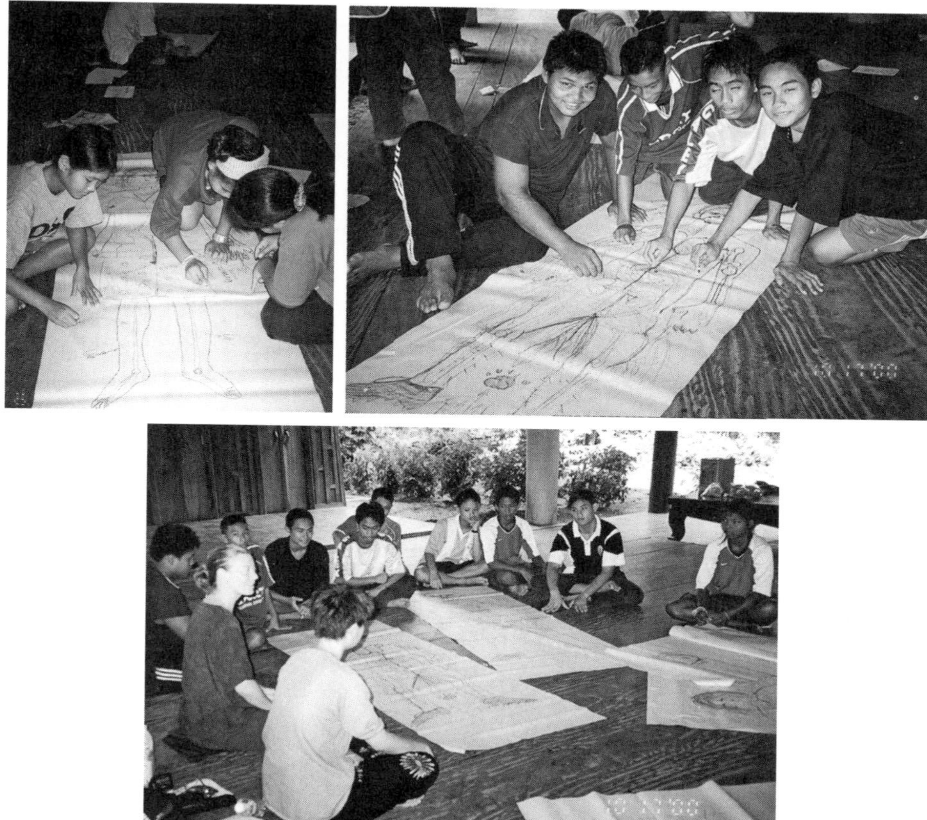

Fig. 8.1a, b, c. Teens in Thailand draw their perceptions of what is inside their bodies, then gather together to discuss their drawings.

Exploration: The Mind's Eye and the Body Systems

(30–45 minutes)

PURPOSE. To discover what you know or imagine about your internal body; to enhance awareness of all the body systems; to define the body systems.

Activity

MATERIALS

- Individual sheets of paper
- Drawing supplies, such as crayons, colored pencils, or pastels

Begin with Constructive Rest Position activity. (Take 5 minutes or so for this.) Then proceed with the following guiding directives and questions.

- ❍ As you rest lying down, use your mind's eye to look within your body. Imagine what is inside. What do you notice?
- ❍ What systems make up your body?
- ❍ Which systems can you picture? Which can you feel?
- ❍ What functions does each system have?

After guiding the class to sit up, prompt the class to make drawings with the paper and supplies.

- ❍ Take a few moments to draw your perceptions. What body systems did you see or experience inside your body? *(After students have completed their drawings, they can work in pairs or small groups to share them.)*

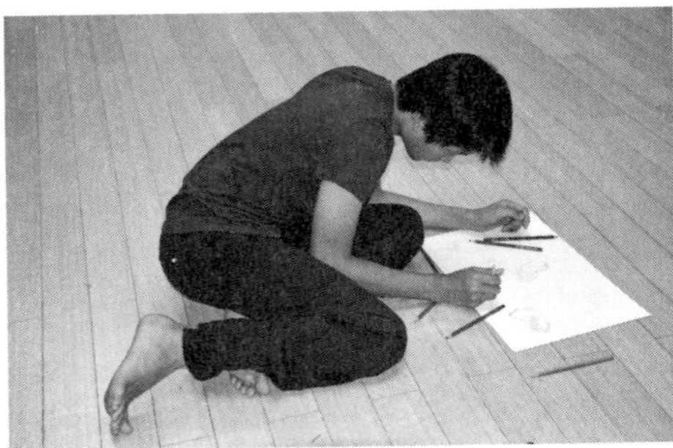

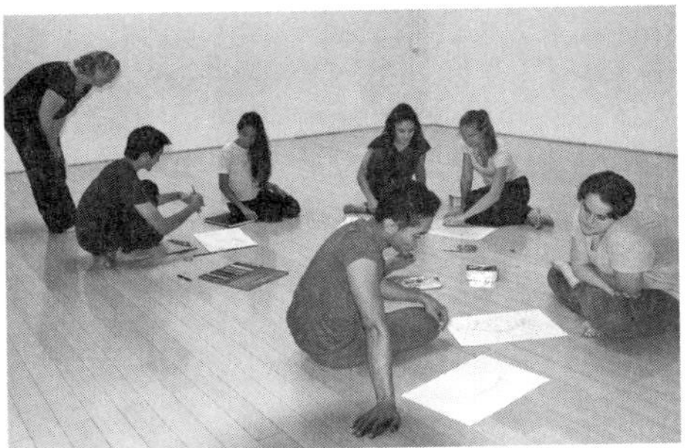

Fig. 8.2a, b. In The Mind's Eye and Body Systems, after looking within while lying in Constructive Rest, teens draw their impressions of what is inside their bodies (a), and then share their drawings in partners (b).

Museum: Students can then put all the drawings in a circle, and stand and walk around the outside perimeter of the circle to look at each other's drawings. This activity serves as a museum tour of their collective understandings and perceptions *(Fig. 8.2c)*.

Discussion

- What did you picture inside your body? What did you notice? What systems could you "see"? What could you feel? Were there any systems you could identify but couldn't see in your mind's eye?
- What are the functions of these systems? What did you learn from looking within your body? What did you learn from creating your drawing? What questions do you have?

Tips for Teachers

- Make a list of the body systems that students name, either using the board or newsprint; students can take turns as the "scribe," the person who writes down what other students say, to write this list. Add in any systems that students have omitted. You can also refer to their anatomy coloring plates or an organ model.

HOME PRACTICE

- Students can color the anatomy plates associated with each system.

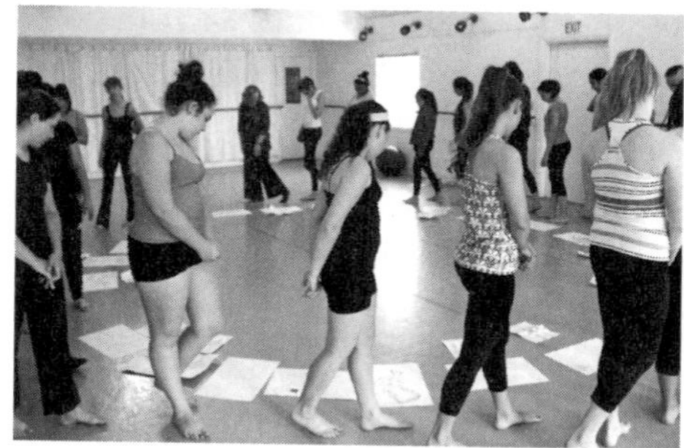

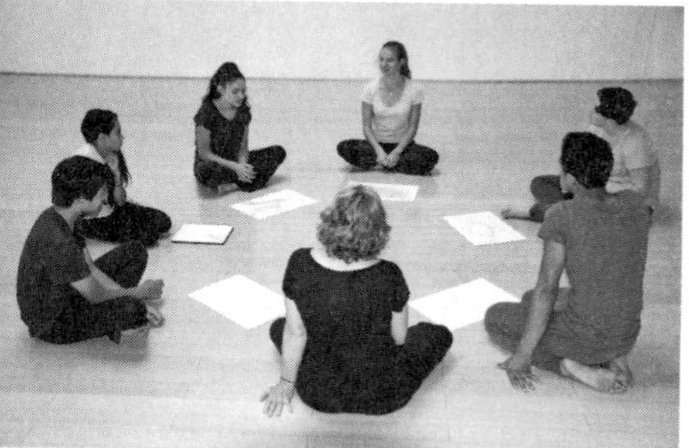

Fig. 8.2c, d. In Mind's Eye and Body Systems, teens view each others drawings in a "museum circle" (c) and then discuss their experiences in the full group (d).

The Cultural Body

In this next exploration, called Body Systems and Perception, rather than directing students to focus on specific body systems they are guided to simply *look within* and see what they feel or perceive, again followed by drawing their perceptions and then participating in a discussion. You can use this activity, instead of the previous one, either with an older group or when there is more time to facilitate this longer version. I developed this more open-ended activity over time, as it invites a broader variety of both *subjective and objective* observations, which inevitably leads to a rich individual experience and lively group discussion.

For example, as students look within their own bodies and bring attention to their sensations, it is often their subjective experience that emerges most vividly—as they notice areas of tension, pain, openness, warmth or feelings of apprehension, fear, or aliveness. In discussing their experience after the activity, they may use such words as "gross," "bright," "dark," "heavy," "swirling," or "tingling"; their drawings also often reflect these varied perceptions with abstract images, such as dark spots, bright areas, or twisted lines. As they come to see, we are not just a collection of tissues and body systems; we also have our lived experience of our bodies: our *soma.* This activity welcomes each person's subjective experience—even if it differs from the experience of others in the group—as an authentic starting point. Once this personal connection is made, students' motivation to learn more about their own bodies inevitably increases.

By sharing their perceptions in a group discussion, they begin to recognize the wide variety of our embodied experience. To see the whole, we need to understand the experience of *each person* within the collective. When you model this inclusive approach early on in the process of working with your group, you lay the foundation for this experiential anatomy approach by setting a tone that values each individual's contribution as essential.

The discussion after this activity can be used to process both these personal observations and more didactic learning. For instance, to increase students' knowledge of anatomy they can define the various body systems, as in the previous exploration, since inevitably students will also mention actual anatomical structures they have experienced or drawn, including bones, muscles, blood, tendons, or specific organs, such as the lungs, heart, or stomach. By relating to the words they offer, you can then guide the group by, for example, helping them to name the specific bones that make up the skeletal system, or listing the particular organs associated with our cardiovascular or digestive systems, and so forth.

In some cases, students may also discuss and/or draw aspects not directly related to physical anatomy, such as *atoms, meridians, chi,* or *chakras.* Such words relate to various cultural paradigms, such as Western physics and neuroscience (atoms make up all matter), Eastern medicine (meridians are used in acupuncture, which encourages the flow of chi or vital energy in the body), or certain religious and spiritual traditions (chakras are considered energy centers in many cultures' view of the body). Discussing these terms expands the perspective of how a "body" may be conceptualized cross-culturally, while bringing awareness to the fact that *all our perceptions are culturally influenced.* This important concept will be explored further throughout the curriculum.

While you may be surprised to discover that students include such nonmedical concepts, many students have been exposed to various body paradigms in one way or another. For instance, one student who drew meridians had a relative who was an acupuncturist, while another who drew the body as atoms was studying physics. Another student drew lines of chi that they had learned about by practicing aikido after school, while another who drew the image of a halo at the top of the head (or crown chakra) based it on a religious drawing seen in church. Encouraging students' own perspectives to come forth is an essential aspect of this experiential study.

You can also choose to introduce specific alternative cultural paradigms for viewing the body, even if the group has not mentioned them, to begin a discussion about cultural perception.

The concept of chi for instance, is a particularly relevant topic to discuss. This energy flow—called *chi* or *qi* by the Chinese—is understood in various cultures and is drawn upon in healing practices, such as acupuncture, as well as in certain forms of dance and martial arts. Concepts similar to *chi* found in other cultures include *prana* in the Hindu religion of India, *mana* in Hawaiian culture, *lung* in Tibetan Buddhism, and *vital energy* in Western philosophy. Although an in-depth study of chi is not necessarily part of this curriculum, learning to shift your movement or encouraging new movement patterns is not an unrelated phenomenon. This can be explained scientifically, related to activation of the neuromuscular system as explored in the principles of Ideokinesis, or can likewise be related to the concept of chi or vital energy.

To study this in more depth, students can engage in movement practices that focus specifically on the movement of chi, such as t'ai chi, qi gong, or aikido. Engaging in such practices—or as a start even discussing them—can expand students' perceptions of their moving bodies, while inviting greater cultural sensitivity. Students can also explore specific paradigms for viewing the body through corresponding units in other courses or through student-designed projects—giving them an avenue to satisfy their own curiosity.

Exploration: Body Systems and Perception

(45–60 minutes)

PURPOSE. To discover what you know or imagine about your internal body; to enhance awareness of all your body systems; to define the body systems; to recognize both objective and subjective experience and learn to distinguish between the two; to validate the inclusion of subjective experience related to a study of the body; to enhance awareness of various cultural paradigms of the body.

Activity

MATERIALS

- Individual sheets of paper
- Drawing supplies, such as crayons, colored pencils, or pastels

Begin the first part of the activity in Constructive Rest.

- ❍ As you are lying down, begin to feel your weight on the floor. Relax and let yourself be supported by the earth. Take a few deep breaths, in and out. Bring your awareness to the parts of your body that are touching the floor. How heavy are they? Where do you feel your weight the most?
- ❍ Then begin to bring your awareness to the outermost layer of your body: your skin.... What is the temperature of the floor against your skin? Or the temperature of the air around your body on the parts that are not touching the floor? Can you feel the texture of your clothes on your body? Your hair against your neck or face?
- ❍ Now use your mind's eye to go even deeper, below the layer of your skin. Use your mind's eye to look within your body. What is inside your body? What can you imagine, what do you feel, what do you experience, what can you see?... Take some time and look around; notice what you feel or imagine. *(Leave a few minutes of silence for this.)*
- ❍ What do you know about what is inside your body? What can you feel? What can you see? What is a *mystery*? *(Leave a few minutes of silence again.)*
- ❍ Now take a last moment on your own.... Is there anywhere you forgot to look? That you cannot feel? *(Silence again.)*
- ❍ Now bring your awareness back to the layer of your skin. Feel your clothes against your skin, the temperature of the floor, of the air around you. Take a few breaths, in and out. Notice your weight on the floor.
- ❍ Take a moment to move or stretch in any way you like. You can stretch your arms or legs, or roll to your side.

- Roll to either side and rest there for a moment. Then you can use your arms to push yourself back up to sitting. Take a walk around the room when you are ready. Notice how you feel.

Set up space for drawing.

- Take a few moments to draw whatever you like from this experience. What did you see inside? What drew your attention? What did you feel like? You can draw anything that helps you to express something about your experience.

After completing their drawings, students can share them with a partner, or form small groups to discuss them before gathering back together for the full group discussion.

Discussion

As students discuss their experiences as a group, make a list of all the words they mention in their comments, using the scribe method; for this exploration it is best to write the words haphazardly rather than in any particular list or order. Then you can begin to group these words together. Begin by circling one of the elements from a system in a particular color, such as the word *bone*.

- What system is that a part of? *(Once you have found all of the words that relate to one system, write the name of that system in the same color. For example, with the skeletal system, write the words* skeletal system *in the same color as the word* bone. *Students can then circle the words that relate to that system using the same color such as* ribs, vertebrae, *and* scapula. *Then use another color to circle words of a different system—for example,* heart, veins, arteries, *as part of the circulatory system—and again write the name of that system in the new color. Alternately, you can use different shapes to highlight words related to each system, such as using a circle for the skeletal system words, a rectangle for words related to the digestive system, and so on.) (Fig. 8.3b.)*
- What other systems are there ... have we missed any of them? *(Add any systems that the students have missed on their own. Define these systems as the Western model of anatomy, which divides the body into twelve different major body systems.)*
- Depending upon the level of the group and context of the class, you may also add: *What are the functions of each of these systems?* (Discuss ways in which these systems function interdependently in our bodies.)

Other words listed may be more subjective; you can focus on these when they are noticed by the group, or choose to highlight these first or last. Here is an example of how this might be facilitated:

- What about these words you mentioned, like *gushy*, *tight*, *grounded*, or *bright*? *(Circle these in another color.)* Would someone who offered one of these words like to tell us why you said that? What was your experience? *(You can do this for a few of the words.)*

This can initiate a discussion of subjective experience. As part of this discussion, you can work with the group to define the term *subjective* and distinguish it from *objective*. Objective information relates to measurable facts, while subjective information is based on experience that varies from person to person based on one's own perception. You can also use dictionary definitions, by providing them or having students research this on their own.

Emphasize that this exploration of our bodies will include both one's own experience as well as factual information about our bodies as *equally valid methods of research and learning*.

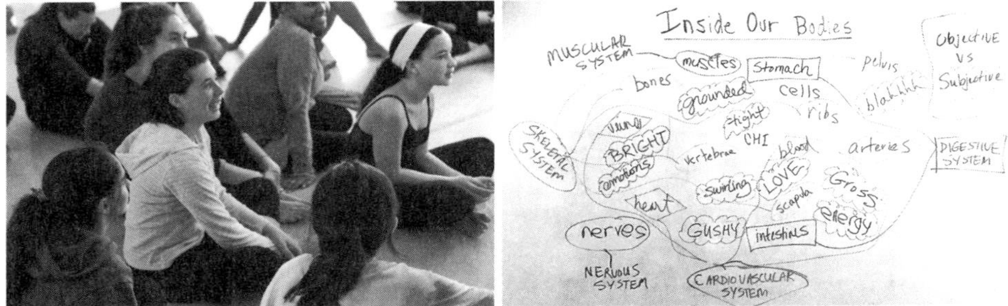

Fig. 8.3a, b. The whiteboard shows words students shared during the discussion section of Body Systems and Perception. By using various shapes and colors, they can group words into body systems and also add a category for their more subjective perceptions; students engage when given time to share their perspectives and hear from each other.

Tips for Teachers

- To determine how long students may need for a certain part of this visualization activity when lying in Constructive Rest, you can say, "When you've had enough time, wiggle your fingers (or toes) so I know you are ready to move on." This also gives you a measure of who is paying attention, or who may have fallen asleep. In that case, you can gently speak to or tap a person who may be asleep to invite them back into the activity.

- You can also use this activity as an opportunity to discuss different approaches to studying the body—such as allopathic or homeopathic medicine, physical therapy, sports medicine, and so on—which each have different purposes. If you haven't already done so, introduce the term *soma*—the lived body as a holistic process and experience—as opposed to the purely physical body, in discussing these varying approaches. Depending on the context of the class, this can also initiate a discussion of the terms *somatics* and *somatic movement education*, which can include definitions of these words along with some introductory historical background on these fields. This helps students to orient to the approach they are involved in, as well as to learn about the extensive lineage of the field.

HOME PROJECTS

- Students can color *The Anatomy Coloring Book* plates associated with the body systems, starting with the one that provides an overview of each of the twelve systems. They can also do further scientific research on specific body systems, or of various cultural paradigms for viewing the body.

Below are sample student drawings. When they draw about their experiences, a wide range of responses emerges. Some students picture themselves resting in nature—even though no reference is made in the exploration itself, other than to suggest they rest on the earth. Such relaxation seems to conjure up past memories of enjoyable and peaceful images (such as water and flowers), sounds (such as birds singing), or sensations (such as walking in cool grass or lying in the warm sun). *(Fig. 8.4a, b.)*

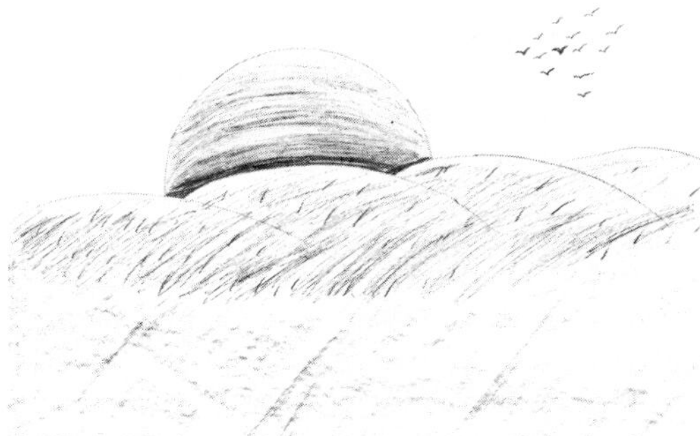

I felt strong, I felt smooth
I could sway in the wind
While my mind went blank
I felt the water raise against
my back while my feet were
soothed dry grass in the mountains.
The sun drying me off while I can
hear the birds singing acres away
from me.
I am relaxed
I am strong
I am smooth

Fig. 8.4a. Student drawing done in the Body Systems and Perception exploration, along with a brief journal entry written about the drawing. *(Cristiano, age seventeen)*

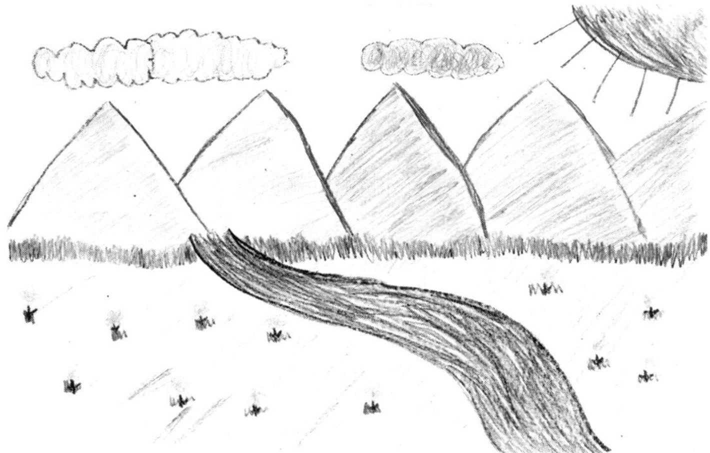

Fig. 8.4b. "This is about a place that I felt a lot of peace in. There is water flowing because I had alot of thoughts flowing and going through my mind. I just felt warm and happy so I drew the sun and the flowers. I felt like peaceful like I was in a place alone and felt very relaxed." *(Giuliana, age fifteen)*

Other students may reference particular organs, like the heart, or sensations like feeling their blood moving through their veins *(Fig. 8.4c)*. Still others become more contemplative, and reflect on the miracle of the human body or the feeling of being part of something larger than themselves through the experience in the class *(Fig. 8.4d, e)*.

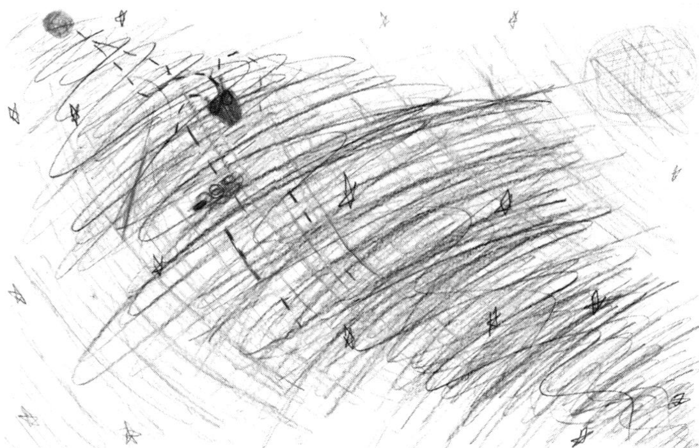

Fig. 8.4c. "The blue is calming + relaxation. The yellow is the sunny, warm, happy feeling. The stars are because I get dizzy and because it was relaxing like sleeping at night. The other shapes are the organs in my body that I thought about and the blood rushing through me. I also included surfaces of my arms and legs and neck because I thought about that too." *(Cally, age eighteen)*

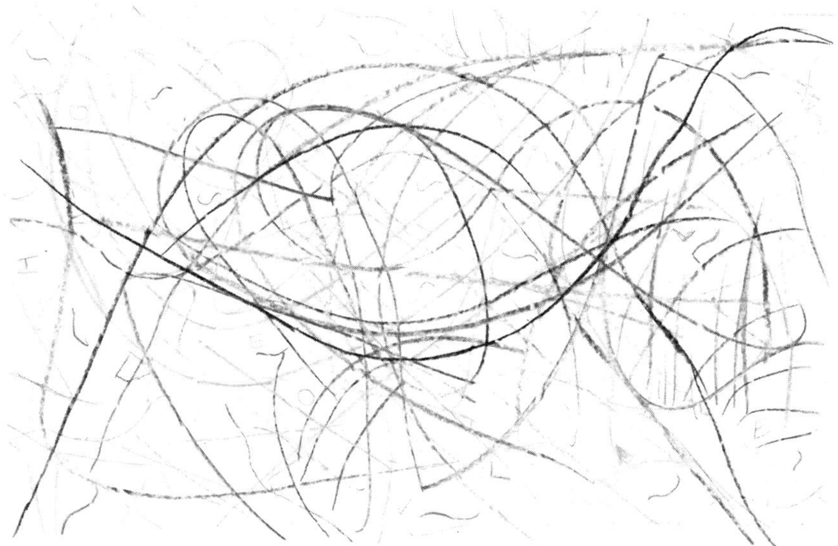

Fig. 8.4d. "The purpose of my drawing was to explain the human body through analogy. You see different colors and shapes separately, and their beauty. You also witness how they come together to become something whole. Which is how I think we can view our bodies. All the different parts are unique and beautiful, but they come together to make something more beautiful: us." *(Cameron, age fourteen)*

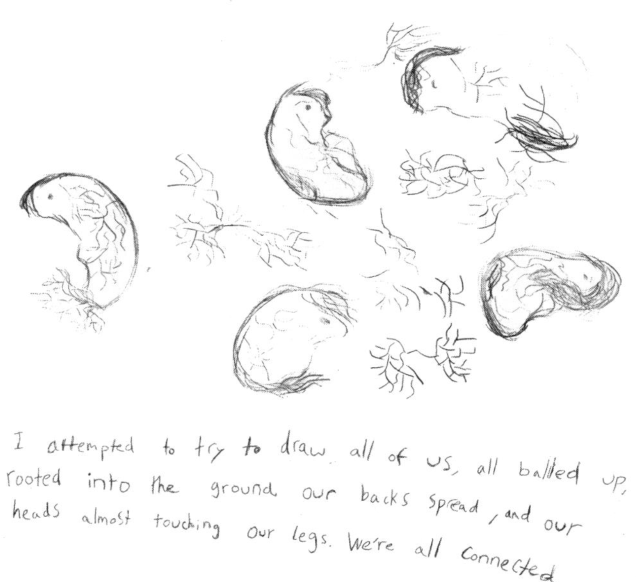

Fig. 8.4e. "I attempted to try to draw all of us, all balled up, rooted into the ground. Our backs spread, and our heads almost touching our legs. We're all connected." (*Jonathan, age sixteen*)

Movement Integration and Dedications

Now that students have some experience with basic mindfulness and embodiment techniques, they can begin to apply these to more full-bodied movement sequences through what I call integrative movement phrases. These phrases can be added to the movement matrix, and may be drawn from yoga, martial arts, or specific somatic practices like the Bartenieff Fundamentals, depending upon your own background. Such movement activities provide a means for students to practice and integrate their embodied learning as various body systems are explored throughout the curriculum.

One phrase I like to use for this purpose is called The Sun Salutation, also known as *Surya Namaskar,* which is a yoga exercise from India that is traditionally done outdoors in the morning *(see Fig. 8.5)*. Yoga is a Sanskrit word that means "union," "gathering," or "bringing together." In this broader sense, yoga relates to our inner awareness and how we conduct ourselves, and goes far beyond stretching or holding poses, as will be discussed further in the upcoming section on dedications.

For the purpose of this curriculum, repeating the Sun Salutation sequence several times in consecutive classes can help students integrate their newfound somatic awareness. For instance, when studying the skeletal system, they can do the phrase with a focus on supporting weight through the bones and joints; when studying alignment you may add a focus on alignment of the head, spine, and pelvis; further topics can include coordinating the flow of movement and the breath, or on lengthening the muscles, or on supporting the movements from the organs, or on feeling the flow of energy created by the series of movements. You can integrate these various aspects cumulatively as each topic is explored in the curriculum. As students become familiar with the phrase and their movements become more integrated, you can also focus on doing the phrase progressively faster to increase cardiovascular activity, which is traditionally one of the goals of this sequence.

Students can also do the Sun Salutation phrase as one of the check-in activities at the beginning and again at the end of a class, or it can serve as a structured movement sequence later in the warm-up formula described in chapter 16. When they do it as a check-in activity, students can see how it feels to do a simple yoga phrase before and after the explorations to measure changes in aspects like their breathing, focus, and flexibility. It can also be done as one of the structured sequences with a focus on establishing core connection and full body integration, as also discussed in chapter 16.

Dedications

The Sun Salutation can be seen as a warm-up, a stretch, an offering, and a prayer. Within the culture of India in which yoga developed, prayer and warm-up are not mutually exclusive—with the Sun Salutation phrase seen as a gathering inward and extending outward of energy, whether of the sun, of one's inner source of energy, or of a sense of the spirit. Any movement can become a "prayer"—a living affirmation of life and our connection to the world—but the Sun Salutation has a particularly long history of being applied in this way. Simply discussing these perceptions can broaden students' experience of this movement and their perception of movement in general.

As an alternative to the concept of prayer, the phrase can be used as a dedication, with students dedicating their practice to whatever person or situation they may choose. Dedications may be distinctly personal (the successful completion of an academic project, or doing well in an upcoming play or musical performance), or more community-oriented (the well-being of your family), or even global (such as dedicating to the benefit of a community which has recently experienced a natural disaster). Teenagers are generally very enthusiastic about these dedications. They especially appreciate this as a chance to dedicate their movement to a person in need, such as an ill relative or pet, which gives them a sense of agency and helps to ease their anxiety. Students also may choose to dedicate their practice to a friend or family member who has recently died. Students can share their dedications with the group or keep them to themselves.

Dedications can also be done as a group, with students choosing a single purpose for their movement on a given day. This has been especially helpful when they are upset about a particular issue of local or global concern, such as a fire in the community or a natural disaster in the news. Dedications enhance your feeling of movement as an "offering" and strengthen the bond you feel with others—as you move in service of yourself as well as of the larger community.

Exploration: Integration—Sun Salutation

(10–30 minutes; time can vary with purpose)

PURPOSE. To provide a structured movement phrase that can be repeated throughout the class with a variety of focuses; to integrate all of the body systems; to experience movement as a flow of energy as well as a series of positions; to gain a physical experience of yoga related to embodied anatomy; to consider and experience movement as an offering or a dedication.

Activity

The first time you present this activity, give a brief introduction to the origin and purpose of the Sun Salutation. Begin by pooling students' own knowledge, either of this particular yoga phrase, or of yoga in general, and then adding any relevant information, such as the cultural context, the definition and roots of the word itself, along with basic principles of yoga that are familiar to you.

- Have any of you done yoga before? What is yoga? Does anyone know what the word means, or where it is from? What contexts have you done yoga in before? What was your experience like?

Introduce this movement phrase with minimal verbal instructions at first, so students can just get an initial experience of the movement patterns as they follow along with you. You can incorporate instructions in the following text as appropriate.

- *(See Fig.8.5, drawing a.)* Stand with your feet slightly apart. Close your eyes. Take a moment to feel your feet on the earth, to feel the texture of the floor against your feet, to feel the weight of your body through your feet supported by the earth.
- Now place the palms of your hands together. Feel the heat from one hand to the other, the light touch of your skin, the connection from one hand to the other in a circle around your arms and torso.
- Now feel the soles of your feet against the earth and the palms of your hands together. Take a breath in ... and out. Feel the length through your spine as your energy spirals up from the earth to the sky while you feel your weight spirals down to the earth.
- (b) Inhale, reach your arms up above your head. Feel the stretch all the way from your feet to the tips of your fingers. *(Watch that the pelvis is not pushed forward, as this strains the lower back. Remind students to keep the pelvis centered over the feet.)*
- (c) Exhale, reach forward from the top of your head and forward through your fingertips. Let your head hang over, releasing the muscles of your neck. Bend your knees slightly if you feel any pain in your joints.
- (d) Inhale, place your hands on the floor and reach back with your left leg. Place your knee on the ground and curl your toes under. Keep your hips parallel and lift through the length of your spine. Relax your shoulders down; open through the front and back of your torso. Keep your spine and head in alignment as you look forward by lengthening the back of your neck.
- (e) Exhale, lift up from your sitz bones, bringing your right foot back beside the left foot, feet slightly apart and parallel. Extend your sitz bones toward the ceiling to lengthen your spine. Keep your knees straight and reach your heels toward the floor. Press your hands into the floor and press up and out of your shoulders, lifting your sternum towards your belly.
- (f) Breathe out, drop your knees to the floor, then lower your chest to the floor between your hands.

- ❍ (g) Inhale, straighten your arms, and reach forward and out through the top of your head; lift through your spine and relax your shoulders down.
- ❍ (h) Exhale, lift your sitz bones toward the ceiling to extend your spine, and press through your hands.
- ❍ (i) Inhale, place your hands on the floor and step forward with your left leg, and reach back with your right leg.
- ❍ (j) Exhale, bring your right foot forward beside your left foot, and reach your sitz bones toward the ceiling. Let your head hang over.
- ❍ (k) Inhale, reach out through the top of your head to lengthen through your spine, reach your hands forward and up until you are back to standing; keep reaching your arms up and over your head.
- ❍ (l) Exhale, lower your arms, and bring your hands together. Soften your focus with your eyes and draw your attention inward. Notice the sensations taking place within your body. Bring your awareness to your palms touching, feel the feet on the floor, the length of the spine. Inhale ... exhale.

Repeat this full phrase a few times.

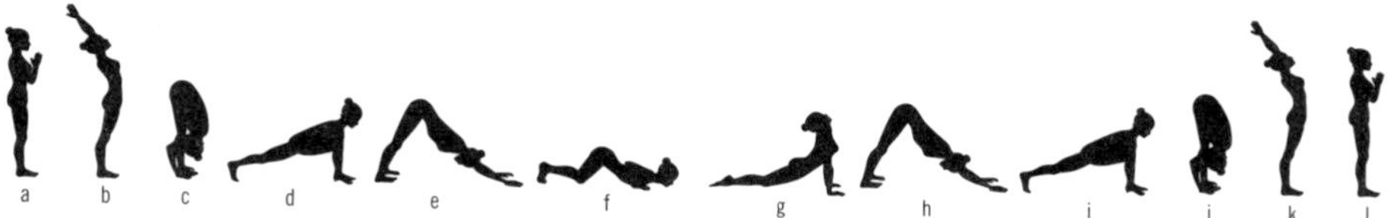

Fig. 8.5. Movement sequence associated with the Sun Salutation phrase.

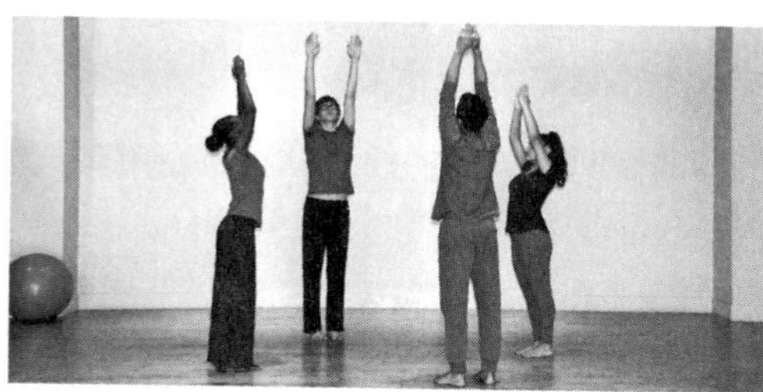

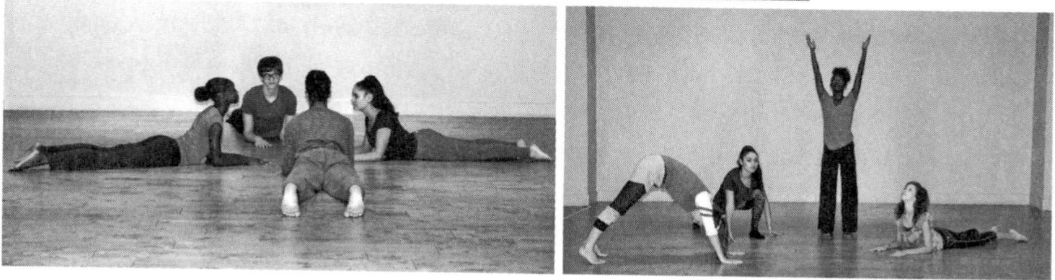

Fig. 8.6a, b, c. Teens engage in the Sun Salutation, first learning it together in unison (a and b), and then practicing it together by each following their own timing (c).

Variations

Body Systems: Repeat this phrase with a focus on specific body systems, such as feeling the support of the bones, the length of the fascia, or the full-bodied presence of the organs; you can integrate this into the curriculum cumulatively as each topic is explored (see the corresponding chapters for more detail).

Dedications: Repeat this phrase as a dedication, by first asking students to close their eyes, and imagine someone or something they would like to dedicate their practice to, such as a specific person, pet, or situation. Students can also decide on a group dedication, and all engage in the movement for a shared purpose. You can lead this in a way that feels comfortable to you. Here are a few examples that you might draw upon:

- *(With students standing and ready to begin the phrase)* Now let's take a moment and close our eyes. Before you begin, I'm going to invite you to dedicate your movement today to anything you would like to dedicate it to. All of your participation—in this and in any activity—takes your effort, your willingness to participate, and your focused intention. We can dedicate all that effort toward anything we like.
- What would you like to dedicate your movement practice to today? You can dedicate it to yourself, to do well in your test or an upcoming sports game, or to cultivating a quality you would like to have, like more patience or determination. Or maybe you want to dedicate it to another person, like a friend or family member who needs some support, or even to your favorite pet. You can even dedicate your efforts to a global situation, like a struggling community you've seen in the news recently, or toward an ideal you'd like to see achieved, like a clean planet or world peace.
- Just see what comes to you today, and take a moment to dedicate your practice if you like right now. *(Pause.)*

Or on another day you might suggest students choose a group dedication:

- Let's close [or begin] today by doing the Sun Salutation again. But this time, instead of doing our individual dedications, maybe we can check in together and see if there's something you'd like to dedicate it to together. Does anyone have any ideas?

There are many ways to do this, depending on how extensively you want to focus on this dedication process: students can share ideas in a full group, or you can take a moment to let them talk in small groups and come up with ideas; or students can pool their ideas and write them on a paper or whiteboard, choosing one and saving the rest for next time.

Or, if there is an issue you think is upsetting students, like a recent flood or other natural disaster in the community, you might propose an idea yourself, suggesting they dedicate it to those who have suffered in that situation.

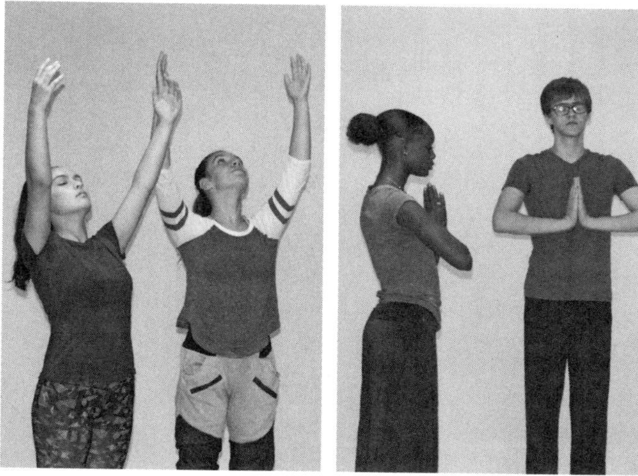

Fig. 8.7a, b. Teenagers practicing Sun Salutation as a dedication, by first identifying a particular purpose to which they would like to offer their movement practice and dedicate their efforts.

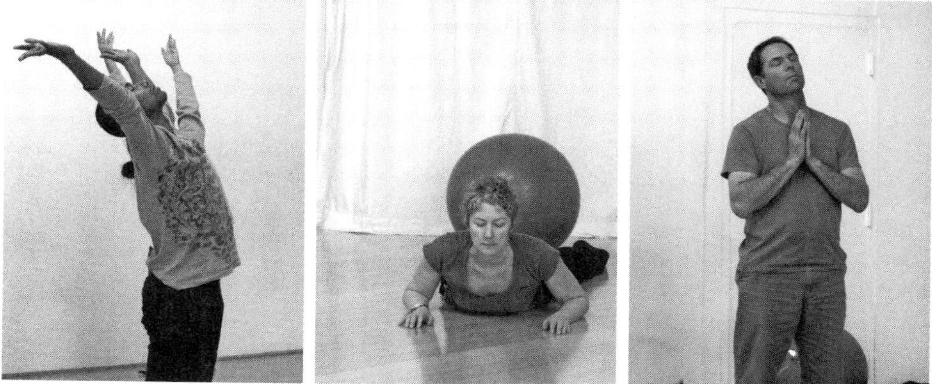

Fig. 8.8a, b, c. Adults practicing the Sun Salutation as a dedication; dedications can be deeply personal or done as a group for a common purpose.

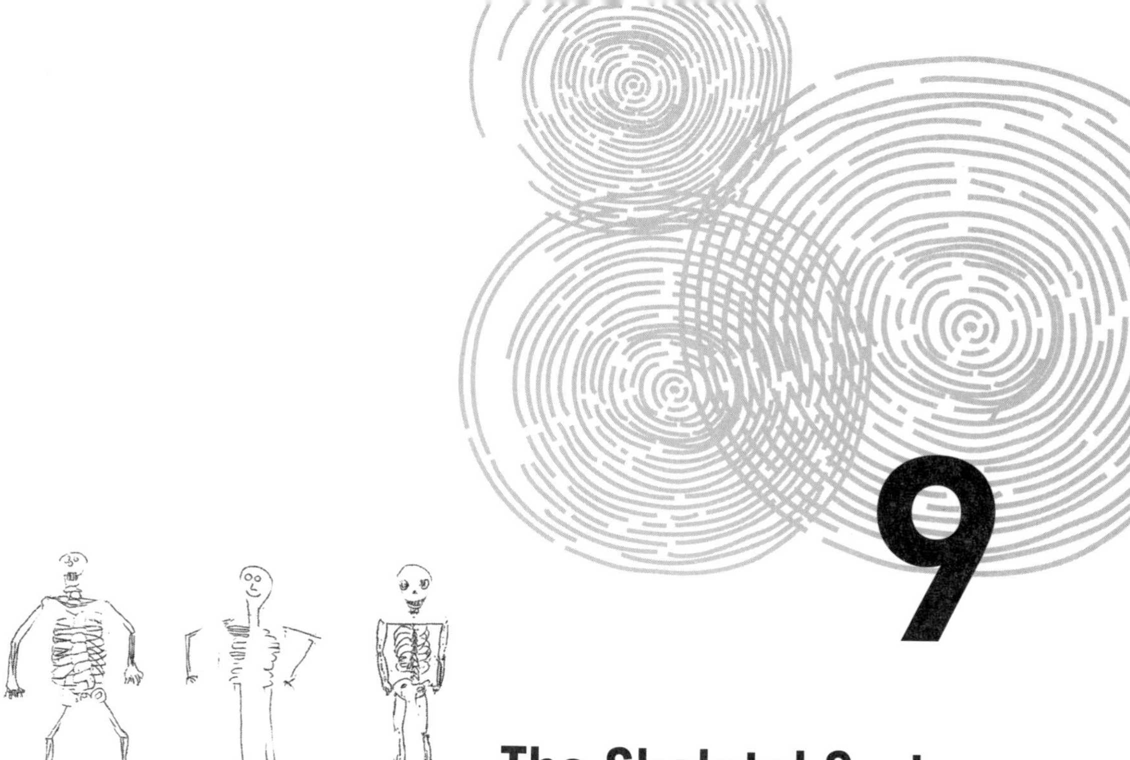

9

The Skeletal System

To begin studying and embodying the various body systems, we begin with the bones. The skeletal system is often the most familiar and accessible of the body systems for students, primarily because of the physical concreteness of the bones. Students can also usually visualize at least some version of the skeleton, as we often see it as an image throughout our culture, such as at Halloween or at the doctor's office. To introduce the study of the skeletal system, students visualize and then draw their skeletal structure. Their drawings help them recognize what they *know,* or *may not know,* about their bodies' structures. From drawing the skeleton, they often become motivated to understand the workings of their bodies—as they begin to realize how much there is to know.

Perceptions of the Skeleton

After completing their drawings, students reflect on them, first personally and then as a group. Students often find it fascinating to compare their perceptions, as Anna mentioned in her journal entry for that class:

> *I love that drawing is part of this class. As an artist, I think about things visually, so I liked doing the skeleton drawing. It is also interesting to see what the rest of the class drew. Some skeletons were too large for the page, some too small, some*

disproportioned, but overall everyone had the same general idea of a skeleton from our common knowledge of what we look like and pictures we have seen.

Students also often realize it is not so easy to visualize your own skeleton, nor to draw it, as expressed in this journal entry by another student:

> *As we put on our "x-ray glasses" to look at our own skeletal system, I had a hard time imagining the bones in my own body. I found myself picturing some other naked skeleton out there somewhere. And, of course, what I could picture was probably not even that correct. I would really like to get a better body-mind awareness of my body that is grounded in fact.*

Amazingly, here is the journal entry written by this same student just one month later: "I've been finding it much easier to imagine my body within than when we first started. It's real: my skeleton, muscles, and organs are unique and actually exist inside of me." Many students similarly find that it takes some time to make the tangible connection from picturing an outside skeleton to visualizing and feeling their *own* bodies.

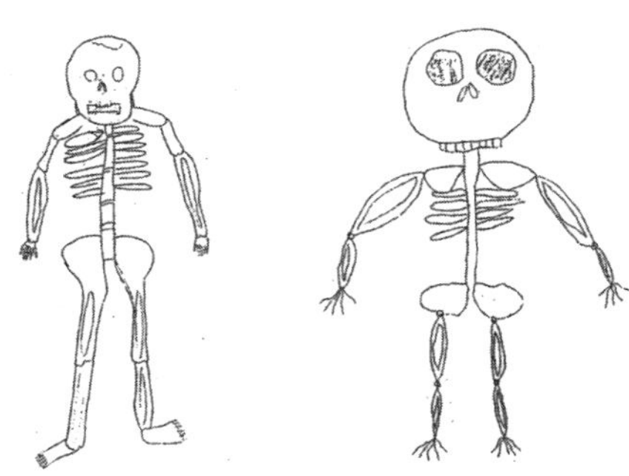

Fig. 9.1a, b.

For the facilitator and the student alike, drawings provide valuable information about a person's perceptions of the body in general and of his or her body specifically. Often correlations between a student's body and his or her drawing become evident. For instance, a student who has tense shoulders that stay hunched up may draw the head without a neck; another who is short and has wide hips may draw a short skeleton with a pelvis wider than the shoulders *(Fig. 9.1a, b)*.

Drawings may also correspond to particular physical or emotional challenges. For example, the boy who draws a tiny skeleton in a bottom corner of the page is the tall and lanky adolescent who has sprung up to six feet before his friends have; the girl who draws a skeleton without feet, we later learn, has sprained both ankles several times *(Fig. 9.2a, b)*.

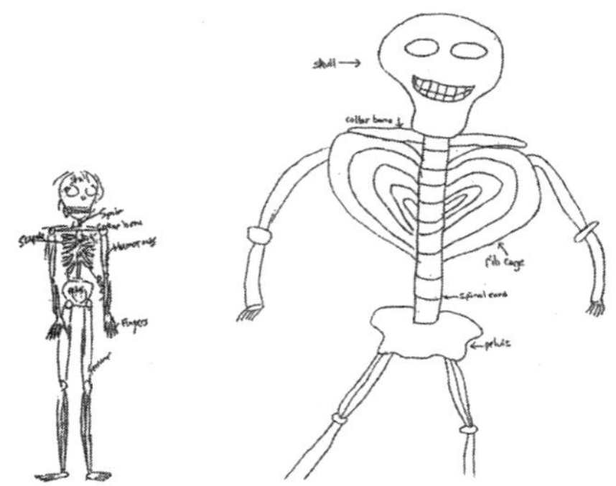

Fig. 9.2a, b.

And another student, who was missing a limb on the left side, had this to say in her journal about her own drawing:

One relationship between my skeletal portrait and me is that I didn't draw the left side. I think, unconsciously, I feel normal like everyone else but different at the same time. So, I drew a normal skeleton without a left side (still normal to me!).

The images we hold, whether we are conscious of them or not, affect our posture, our movement, and our perceptions of ourselves. These perceptions are often revealed in students' drawings.

Drawings may also reveal general misperceptions about the structure of the body. For instance, many students draw the arms as connecting directly into the rib cage, and may not include the shoulder girdle of the clavicles and scapulae at all in their drawings. Others draw just a single bone in both the upper and lower leg, though the upper leg has one bone (the femur) and the lower leg has two bones (the tibia and fibula). In another example, most students imagine their legs to project straight up into their hip sockets, such that they draw the femur (thigh bone) inserting up at a straight angle into the hip socket or acetabulum *(Fig. 9.3a, see also 9.1 and 9.2)*, when actually the femur bone angles slightly out and the head of the femur (the top portion) angles inward, creating more of a sturdy triangle of support *(Fig. 9.3b)*.

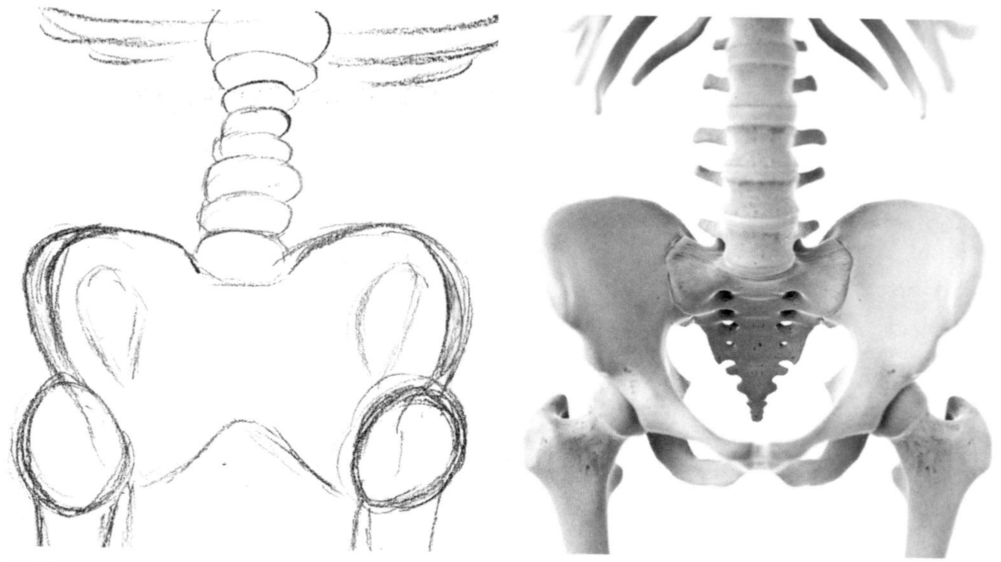

Fig. 9.3a, b. Student drawings often reveal their misperceptions, such as about the angle of the femur, or the opening of the pelvis, both shown here.

Why do youth have such misperceptions of their bodies? We tend to use generalized words, such as "shoulder," "legs," and "hips" for these parts of the body, with little education as to the complex physical structures to which those terms actually refer. This initiates a perception of certain parts of the body as one stationary "block," instead of an interface of bones and joints with intricate mobility. These misperceptions inevitably affect students' bodies and their movement—often limiting their full range of motion. As students reflect on their own drawings and share them with their peers, they become more conscious of the way they perceive various parts of the body. These realizations have many practical, physical benefits. As they learn to visualize their bodies more accurately, they can move with more clarity and ease. Students begin to discover that their perceptions shape how they experience their own bodies and how they move.

As students recognize that we all share this same common structure of the skeletal system, they also gain insight into our collectively shared humanity. This insight develops a core level of comfort, self-respect, and compassion for themselves and others. One tenth-grade girl named Jeanne wrote: "The fact that I have a complete skeleton amazes me, as I think that everyone has the same structure as me, that we all have something in common!" The impact of such profound realizations should not be underestimated. Reflecting that we all "have something in common," such as our skeletal system, we gain a level of respect for all other human beings. These profound insights can help teens to gain compassion for their peers—learning to look beyond their preconceived ideas and to treat each other with more kindness, despite perceived differences. Such a deepened awareness of our common humanity allows them to look beyond their conditioned responses, prejudices, and assumptions. Imagine the level of kindness and wisdom that would emerge if we could all hold this deeper perspective?

When studying the body so personally, students also inevitably discuss the topic of their own mortality—especially when focused on the skeletal system, which often serves as a symbol of a dead body. As His Holiness the Dalai Lama has reflected, "We all have the same body, the same human flesh, and therefore we will all die." Regardless of our religious or spiritual beliefs, by reflecting upon death we can deepen our appreciation of the sacredness of this life—both our own and that of all other living beings. When personalized through such experiential learning, this perspective can begin to permeate students' interpersonal and intrapersonal relationships and positively impact all aspects of their lives.

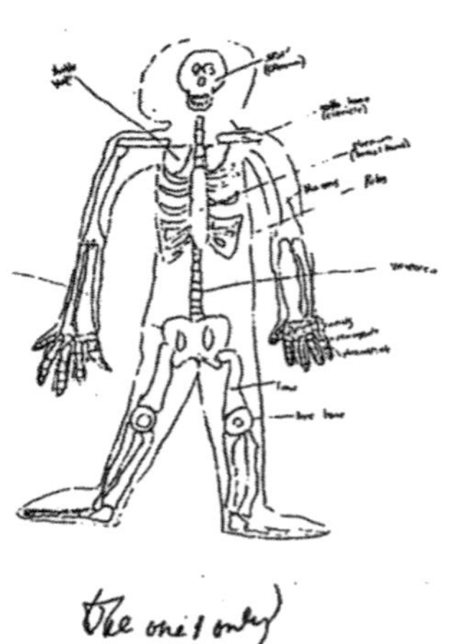

At the same time that students recognize their commonalities, they also begin to appreciate their *individual uniqueness* as well. This was duly noted, for instance, by one eighth-grade boy who boldly wrote the phrase "The one and only!" prominently under his skeletal drawing. And of course, he is correct! For while we all share a common structure, each of our skeletons is also unique—as our bones develop and change over our lifetimes in response to many factors such as heredity, as well as how we live and move. This understanding can lead to increased self-esteem, as students appreciate their own individuality. The discussions led after the drawings allow time for such student insights, as well as for sharing and processing their perceptions as a group.

Exploration: Visualizing and Drawing the Skeleton

(45–60 minutes)

PURPOSE. To give form to the image in your mind of your skeleton; to increase awareness of known and unknown areas of your skeleton; to discover what you know or imagine about your skeleton, including both size and shape of bones and joint structures; to discover how you imagine specific body parts to be connected to each other; to collectively share our perceptions.

Activity

MATERIALS

- Large newsprint paper
- Pencils with erasers

The following directions assume previous experience with both body scanning and Constructive Rest, as described in chapter 7.

- ❍ Stand and notice how you feel. Close your eyes, and do your body scan in this position. Then when you've completed your body scan, you can go to the floor and settle in to Constructive Rest.
- ❍ As you lie down, feel the weight of your whole body, resting on the earth. Take a few deep breaths, in and out, and allow yourself to be supported by the floor.
- ❍ We'll be doing the body scan again in this position. But this time as you bring your awareness to each part of your body, I invite you to put on your "X-ray" glasses so you can use your mind's eye to see just the bones in your body.
- ❍ Bring your awareness first to your feet. Feel the bones of your feet resting on the earth. How heavy are they? What bones are in your feet? What can you picture? What can you feel? How many of them are there? What shape do they have?
- ❍ Then bring your awareness to your ankles.... What is an "ankle"? How do your feet connect to your body? What can you see? What do you know about this place in your body?

- Now bring your awareness to your lower legs. How do your feet connect to your lower legs? What bones are in your lower legs? How many of them are there? Feel the weight of your lower legs releasing down into your ankles and feet.
- Now bring your awareness to your knees.... What is a "knee"? How do your lower legs connect to your upper legs? What can you picture? What can you feel? What is a *mystery*?
- Feel the bones of your thighs. What can you picture; what can you feel? Feel the weight of your upper thighs releasing down into your hips. What is a "hip"? How do your legs connect to the rest of your body?
- Bring your awareness to your lower torso, your pelvis. What is a "pelvis"? What bones are in this area? What can you picture, what can you feel? How heavy is this area on the floor? How does your lower torso connect to your upper torso?

Progress up through the body in this same manner, in other words by first asking that students bring awareness to the new area, then that they feel their weight and aspire to release it into gravity, and then that they visualize the bones in that part of the body. Also invite them to inquire into colloquial expressions related to anatomy. Particular words to point out and ask "What is a ___?" include ones that indicate a complex joint or bone structure with several parts that are commonly given a single name, such as hip, neck, shoulder, or elbow. Continue all the way to the skull, and then end with sensing the full skeletal structure.

- Now feel your whole skeleton resting on the earth and being supported by the earth. *(Pause for a few moments.)* Take a deep breath, in and out. Now let's do that again, this time letting out any sigh or sound on your exhale. Ready, breathe in, and out.
- Take a moment to roll to one side, and rest there for a moment. *(Pause.)* Keeping your eyes closed, use the bones of your arms to support your weight as you push yourself up to sitting. *(Pause.)*
- Take your time to bring yourself back up to standing, still keeping your eyes closed. When you come to standing, take a few moments to do your body scan again, and just notice what you feel. Does this feel the same as or different from when you stood at the beginning before lying down?
- Now take a moment to walk around, or move in any way you would like. How does this feel?

You can progress to the drawings from here, or gather in a circle first to briefly share a few perceptions of this experience as a group.

- How do you feel? What did you experience when doing your body scan at the end? *(Often students will notice a wide variety of changes, from feeling more grounded and heavy to feeling taller and lighter. Allow for this variety by taking the time to hear from several students, and then eventually asking the following question.)* Did anyone have a different experience?

Move on to doing drawings.

❍ Now I'm going to invite you to draw the skeletal system. Include as much detail as you can. Draw the skeleton from a front view. When you are done, also draw a side view of just the head and spine. *(Students can draw the head and spine on the other side of the paper and use this drawing in a subsequent exploration; alternatively, students can do this second drawing on another day, when they repeat this activity.)*

After students have completed their drawings, they can work in pairs or small groups to share their drawings, or proceed straight to the museum observation circle.

Museum: Students can put all the drawings in a circle, with the heads placed toward the center, and walk around the outside perimeter of the circle to look at each other's drawings, observing their collective understandings and perceptions. Then proceed to the discussion, with students referring to their own drawing.

Discussion

- Could you picture your skeleton inside your body? What was easiest to see? What was more difficult? Why do you think that was? Were some areas easier to visualize? Were the same areas that were easy to visualize also easier to draw? Were some areas harder to visualize? Were the places that were more difficult to picture also harder to draw?
- Look at your drawing. What do you notice most about it, what do you see? What did you learn from doing your drawing? Were there some areas of your skeleton you knew more about than other areas?
- What did you notice about our collective drawings?
- Do you notice anything about your drawing that seems to relate to the structure of your own body?

In subsequent classes students can use their drawings to compare their perceptions with specific aspects of the skeletal structure they are learning about, referring to a skeletal model or anatomy plates and reflect on what they notice about their own drawings in relation to the actual structure of the skeleton.

Tips for Teachers

◆ When you ask students to draw the skeleton, students may initially feel anxious and "put on the spot" by being asked to draw, as they anticipate that they are supposed to produce a quality piece of artwork. Assure them that this process is meant to help them to get a sense of what they may know or picture about the bones of the skeletal system, rather than to judge their artistic ability. Also acknowledge that they likely have never been asked to draw a skeleton before, and so you don't expect them to know more than they already do—and neither should they! To help keep this feeling informal, you can put on some background music while they are drawing, using a few short instrumental musical selections that vary in rhythm and tone for variety, or have students provide some music of their own.

- If some students have finished their drawings before others, invite them to label their skeletal drawings using any words they know for the bones. (These words can be colloquial, such as "funny bone," or lay language, such as "hips," or can be the actual anatomical names of bones.) Once you see that any two students are finished, suggest that they sit together and share their drawings and insights. These adaptations help to keep all students engaged during the full activity time. Once all students have had time to finish drawing and share in partners, proceed to the Museum circle.

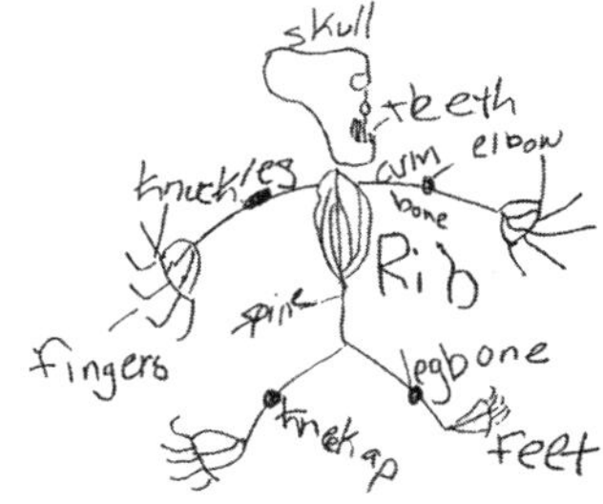

The Nature of Bone

Bone is dynamic living tissue. This concept may be foreign to students, as they often view bones as solid, dry, and unchanging. Although they generally recognize that aspects of their structure (such as their height or build) are influenced by heredity, they often believe that their skeletal systems remain the same once they reach their full height. Of all the systems, the skeletal system feels the most solid to the touch, but bone, just like other living tissue, is constantly changing. Through these explorations, students discover that their skeletal systems—like each of the body systems—evolve over time, and transform within their lifetimes.

The skeletons you see in museums and classrooms, in fact, are actually mineral salts, representing only 65 percent of the weight of the bones; this is the part that remains long after death. Living bone also consists of blood vessels and nerves in a watery base substance. In addition to producing blood cells, bones function to align and support the body as our weight is transferred to the earth; to protect the organs of the rib cage and pelvic girdle, as well as to protect the brain in the skull; to absorb shock from the impact of locomotion; and to provide a bony framework as sites of attachment for muscles, tendons, and ligaments to facilitate movement.

Bone tissue, with its hard outer layer and soft inner core, responds to the forces of gravity by building up and breaking down; the shape of our bones is affected by the forces exerted by muscles and tendons. Bones also respond to our diet, by storing or releasing calcium into the bloodstream as needed. How we live in our bodies through our habitual movement patterns, specific physical activities, diet, and emotional responses affects our structures on an ongoing basis. This information can be life-changing for students, as they realize that *the way they live and the choices they make* continuously affect their bodies—even down to their bones.

To begin to learn about bones, students first practice using touch to differentiate soft tissue from bone in their own arms. Having developed this "bone touch" skill, students then trace their own bones throughout the rest of their bodies. This gives them a way of "knowing" their bones through touch, which often leaves them feeling that the areas they touched feel more articulate and "alive." They also discover more about the anatomy and functions of bones themselves through specific movement activities and discussions. They also learn the anatomical names of their bones. When we know the name of something, we develop a greater intimacy with it. To make this point, you might ask your students to imagine how they might feel if by the second week of classes you still didn't know their names! Naming brings specificity and familiarity. As students learn to name and embody the bones, they often feel an increased sense of stability and groundedness. In their complex lives, coming back to these embodiment basics can feel relieving and simplifying.

Exploration: Bone Touch

(10–15 minutes)

PURPOSE. To clarify how to define your bones using touch; to practice bone touch; to experience the effect of bone touch on your body awareness and your movement.

Activity

This activity can be done sitting or standing.

- Take a moment to move your arms in any way you would like. Just notice how that feels. You might want to close your eyes to focus on the movement and see what you notice. OK, now just rest your arms at your sides.
- Place the palms of your hands together and close your eyes. Feel your hands touching each other.
- Bring your awareness to your skin, the skin of each hand touching the skin of the other hand.
- Bring your awareness to the layer beneath your skin, to your bones. Feel the bones of one hand touching the bones of the other hand.
- Now curl your fingers so you can place the tips of your fingers together, with your palms slightly separating. Feel the bones of the fingers of one hand touching the bones of the fingers of the other hand. *(Fig. 9.4a.)*

- Use the bones of your fingers of one hand to touch your arm. Press in slightly and gently, to feel the bones of your arm with the bones of your fingers. Where do you feel the hardness of the bones most directly? You may want to touch at your wrist or at the sides of your arm. *(Fig. 9.4b.)*
- With your palm facing up, press your fingers gently into the tissue in between the bones. Can you feel the difference between the hardness of the bones and the softness of the tissue? *(Fig. 9.4c.)*
- Now trace the full length of the bones in your arm.
- Now move the arm that you touched in any way you like. Then move the arm you didn't touch ... does it feel the same or different? You can also try this with your eyes closed. What do you experience?

Take a moment to have students share their experiences as a group; then repeat on the other arm, with both the bone touch and moving the arm.

- Come back to stillness. Close your eyes and place both hands together again. Feel the bones touching the bones, the skin touching the skin. Open your eyes when you are ready.

Discussion

- What did you experience? Could you feel the bones? What did that feel like?
- Is it different from other types of touch? How?
- How did it feel to move your arm after you had touched it with the bone touch? Was it the same as or different from your experience of moving the arm you didn't touch? What did you experience?
- What do you notice now when you move both arms? Is this the same as or different from when we did this before?

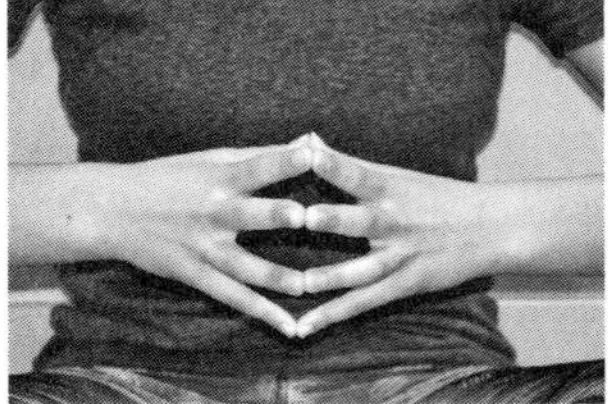
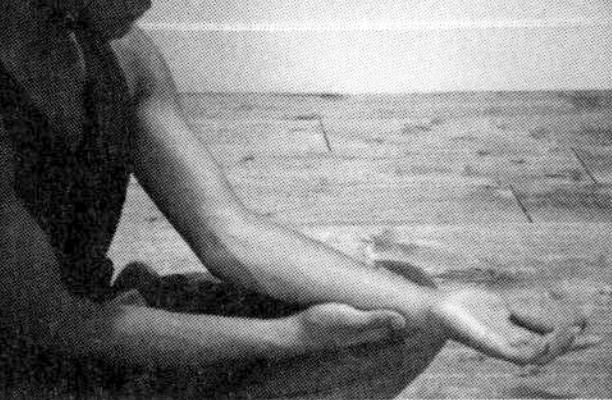
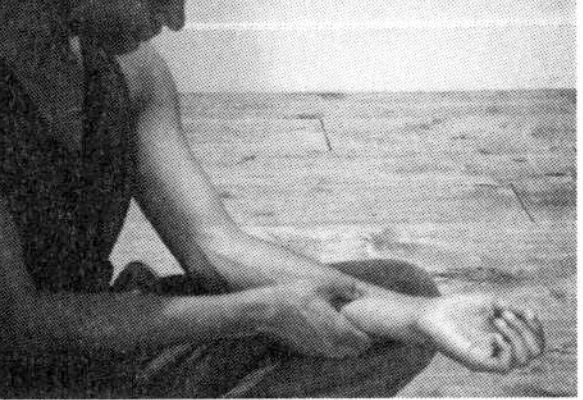

Fig. 9.4a, b, c. In the Bone Touch exploration, students first feel "bone to bone" touch through their fingers (a), then touch their own forearm to feel the difference between the hardness of the bones (b), and the softer tissue between the bones (c).

Variation: Further Discussion and Activity

To help put this activity into a context that may be more familiar to students, you can discuss associations students may have with specific qualities of touch. Here is one example of how this might be facilitated:

- What we just explored is called "bone touch," using our bones to locate and touch our bones, but there are many types of touch. For instance, now use one hand to gently squish the muscles of your other arm. *(Demonstrate this while you speak.)* What type of touch does this remind you of? *(Such kneading of the muscles is often associated with massage, which students will generally mention.)* Yes, like in massage, in this quality of touch you are engaging more of your muscles of your hand, and are touching the muscles of your arm. We might call this a more "muscular touch."

You can review three types of touch: bone to bone, muscle to muscle, or bone to muscle, and explain that they'll be using all three of these at different times in other activities as well.

Tips for Teachers

- The Bone Touch activity is an important precursor to the few other self-touch and touch-based partner exercises in the curriculum. It helps students to be specific in their manner of touch, while providing a common vocabulary to describe touch in further activities. For instance, when students do the bone tracing activity by tracing the bones of the feet later in the curriculum, they often resort to a more common "muscle touch" approach (by massaging the feet) and end up using much more pressure than is needed to trace the bones themselves. At that point, you will be able to remind them to use their "bone touch," rather than a "muscle touch" approach. You can also remind them that the point is to touch the bones rather than to massage the muscles. Differentiations between types of tissue such as bones, muscles, and fascia will also be explored further in chapter 12 on fascia.

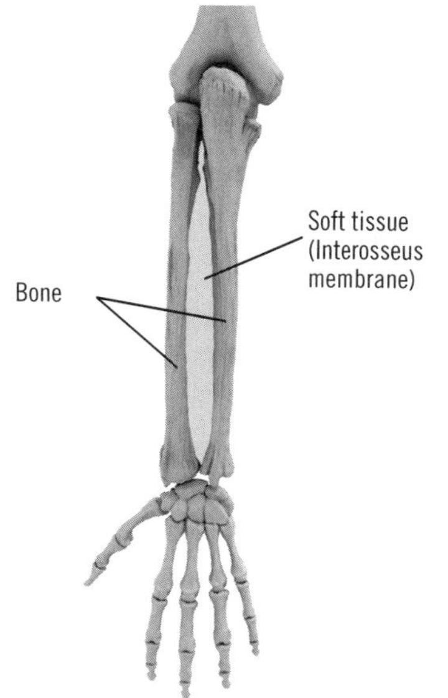

Fig. 9.5. Here the bones of the ulna and radius in the forearm are in supination; in pronation the bones cross and it is more difficult to clearly locate the bones and feel the distinction between soft tissue and bone.

Exploration: Bone Tracing

(20–30 minutes; 45–60 minutes with variations)

PURPOSE. To clarify and internalize the structure of your skeletal system; to activate physical awareness of your bones through touch; to learn about the shape of bones; to understand the relationship of bone health to your physical health and well-being; to create an experiential process to learn the names of your bones.

Activity

This activity is done first standing and then sitting in a circle.

- Take a walk around. Now stand and close your eyes. Notice how you feel, what you experience. Take a moment to do your body scan.

Then gather back in a circle, with the students sitting.

Invite students to use the bone touch when doing this activity.

Start with the feet and trace the major bones of the body: feet (tarsals, metatarsals, phalanges); lower leg (tibia, fibula); thigh (femur); pelvis (top ridges of the ilium, base or "sitz bones" of the ischium, pubic bones); spine (vertebrae); skull (cranium and facial bones); rib cage (ribs, sternum); shoulder girdle (clavicles, scapulae); upper arm (humerus); lower arm (radius, ulna); and fingers (carpals, metacarpals, phalanges). Refer to the skeleton and have students name the bones as you go. *(See Fig.9.7 as a reference.)* While not all areas are accessible through self-touch, such as the full length of the spine or the scapula, students can trace bones that are easily accessible.

Students' main focus should be on *feeling their own structures with bone touch* in a general way; further detail about the bones in each area of the body will be addressed later in the curriculum, and is not necessary to focus on here. For instance, you can have students try to name the bones during this activity, or save that for another day and just focus on them feeling the bones first. In this case, you would just use the lay words, such as "feet" or "lower legs," rather than naming specific bones.

Remind them to use their "bone touch" as they trace each area, especially if you perceive they are using more effort or force than necessary.

- Now stand to feel all your bones supporting your weight. Close your eyes. What do you notice?
- Open your eyes and walk around the room. How do you feel? What do you notice?

Discussion

- What did you feel *(in your arm, leg, and so on)*? Is this what you expected to find? How did it feel to stand after you had traced all the bones? Are there any areas you felt particularly aware of? What was new to you?
- How did you feel after doing this and walking around? What did you notice?
- What do you know about bones? What are they made of? What are some of the ways bones function in our bodies?

Discuss the structure and function of bones by first drawing upon the collective knowledge of the group, using student scribes to record their comments for the full group to see. Then add any relevant information in response to students' questions.

Functions include producing blood cells, aligning and supporting the body, transferring weight, protecting the organs, absorbing shock from the impact of locomotion, and providing a bony framework as sites of attachment for muscles, tendons, and ligaments in order to facilitate movement.

Also, relate this study of bone structure and function to general health, as discussed in the previous introductory text.

Variations

After learning about various anatomical and physiological functions of bones, students can explore these through movement improvisation. For instance, to explore skeletal support and levering, they can take weight on different parts of the body, share weight with a partner, or try a variety of balance positions to support weight through the solidity of the bones.

If you are using the Sun Salutation or some other set form of movement with your group (see chapter 8), you may guide students to move with a focus on supporting the poses through their bones. This can help to bring spatial clarity to the movements, as well as to invite an ease of movement by releasing excess muscular effort.

Tips for Teachers

- To review the names of the bones in subsequent classes, students can get into groups of three or four and be given a small skeletal model or skeletal drawing. Each person can take turns naming all the bones, with the other students helping out as needed. *(Fig.9.6.)* They can also name the bones by referring to their own bodies, though using the models provides more visual specificity. In any case, by using this fun activity you can be sure that by the end of three or four rounds, students will have learned most of the names through repetition!

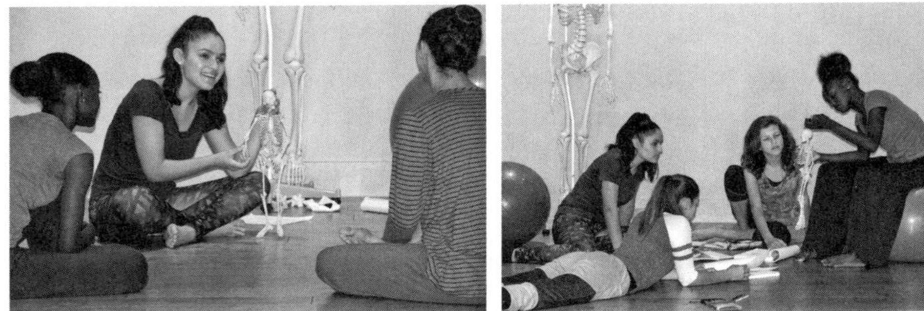

Fig. 9.6a, b. Taking turns to name all the bones of the body is a fun way to learn them through repetition. Students can be free to sit or lie in whatever way is most comfortable, and to change their positions as needed.

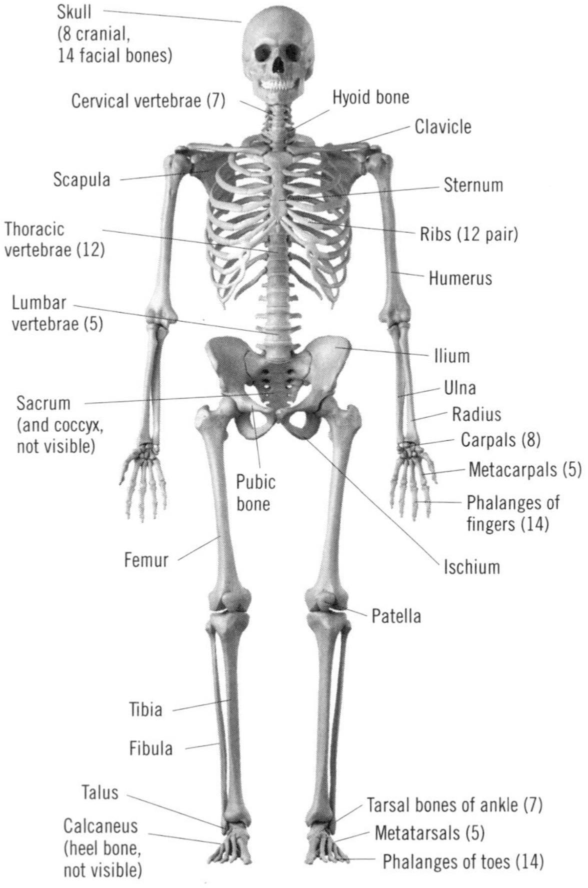

Fig. 9.7. Skeleton, anterior view with names of bones.

Bone Tracing and Movement

By clarifying the shapes of your bones through touch, you increase the proprioceptive awareness of their shapes and experience each of the bones more distinctly. As you awaken this differentiation, you also often increase the *articulation of your movement.* This can be discovered in any part of the body. One place you can experience this quite dramatically, for example, is in your feet.

Bone Tracing: The Feet

Although the arches of the feet provide necessary *stability* in the feet, the aspect of mobility is equally important. Yet many of us spend most of our waking hours with our feet confined in socks and shoes, giving us both an *image of* and a *physical sensation of* each foot as being one "solid block." But in fact there are twenty-six bones in each foot. Additionally, each foot has thirty-three joints—twenty of which are classified as actively movable—and more than one hundred muscles, tendons, and ligaments, allowing for a wide range of articulation. To learn about the bones of the feet, students are guided in touching or "tracing" them, as well as to feel the difference between the solidity of the bones and the softness of the tissue in the spaces *between* the bones. This helps them to regain the articulation of the many joints in the foot. They also gain a more accurate image of the structure of their feet, which also changes the way they use them.

For instance, students often think of their toes as beginning where the fleshy part of their foot ends, which means they are regarding their phalanges as the separate "toes," and the rest of the foot as one solid block. They are often surprised to discover that as well as having space between the phalanges of the feet, which they can visually perceive, though hidden beneath the skin there is also space between the metatarsal bones. A variation of the bone tracing exploration guides students in comparing the bones of their hands with those of their feet. This helps them to gain a more realistic understanding of the feet and to increase their mobility.

The exploration done with the feet is just one example of bone tracing in a specific area of the body that creates awareness, articulation, and increased movement potential. As students often find, tracing the bones of the feet brings a sense of groundedness and resilience, as with more articulate and adaptive feet we feel the ground beneath us more solidly. Students usually love the grounded feeling they get from tracing the bones of their feet; many of them choose to do this on their own—in the morning, before a sports game, or at night at the end of a long, active day. Bone tracing becomes another important self-care tool that students begin to integrate into their lives.

Exploration: Bone Tracing—The Feet

(20–30 minutes)

PURPOSE. To clarify and internalize the bone structure of your feet; to activate physical awareness of all the small bones of your feet through touch; to increase proprioceptive awareness and movement potential in your feet; to learn the names of the bones of your feet.

Activity

Students will need to take their socks off for this activity.

- Stand and feel your weight supporting you. Just see what you notice as you stand on the earth today.
- Now let's sit down. Today we're going to trace the bones of our feet using "bone touch." *(Here you refer to the skeletal model or students' anatomy plates of the feet. Review each of the bones, their names, and their locations in the feet.)*

Have students trace the bones of the feet as you guide the exploration verbally. You might begin with the talus and calcaneus, which are larger bones and can be easier to touch, and then move to the tarsals, metatarsals, and phalanges. Refer to the skeletal model and drawings as you go. Students' main focus should be on feeling their own structure. *(Fig. 9.8.)*

- Once you have finished, move the foot you touched. How does it feel?
- Stand again and see how that feels. Close your eyes and just notice what you become aware of. Is it similar to or different from when you were standing before? How? What do you notice? Do you notice any difference between your feet? Or between one side of your body and the other?

Take a few moments for students to share their perceptions, either in partners or as a full group. Students can then sit and repeat the bone tracing on the other foot.

- Once you have finished, move your feet and the toes of the foot that you just touched. How do they feel?
- Stand again and see how that feels. Close your eyes and just notice what you become aware of. Is it similar to or different from when you were standing before? How? What do you notice?
- Now open your eyes and walk around the room. How do you feel? What do you notice?

Variation (Fig. 9.9.)

This variation can be done before of after the previous activity, and helps students to visualize the bones of the feet, particularly the long metatarsal bones, as well as to gain further joint mobility. It can help to have a skeletal model of the bones of the feet, or a drawing, to refer to as you do this activity with them.

Have students sit with the left foot in front of them on the floor, and place their left hand next to their foot, on the inside near the medial arch. They can then use their right hand to cover the left hand, placing it perpendicularly so just the top knuckles show. (This is akin to the way the skin covers the metatarsals, leaving just the phalanges exposed as separate bones).

- Put your left foot out, and put your left hand next to your foot on the inside, like this. *(See Fig. 9.9a for a demonstration.)* Now take your right hand and cover your left hand like this. *(Fig. 9.9b.)*

Then, ask them to wiggle their fingers and notice how they can only see the top finger digits moving, when in actuality the whole finger moves. (This is akin to moving the toes, when both the phalanges and metatarsals respond.)

- Now wiggle your fingers, and also wiggle your toes. Do you see how you can only see the top digits of your fingers moving, even though you are moving the full length of your fingers under your hand? *(Fig. 9.9c.)*

Have them place their left hand over their *foot* in that same way as well, and wiggle their toes. Then prompt them to lift their hand up, and wiggle the left toes and the left fingers, so they can imagine how the bones of what they perceive as the toes actually extend further down into the foot.

- Now put your left hand over your left foot instead of over your hand. Now wiggle your toes again. See how you can only see the top digits of your toes moving now? Now lift up your hand, and wiggle your fingers and your toes. Do you see how you can now see the full length of your fingers moving now?
- When you wiggle your toes, the same is happening, you just can't see their full length! *(Then, refer to the skeletal model or drawing.)* Your metatarsal bones actually extend down into the part of your foot covered up by your skin, so they really move more like your fingers in that sense *(Fig. 9.9d).*
- But often, we have our feet all covered up—in socks and shoes—for most of the day, and don't often realize how much they can move! Imagine, for instance, if you had your hands in gloves all day long, and how that might affect your sense of them, or your ability to move them?
- By doing some of these activities, like the bone tracing with your feet that we just did, you can regain some of this movement and the sensation in your feet—that is more of your natural ability.

Repeat this on the other side with the right foot.

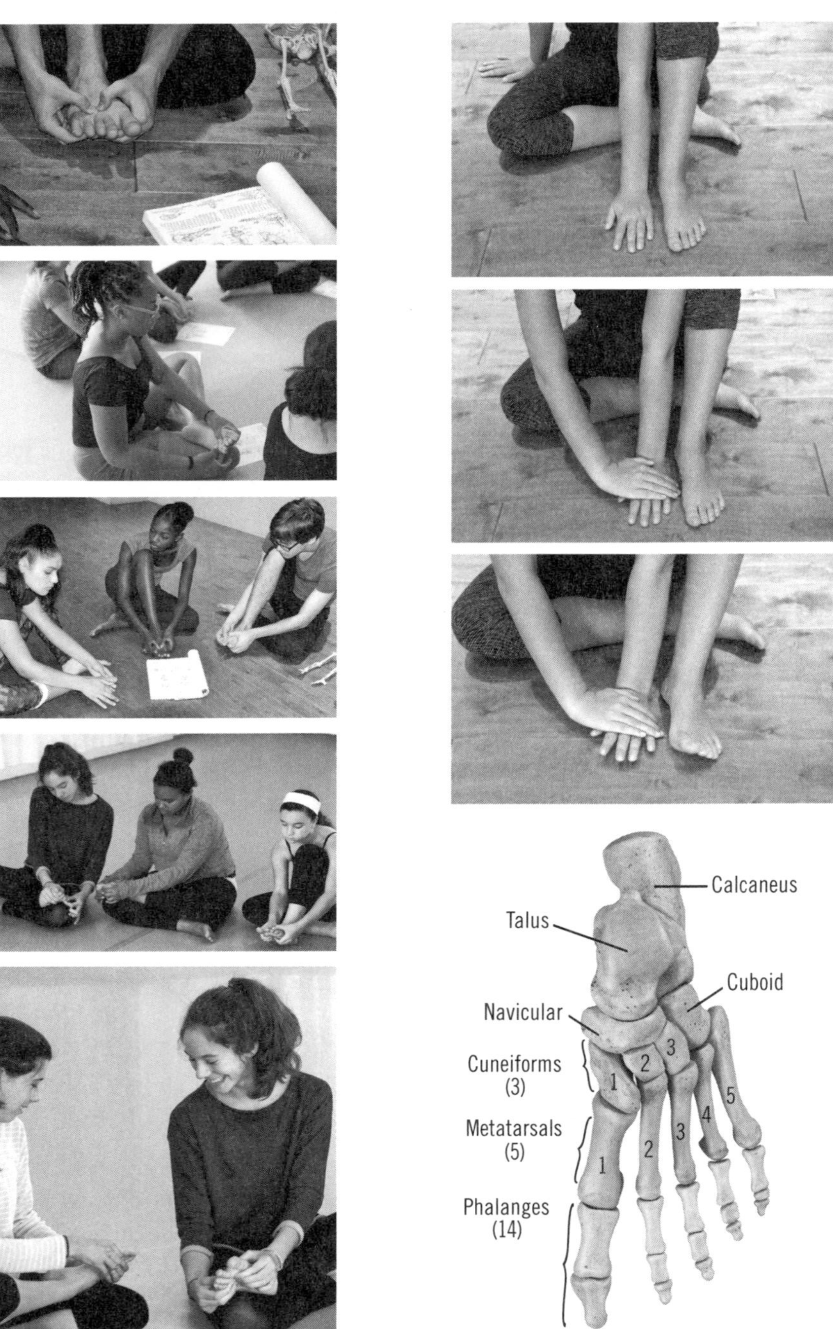

Fig. 9.8a, b, c, d, e. Students touch the bones of their own feet as a way to locate and name them. They can also refer to *The Anatomy Coloring Book* or skeletal models, working individually or in groups.

Fig. 9.9a, b, c, d. Variation: Students compare the bone structure of their hands and feet to gain a more realistic perception of the bones of the feet (a–c), which include spaces between the metatarsal bones, though they are not visually apparent (d).

Discussion

- How did it feel to trace the bones in your feet? What did you feel or notice? How did it feel to stand after you had traced all the bones? What was new to you? When might you do this on your own?
- *(For variation)* Can you feel this difference now in how your feet move? When you trace your feet, can you feel where the metatarsals end and the cuneiforms and cuboid begin?

Tips for Teachers

- Some students may have a particular aversion to touching their feet. Their feet may be sensitive or ticklish, or they may just feel "squeamish" about touching them. These students can do the activity with their socks on at first if necessary. You may find that those who prefer to keep their socks on will be willing to do the activity with bare feet on another day. You can also openly discuss any aversion to this activity, using this as a further opportunity to invite dialogue about touch and personal preferences—either talking privately with an individual student, or discussing this as a full group.
- Related Activities: You can also teach further ways to add proprioceptive feedback to the feet, such as brushing the feet lightly with a soft or firm brush, or stroking or tapping the feet with your hands, and so on. (For more about proprioception, see chapter 10.)
- Students can complete a journal entry using the free-form writing exercise with an entry entitled "My Feet." You can also facilitate this writing activity as part of the class time itself.

HOME PRACTICE

- Invite students to trace the bones of their feet at night before going to bed, or in the morning before beginning the day. They can also write about their experience in their body journals.

Bone Tracing: The Shoulder Girdle

You can also use bone touch to increase the articulation of your movement in the shoulder girdle—an area that, like the feet, is often misperceived as a single unit rather than as an intricate network of distinct bones. Your shoulder girdle is made up of the two clavicles and two scapulae, and is considered part of the appendicular skeleton (along with the pelvis and legs), while the skull, spine, and rib cage are considered the axial skeleton. The shoulder girdle has only two points of attachment to the axial skeleton—on the ventral (front) side at the two sternoclavicular joints (where the clavicles meet the manubrium of the sternum). These fluid-filled synovial joints allow for movement of the shoulder girdle separate from the rib cage.

The two scapulae in the dorsal (back) side of the body have no joint attachment to the axial skeleton and therefore are free to glide along the rib cage in various directions. The scapula each actually only articulate with one bone: the clavicle (at the acromioclavicular joint). Despite this enormous potential for movement, often our movement is quite limited from excess tension in our shoulders and upper back. Exploring the shoulder girdle and scapulae through touch and movement helps increase mobility and ease through the upper body and arms. When the scapulae move, ideally the clavicles also respond by slightly rotating and lifting up or depressing down. You can increase the blood flow to the many muscles of the upper back—an area where many people hold considerable tension—as you move your scapulae with a fuller range of motion.

Two explorations here use bone touch to locate the clavicles and scapulae, while encouraging a wider range of motion and an ease of movement. The first uses self-touch; the second involves partners working together through movement and touch. Be sure you have first introduced the basic self-touch exploration called "Bone Touch" before doing this activity with your group, as well as reviewing the touch guidelines together as discussed in chapter 6. If you prefer not to use touch-based partner activities with your group, you can use the first exploration, Tracing the Shoulder Girdle. The bones of the scapulae, focused on in the second exploration, are harder to define using self-touch alone.

Exploration: Bone Tracing—The Shoulder Girdle

(20–25 minutes)

PURPOSE. To clarify the bones of the shoulder girdle through movement and self-touch; to experience greater range of motion of the shoulder girdle from an ability to feel the shape of the bones more distinctly and to visualize the anatomy more accurately.

Activity

Review the names and shapes of the bones of the shoulder girdle using the skeletal model and/or anatomy plates. You can also discuss the names and types of the joints.

Review the names and shapes again, with each person briefly tracing the bones on his/her own body as you trace them on the skeletal model. Remind students to use their "bone touch."

- *(After tracing each bone you can ask the following:)* Now take a moment to move that area. What do you notice? How do your clavicles move? How do your scapulae move?
- Try this with your eyes closed, and then with them opened. What do you notice now?

Discussion

- What did you experience? Did you notice any difference in your movement from before you traced your shoulder girdle than after? What did you notice? How did it feel to move? Has your movement changed? How?

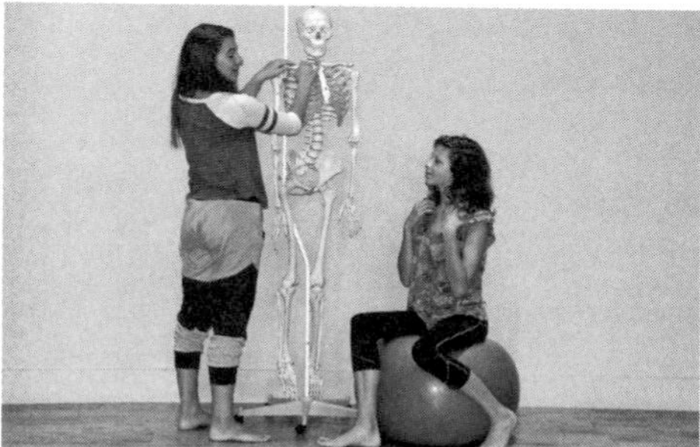
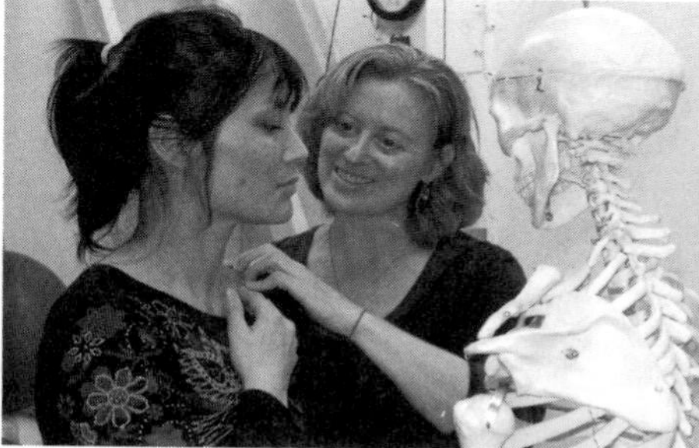

Fig. 9.10a, b. Teens use the skeletal model and self-touch to locate the bones of the shoulder girdle, such as touching the clavicles to feel their shape; photo b shows a dance educator in Embodiment in Education being guided in doing the same.

Exploration: Bone Tracing—The Scapulae, Our Wings

(20–30 minutes)

PURPOSE. To clarify the shape and movement of the scapulae; to recognize these as "free-floating bones"; to explore the full range of motion of the scapulae and differentiate them from the ribs and spine. (This exploration can follow the previous one, Bone Tracing—The Shoulder Girdle.)

Activity

Have the students do this activity in partners with one partner sitting behind another. Partners can sit on the floor, on a physioball, or chair. Any combination can work, as long as both partners are at the same level. Both partners can also stand if preferred.

Review the names and shapes of the bones of the shoulder girdle (the clavicles and scapulae) using the skeletal model and/or anatomy plates if you haven't already done so.

Demonstrate how this partner exercise will work by placing your hands on the scapulae, either demonstrating with a student or using a skeletal model. Place one hand on each scapula, with the palm of your hand at the inferior spinous process, and the fingers at the spine of the scapula.

- Now sit behind your partner. Place your hands on the scapulae, and the person being touched can close your eyes.
- Now slowly begin to initiate movement from your scapulae. Move slowly at first so you can feel what is happening in your body. The partner touching, keep your hands on the scapulae and follow along with your partner's movement, not directing but supporting through your touch. *(You can also suggest that they close their eyes as well, to heighten the focus on sensation through their hands, as they follow their partner's movement with their hands.)*
- (*Person moving*) Now notice what has been happening in your spine as you move. Are you moving your spine also? If so, as you continue, this time stabilize your spine and just move your scapulae. How does this change your movement? Can you feel your scapulae gliding along your rib cage? How many ways can your scapula move?
- Now place your hands on your clavicles as you move your scapulae. Do they move as well?
- Now move your scapulae and let your clavicles, rib cage, and spine respond.[1] Is this the same or different? What happens to your range of motion?
- Keep exploring this for a few moments, and the partners sitting behind can now close their eyes also, if you haven't already done so, and respond by following along with your partner's movement, allowing your body to move as they are moving, whether forward and back, side to side, or however they are moving. Those who are moving, go slowly so your partner can more easily follow along *(Fig. 9.11)*.
- Now complete your movement and pause. When your partner has stopped you can remove your hands. The person being touched can now take a moment to move on your own. You might want to stand or walk around. Notice how you feel and what you notice. Do you feel any changes in your body? Do you notice any difference in your movement?
- Come back together with your partner. *(Partners can take a few minutes to share about the experience before switching roles, or save that for after they have switched roles.)*
- Switch partners. *(Repeat this process.)*

Students can share their perceptions in partners, or you can proceed directly to the group discussion.

Discussion

- What did you notice as you moved? Does this feel the same or different than before you did the partner exercise? How may ways can the scapulae move? What else did you discover? How did it feel to follow your partner's movement with your eyes opened versus with them closed? Did anyone have a different experience?

After the discussion, you can relate students' experience to the anatomical terms for movement of the scapulae here if you want to introduce them—retraction, protraction, elevation, depression, and upward rotation. They can then try these on their own and then work in partners again to feel these specific movements *(Fig. 9.12)*.

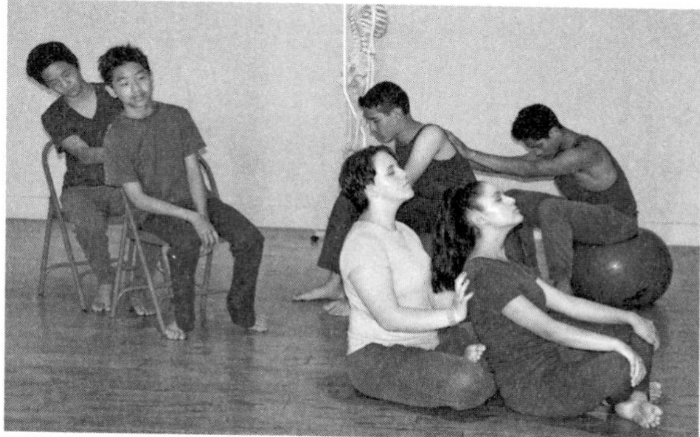

Fig. 9.11. In partners, students find all the ways they can move by initiating movement in the scapulae and letting the spine and head respond as they move. The partner in front initiates the movement, while the partner behind follows the movement through touch. Students can choose to sit in a variety of positions according to what is most comfortable.

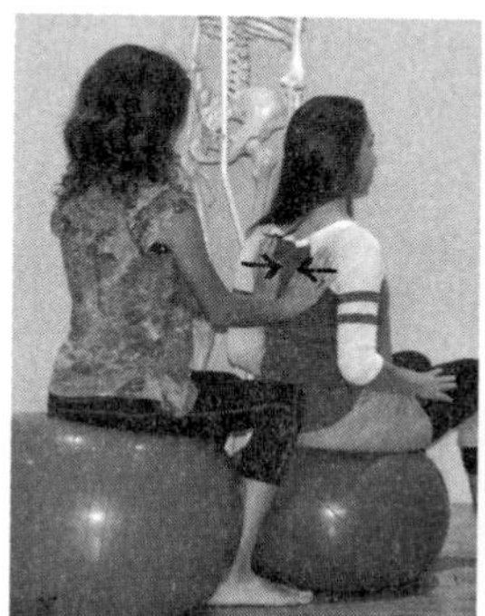

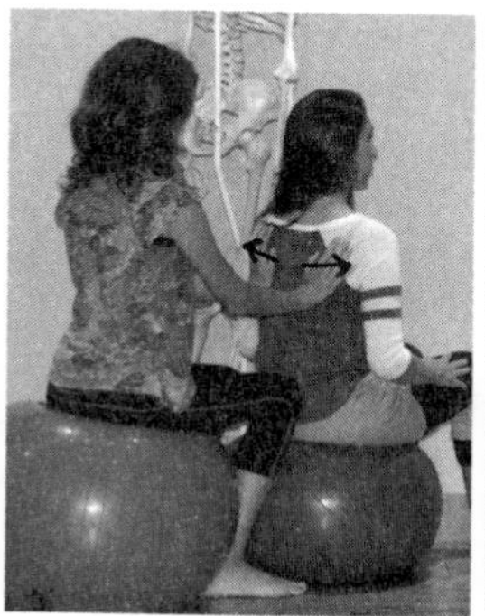

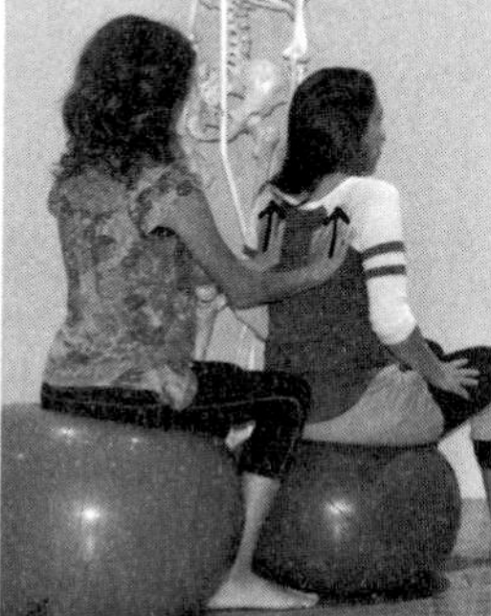

Fig. 9.12a, b, c. Through movement and touch with a partner, students feel the movement of the scapulae. Shown here are retraction (a), protraction (b), and elevation (c). (Depression and upward rotation not shown.)

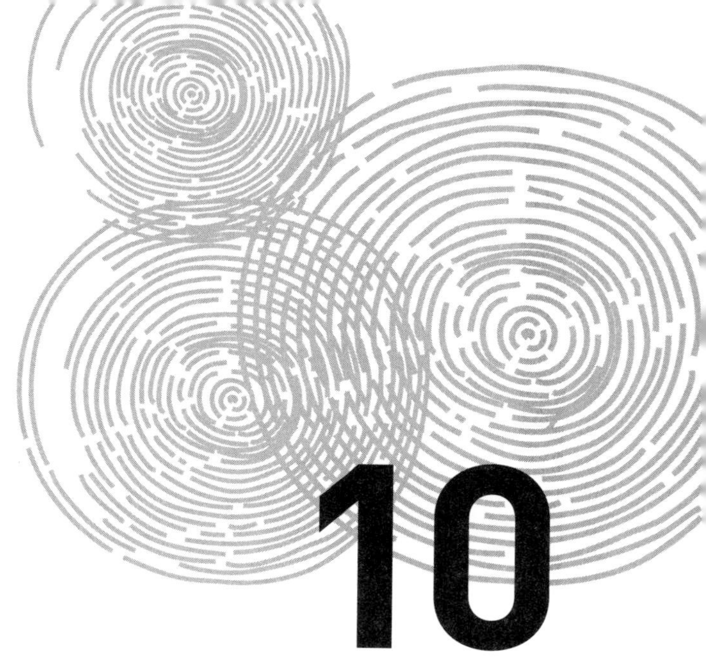

10

Joints, Proprioception, and the Kinesthetic Sense

Being able to perceive where we are in space—as well as the amount of effort we are using to move—is an important first step in inviting more ease in our movement. How do we know where we are in space at any given moment? Try this: notice how you are sitting right now. Hold this position. How can you feel the position of your body? How do you know your body position at any given time? *Proprioceptors* are the specialized nerve cells in your muscles and joints that make this inner knowledge possible. After a moment, change your position (perhaps sit differently, shift your weight, move your legs, or place your arms differently). Notice how this feels. Now, go back to your original position, the one you were just in. Can you do that? Your level of proprioceptive awareness will affect your ability to register your position in space, as well as to perceive your position with enough specificity to easily return to this same position. Developing heightened proprioceptive awareness is an essential step in achieving a solid foundation of body awareness, movement proficiency, and ease.

Body Awareness

Proprioceptors are amazing cells that serve as "self-receivers"—specialized nerve cells whose function it is to *know one another* by receiving sensory information. Located in the muscles, tendons, and joints, these nerve cells help to provide us with an inner body awareness by registering muscle and ligament length, muscle force, and pressure or weight bearing at the joints. This lets us sense, for instance, if there is more weight on one foot than the other when we stand, or where the weight of the body is heaviest when lying down.

Proprioceptors also help us register our position in space—even with our eyes closed, we can tell the position we are in with specificity. This is because our proprioceptive sense is not contingent on our primary senses of taste (mouth), hearing (ears), smell (nose), sight (eyes), or touch (skin). For instance, someone who is blind or deaf would not lose awareness of his or her body position in space; in fact, this sense of body awareness might be heightened due to a lack of distraction by other senses. Along with our interoceptors, which sense our inner bodily organs, proprioceptors contribute to our body awareness.

All these sensory receptors, combined with the equilibrium sensors in the inner ear (also proprioceptors) and the visual righting reflex of the eyes, provide our spatial awareness and help us to move and maintain our balance. Proprioceptive awareness thereby contributes to our *kinesthetic sense,* or *kinesthesia*—our awareness of our bodies when we are in motion. Specific proprioceptive receptors can be found in our muscles (muscle spindles, which register muscle length), tendons (Golgi tendon organs, which sense muscle tension and register the pull on tendon tissue), joints (joint receptors, which measure joint compression), and our inner ear (maculae and cristae, which register inner ear equilibrium to feel where our head is in relation to gravity). The kinesthetic sense is developed through *movement,* which stimulates all these receptors. New movement encourages awakened sensation. Any highly refined movement skill requires a highly developed proprioceptive system.

I have a favorite way of demonstrating what is happening during this type of proprioceptive reawakening from experiencing new movement, using a pink pen with a top half made of clear plastic with multicolored glitter floating around inside. When you put the pen to paper and just pretend to write with it, you see the pen and glitter moving around. This is like moving with your current baseline level of body awareness. Then, when you press down on the pen to actually write on the paper, the inside of the clear glitter section *lights up* with a bright pink glow from a small flashlight inside! This moment is similar to when the proprioceptors and interoceptors—your self-receivers—discover themselves, such as when you move in a new way that elicits a fresh awareness. As you continue to move in new ways, you can deepen and expand your body awareness. Eventually, your whole body lights up from within!

Another way to explain and demonstrate the moment of proprioceptive awareness is to use the metaphor of meeting a new person. When we first greet each other and make an initial connection, we often shake hands. Through touch, we can feel: *Here we are.* Then as we talk and relate, we may come closer together with more of a sense of intimacy. These demonstrations help students to understand the concept of proprioceptive awareness more personally.

Why is proprioceptive awareness so essential? At a basic level, we need new sensory perception to grow, change, and adapt with ease. This helps us to shift from our habitual patterns, and even—as will be explored later in the curriculum—to develop a healthy body image. Caryn McHose explains this relationship between sensation, body awareness, and body image in this way:

> If the exploration is supplied with meaning, imagination, breath, and attention to sensation, we will have accidents of perception that allow the body to do something new.... Whenever we give birth to a new movement from orientation and sense impression, we loosen the hold of body image over our movement ... it is sensory perception that helps to unlock the body image.[1]

The activities in this section help students to learn about their proprioceptive senses—the basis of their kinesthetic intelligence—and to further develop them as a further step in building a foundation of somatic awareness. Later this ability to sense their bodies with greater specificity will also contribute to enhance sensory perception and adaptability as they explore body image more directly.

Joints and Proprioception

To understand this relationship of joints and proprioception to kinesthetic awareness, students first learn about the structure and function of different types of joints through movement and discussion. As a starting point, they move, locate, and name the various joints in their bodies. A main focus is on the highly movable synovial joints, such as those found in the arms (at the shoulders, elbows, and wrists) and legs (at the hips, knees, and ankles). In addition to helping students increase their mobility, this experiential knowledge of synovial joints is essential to an understanding of why movement is needed as a precursor to stretching. (This will be covered further in the section on warm-up in chapter 16.)

At the synovial joints, cartilage-capped bones are surrounded by a fibrous capsule with an inner membrane that secretes synovial fluid. This viscous fluid serves to both cushion the bones and absorb the heat of friction during movement. Movement at these joints increases the *amount of fluid* in the joints and also *raises its temperature.* At a subtle level you can feel this. You can also learn to distinguish among various types of joint movement, differentiating, for example, movement initiated from the bones of the joints from that initiated from the fluid within the joints, as investigated through an exploration called Movement of Joints.

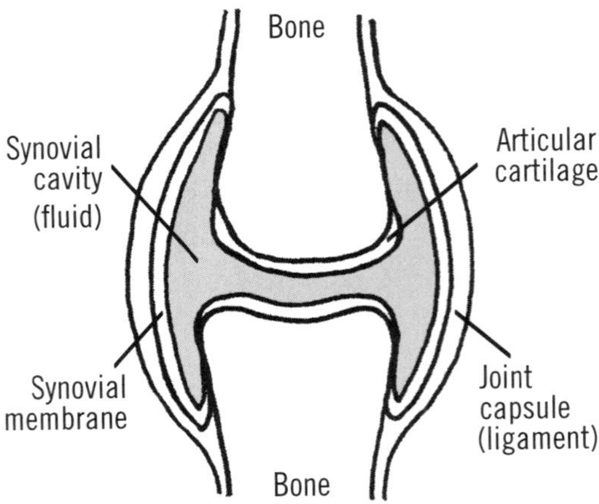

Fig. 10.1. Structure of a synovial joint, which provides for mobility and cushioning provided by synovial fluid within the joint.

A next exploration, called Shapes, provides a movement game that helps students to learn about proprioception and recognize the amazing specificity with which they know their position in space. In this activity, students change their positions multiple times and then recreate their positions (in the same way that you were guided to do in the introduction to this chapter), and then discuss how they were able to know their position. This discussion inevitably gets students enthusiastically involved in trying to describe *how they know what they know* at a body level—inviting a lively discussion of body awareness and, eventually, of proprioception.

Benefits of Learning about Proprioception

In learning about proprioception, students discover that body awareness is a developmental skill that can be learned—and improved upon. In the current paradigm of physical education, particularly as youth enter the preteen and teen years, their progress is generally measured in terms of gross motor skill development. Often those who do well develop confidence in their movement abilities, while those who struggle end up feeling less confident and perhaps even frustrated with their bodies and discouraged with themselves. When we help students to develop *foundational skills,* such as proprioceptive awareness, they recognize that they can improve—from whatever baseline they already have. While some may naturally have a higher level of kinesthetic ability than others, no one is forever either "good" or "bad" at movement, "coordinated" or "uncoordinated." From the vantage point of proprioception, students begin to see that each person can enhance their gross motor abilities by increasing their proprioceptive awareness. Proprioceptive awareness becomes the foundation for further movement skills, helping teens increase their aptitude in a variety of activities—ranging from skateboarding, riding bikes, and dancing to skill-building in yoga or sports. Increased proprioceptive awareness can support adolescents to feel less self-conscious and more confident as movers, while increasing their sense of inner aliveness.

They can also begin to understand why training in one physical activity, such as weight-lifting, yoga, or hip-hop dance—if practiced to the exclusion of other physical practices—doesn't necessarily translate into skill in a new activity. This can keep them from getting discouraged when trying a new activity and feeling like a "beginner," even though they are quite skilled in another area. High level of skill in one area may actually *limit* ability to learn another movement form or even to further develop the proprioceptive system. There are several reasons for this.

In training in a particular movement form, certain nervous system pathways become developed, to the exclusion of others. This gives us the feeling of being good at certain movements we have perfected (such as a particular yoga pose or tennis swing) and awkward at other movements we have practiced less often or have never experienced. As a learned pathway becomes known, it also becomes patterned in the nervous system and can inhibit new learning. This occurs both physically and psychologically, as we may tend to prefer to do what we are good at. Physical movements that fall outside the range of our previous experience (and thus stimulate *new* proprioceptors) may be registered as awkward, uncomfortable, or even weird, and therefore we might avoid them. As you can imagine, this is even truer for adolescents, who are particularly sensitive to how they may appear in front of teachers, other adults, and especially their peers.

To develop new patterns, however, *we need to invite new experience.* This necessitates stepping outside our comfort zones and allowing for a sense of disorientation and newness as part of the learning process. Discussing this explicitly opens teens to the inevitable vulnerability it can take to engage in these experiences. Disorientation is actually a precursor to learning; you need to become disoriented in order to reorient. It is important to help students understand this phenomenon as it relates to proprioception—particularly as they engage in these exercises that may seem so simple and basic, yet feel so strange and new! In fact, one underlying goal of the curriculum is to begin to disorient the nervous system—our way of moving and relating to gravity—to prepare us to open to new movement experience. To repeat the words of Bonnie Bainbridge Cohen: "Training isn't a matter of repeating the same thing for one week or two months and then expecting a result. Each moment should be a dialogue of response and change."[2]

Approaching movement in a way that is responsive in the present moment also initiates *beginner's mind,* in which you ease into an inspiring mode of open curiosity, as one of my college students reflected upon in her final body journal entry for the class:

> *During this course, my movement has really changed! At first I was very shy and unwilling to try some of these things, especially the small and sensitive movements, but now I am more vulnerable and willing to explore. Each class experience provided vital information about my body that challenged me to investigate*

my personal and internal well-being in new ways. It's like I have been given an extra push in my maturity level, like I'm more open to allowing new textures in my life too.

Our ways of moving affect—and are often reflected in—our ways of being in the world. These are just some of the many benefits of staying engaged and open to new experiences. Discussing proprioception and all of these related concepts helps students gain their own insights, as well as to understand the context of the class and the underlying purpose of many of the related activities.

Exploration: Movement of Joints

(20 minutes)

PURPOSE. To explore the movement of the joints; to differentiate between types of joints and their related movements; to experience the wide range of movement in your synovial joints; to learn about the structure and function of synovial joints.

Activity

Repeat the bone tracing activity done in chapter 10, giving the following directions.

- As you locate specific bones, move them with your hand. Then move them on their own. What type of movement is possible at each of the joints? *(Begin with the bones of the feet and progress to the head. Refer to the skeleton to discuss different types of joints and their related movements as you go.)*

Move to standing. Have your students stand in the space in a circle or in whatever arrangement is comfortable for them.

- Close your eyes and notice how you feel. Take a moment to do your body scan.
- Now move the bones of your hands. Then instead of moving the bones, feel the space in between the bones of your hands and those in your lower arm: your wrist. Move from that space in your wrists.
- Now this time, instead of moving to feel the spaces, feel the synovial fluid inside the spaces between the bones. Move the fluid around in the spaces. As you move, the membranes surrounding these joints actually produce more fluid, so you'll have even more cushioning to support you in your movement.

- ❍ Feel your bones supporting your weight. Feel the joint spaces between the bones. Imagine the fluid-filled sacs in each of the synovial joints cushioning your bones. Try this in other parts of your body: move the bones, and then the spaces between the bones, and then the synovial fluid. What are the differences?

Guide students to try this with each area: the elbows, shoulders, ankles, knees, and hips. This can be done with eyes closed or opened, depending on what you perceive as the comfort level and preference of the group.

- ❍ Explore this on your own for a few minutes.

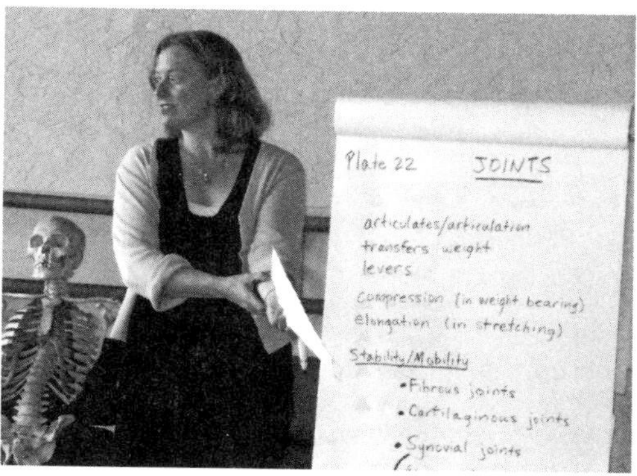
Plate 22
JOINTS
articulates/articulation
transfers weight
levers
Compression (in weight bearing)
Elongation (in stretching)
Stability/Mobility
•Fibrous joints
•Cartilaginous joints
•Synovial joints

Fig. 10.2. Reviewing types of joints as referred to in *The Anatomy Coloring Book.* Both cognitive learning and physical movement can help students to explore the material.

Discussion

- What were you aware of as you stood up? Did it feel different from when we just traced the bones? What were the differences between moving from the bones, moving from the spaces, and moving from the fluid? How do you feel now?

Students can refer to the anatomy plates of the joints to learn more about or review specifics about synovial joints and other types of joints.

Students apply this knowledge further in explorations in chapter 16, in which they are guided to consider aspects of a healthy warm-up related to the anatomy and physiology of their bodies.

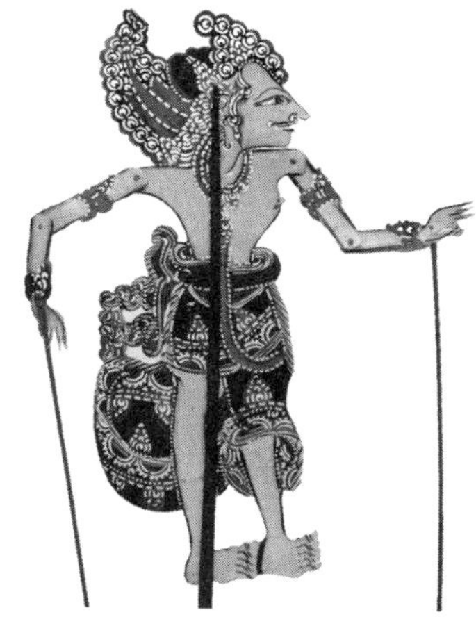

Fig. 10.3. Wayang Kulit puppet of Rama from Bali, Indonesia. Imagine if we could only move in two dimensions. Referring to the way the puppet moves can help students appreciate the incredible mobility of our joints, which give us the benefit of more three-dimensional movement.

Exploration: Shapes

(20–30 minutes)

PURPOSE. To encourage understanding of the proprioceptive system and its function; to explore this experientially; to invite discussion of the anatomy and physiology of proprioception.

Activity

Begin by having students walk throughout the room. Then guide a structured improvisation to elicit a variety of movements; directions such as "shape the space with your arms as you move," and "now explore all levels as you go, moving down to the floor and up again," can be used to encourage a wide range of movement.

- Keep moving, but in a moment I'm going to clap. When you hear me clap, freeze in whatever position you are in. *(Clap.)*
- *(Invite students to close their eyes, and then to bring awareness to all parts of their bodies:)* Feel the shape in your body. Where are your arms, hands, fingers? Are your fingers held together or slightly apart or spread out wide? How about your head—is it tilted to one side or the other? Where is your weight on your feet? *(Fig. 10.4a.)*

Then have them open their eyes and continue to move again, and repeat this one or two more times.

Repeat the clap and freeze direction once more. This time try to clap when you see that most students are in complex shapes and off-balance positions in gravity, such as tilting to the side or upside-down and so on, if possible) *(Fig. 10.4b).* Clap.

- Can you feel this new position you are in? Where is your weight on your feet? Or are you taking weight through your back or belly? Can you feel the angle of your arms? The hair lying against your face? The bend in your legs? *(Then have them move again.)*
- Now when I clap again, return to the exact previous position you were just in, that is, the position in your *body,* not necessarily in the *place in the room* itself. *(Clap.)*
- Can you find that exact position? Check again. Was that where you had your weight on each foot? Was that the angle of your wrist? The tilt of your head? Make any changes to be sure you are in exactly the same position as before. OK, now relax and keep moving.
- Now find an ending position when you are ready, and just rest there.

Discussion

- Were you able to return to the same position? How were you able to remember that position?

Through this discussion, pool the group's knowledge of proprioception. For instance, a student might respond, "I could feel where my weight was on my feet." Then you might ask, "And how could you feel that?" Another student might then offer, "you can feel the pressure in different parts of your feet," and you might ask, "and how do we *feel* pressure in our bodies?" and so on. Lead the conversation by letting other students respond before providing any further information. You might also use the metaphor of meeting a new person, and demonstrate how we can often first connect by shaking hands, and then become more familiar as we converse together. *(Fig. 10.5a, b.)*

As the conversation progresses, mention the relevant information about proprioception that is not yet known or understood.

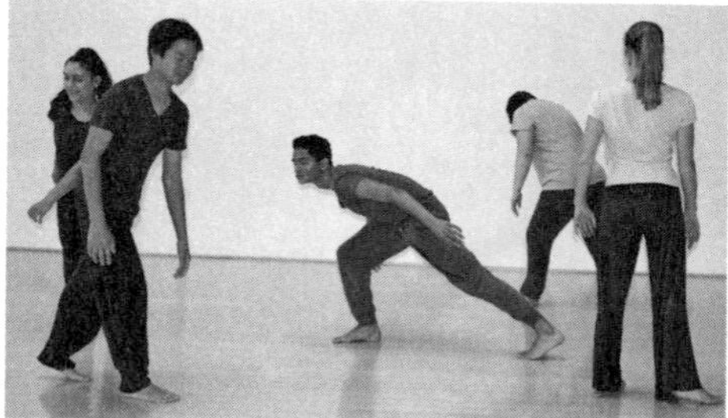

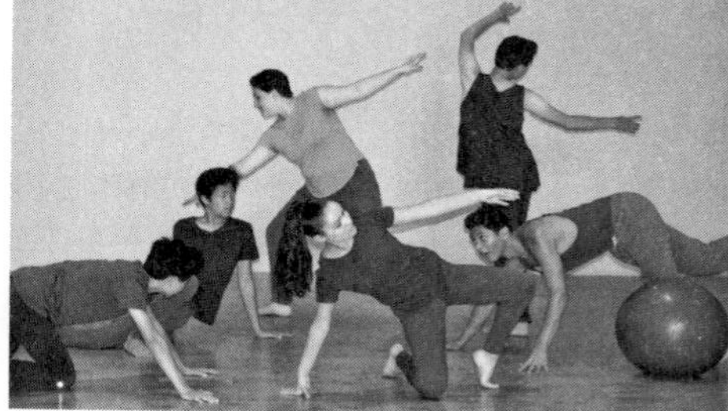

Fig. 10.4a, b. Students pause and close their eyes to feel their position in space (a); then increase the complexity of their shapes by including various levels in space and off-balance positions (b).

Tips for Teachers

- When deciding when to clap to have students "freeze" their movement—particularly when they will be asked to return to that shape—look for a time when most of the students are in a more complex shape. Particularly, shapes that are more "off-balance," like when tilting sideways or upside-down in gravity, give more complex proprioceptive feedback, as this includes subtle distinctions of balance within the vestibular system in the inner ear as well.

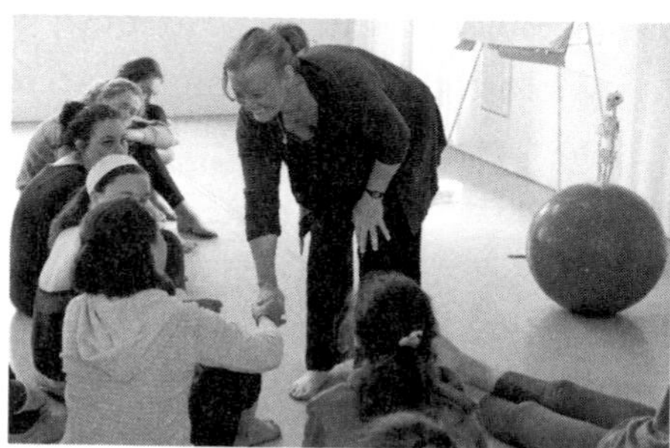

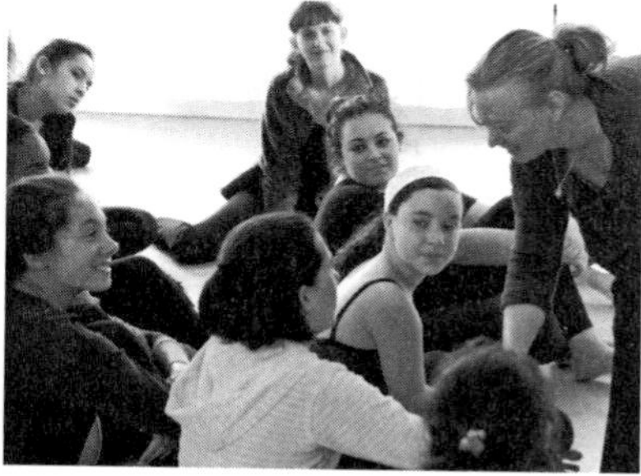

Fig. 10.5a, b. As we gain greater proprioceptive awareness, our bodies feel "more familiar inside." Using the metaphor of meeting a new person can help students to understand this concept; like getting to know a new person, an instant connection can occur, or this can take some time.

Muscles and Movement

Usually we do things the way we know how to do them, and then keep repeating that pattern out of habit—even if it is not most skillful or efficient. We may even be using *more* effort than we need to without realizing it. Although a certain level of muscular activity is always present in the form of tone (the resting state of a muscle before an action takes place), excess tension in the muscles surrounding the joints *restricts proprioceptive awareness in that area.* Such tension also limits mobility and inhibits the readiness of the muscles to respond. Therefore although we develop proprioceptive awareness through movement, depending upon *how* we move, we may in fact be *limiting* the proprioceptive feedback to the body. For this reason it becomes important to be able to distinguish between muscle tone and muscle tension.

To experience this, you can stand up and relax your muscles. You may progressively begin to feel more relaxed while you remain standing, but your muscle tone is still engaged to keep your body upright. If your muscles didn't have this "resting state" of muscle tone, you would just collapse to the floor. Muscle tone supports and enhances our movement, while muscle tension generally restricts it. This is because mobility, the ability of a joint to move, is determined by both the shape and articulation of the bones at the joint *and* the resilience of the surrounding connective tissue. Flexibility, on the other hand, is the range of motion at a joint in relation to the muscle or group of muscles and fascia. Flexibility at any one joint will be affected by the mobility at that joint, just as the mobility at a joint will be affected by the flexibility of surrounding tissues.

To begin to release excess muscle tension, students can focus first on the larger muscle groups. As they release and soften their more external muscles, they rely instead on the deeper, intrinsic muscles of support—moving with more ease and often increasing their range of motion as well. Surprisingly, with *less* effort we feel *more.* This increased proprioceptive sense enhances our kinesthetic awareness and movement proficiency. Developing proprioceptive awareness is often more of a process of *"unlearning"* in order to restore our innate mobility and ease.

In the next exploration, students work in partners to discover the resting state of their muscles, and learn to differentiate between muscle *tone* (which is needed to maintain a position in gravity and to produce efficient movement) and excess muscle *tension* (which inevitably inhibits movement potential). This exploration involves a simple activity of "passive movement" done in Constructive Rest, in which the upper arm rests on the floor while a partner gently moves the lower arm and hand—and then lets go so the arm falls back to the floor. As students quickly discover, this is not necessarily so easy to do! More often than not they will think that they have "let go" of their arm, only to find that when their partner releases it, their arm won't fall to the ground with gravity as it would if they were relaxed. This demonstrates that they are actually still supporting their arm with their own muscular effort. As students recognize that they can hold tension in their bodies *without being conscious of it,* they begin to more consciously release excess muscular tension.

By developing their proprioceptive senses students can also learn to modulate the muscular energy used in any given movement. An exploration called Circles, based on an activity first developed by Mabel Elsworth Todd, uses a simple movement of circling the arms and legs to help sense and release excess tension in the shoulders and hips.[3] As in the previous activity done with the arm, this exploration is done first on one side of the body and then the other, affording students an opportunity to notice the effect of the movement. Students are often surprised at the immediate changes they feel after engaging in these brief activities. After doing the circling activity initially on one side of the body only, students often report that the side they moved feels softer and more relaxed, or sometimes seems heavier and more "sunken down into the floor." In contrast, they often notice that the other side, which may have felt normal to them before, now feels tight and restricted, as they recognize a level of tension in their bodies that had previously gone unnoticed. They then become eager to do the activity on the other side as well!

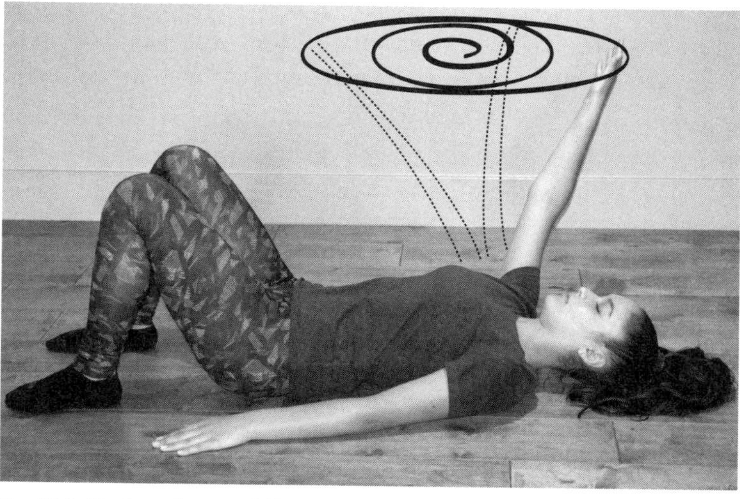

Fig. 10.6. Circles—Arms and Shoulders (See page 188.)

Exploration: Muscle Tension vs. Muscle Tone

(20–30 minutes)

PURPOSE. To observe the resting state of your muscles; to practice focusing your attention; to experience the physical sensation of excess muscular tension, even when "at rest"; to learn to release unnecessary muscular tension; to understand the difference between muscle tension and muscle tone; to understand the relationship of proprioception (sensing) and kinesthetic sense (moving).

Activity

This activity is done with a partner, with one person lying in Constructive Rest and one person sitting to the side. Demonstrate this exploration first by working with one or two students yourself, to let the class observe the variations in responses. Even though you may demonstrate this activity and the students may cognitively understand it, likely many students will still not "succeed" in releasing their excess tension on a first try!

- ❍ *(To the person lying down)* Take a moment to relax and close your eyes. Let the earth support your weight. Take a few deep breaths, in and out.
- ❍ *(To the person sitting)* Touch your partner's arm by the wrist, holding it as demonstrated. When you are ready, gently lift your partner's lower arm until it is resting on the elbow only. *(Fig. 10.7a.)* Then begin to gently toss the lower arm, as demonstrated, occasionally letting go altogether to see what happens. *(Fig. 10.7b, c.)* Does the lower arm remain lifted? Or fall to the floor with gravity? Or hover in the air for a few moments and then release into gravity? Just notice. Repeat this several times. If your partner is having difficulty releasing into gravity, remind him or her verbally a few times to let go and relax the arm down.
- ❍ *(Instruct the person lying down to notice what happens in his or her own body.)* Observe as your partner does this. What do you experience? Can you release your arm, or were you still holding it? Did your response change over time or was it the same each time?
- ❍ *(To the person sitting)* Once you have explored this a few times, move to the other side of your partner, and try this with the other arm. Is the response the same or different on this side?
- ❍ Finish up working with your partner. The person lying down can gently roll to the side and push yourself up to sitting.

Partners can then discuss what they experienced or observed.

- ❍ *(To transition before switching roles, say:)* Take a moment to switch roles; the person sitting can lie down in Constructive Rest and close your eyes, and the person lying down can sit to the side and wait while your partner gets settled.

Repeat with these new roles. Repeat your verbal instructions as they do this again, or let them work on their own.

Partners can then discuss what they experienced or observed.

Discussion

- What did you experience with your partner? What did you notice as you did this several times? Did your experience change over time or stay the same? Did it matter how or where you focused your attention? How were you feeling? What did you notice? As the person lying down? As the sitting observer? What helped you to let go and relax your arm down?
- What is muscle tone? How is this different from muscle tension? *(If students don't readily understand these concepts, explain them, building upon students' comments.)*
- How does exercise develop muscle tone? What happens if you also develop excess muscle tension? How does this affect your body? Your movement? Your sense of yourself?
- How does proprioception relate to how you move?

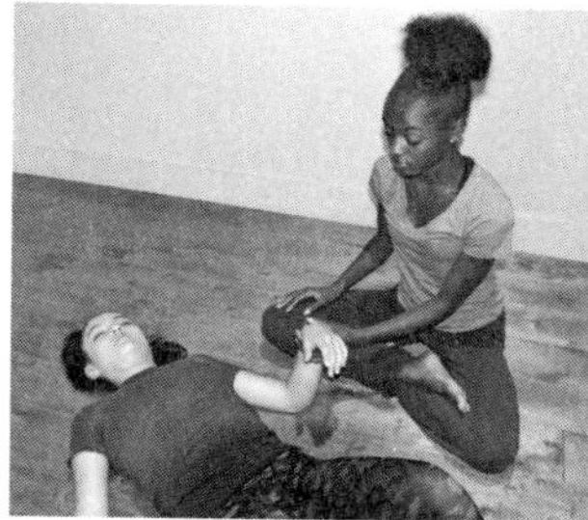
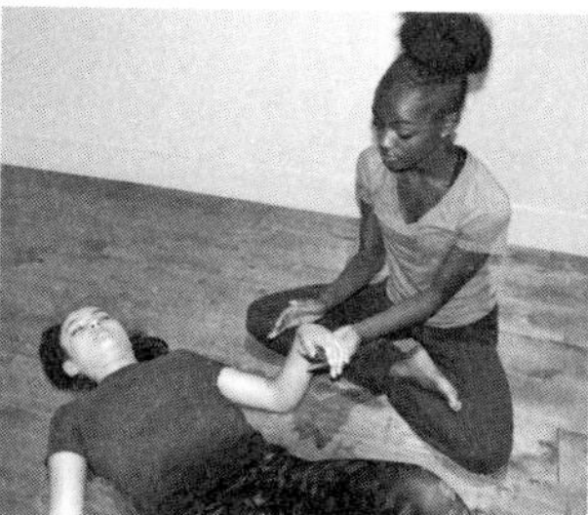
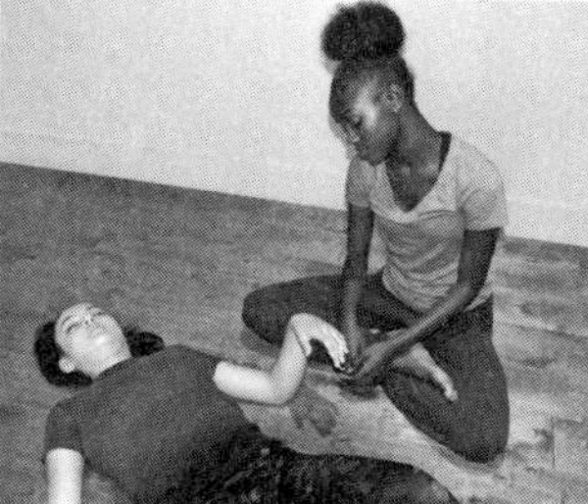

Fig. 10.7a, b, c. To help students test their muscle tension, one partner lifts the other partner's arm (a), then gently tosses it back and forth while they try to relax it (b); then they randomly let go to see if the arm will fall back down to the floor with gravity or remains upright (c).

Tips for Teachers

- You can also introduce the concepts of kinesthesia and the kinesthetic sense here. Discuss the concept of muscle tone vs. muscle tension related to the following: [1] lying in Constructive Rest ("holding" versus "yielding" your weight), and [2] standing alignment (tone needed to remain upright versus tension). Further related topics can include the difference between low tone (limp or flaccid muscles) and high tone (tense, hypotonic, or spastic muscles), which you can include depending upon the context of the class and your own level of knowledge.

Exploration: Circles—Arms and Shoulders

(20 minutes)

PURPOSE. To balance the use of muscles around your joints; to focus your mind through imagery and spatial intent; to recognize the amount of muscular effort being expended in your movements; to learn to regulate your muscular effort; to experience using only the muscular effort needed to produce easy, efficient movement in your shoulders.

Activity

This activity is done in Constructive Rest.

- Rest here and let your body be supported by the earth.
- Now place one arm over your belly. Next you will be lifting that arm toward the ceiling, progressing one by one through the joints of the shoulder, elbow, wrist, hand, and fingers. Begin when you are ready, extending up through your shoulder, elbow, wrist, hand, and last, through your fingers.
- Now reach your fingers to the ceiling so that your shoulder comes up off the floor, reaching up as far as you can go. *(Fig. 10.9a.)* Then let your shoulder relax back down, but keep your fingers still reaching up. *(Fig. 10.9b.)* Can you really let go of the muscles around your shoulder joint? Let the earth support your weight.
- Now imagine that you have a colored crayon or pencil at the tip of your longest finger, and "draw" a tiny circle on the ceiling by circling your arm. Are you still relaxing your shoulder, letting your weight be supported by the floor? See if you can use the least amount of effort necessary as you draw the circle *(Fig. 10.8)*.
- Go slowly, and let your circle get a little bit bigger ... a little bigger ... a little bigger.
- Keep going until you are drawing the largest circle you can. Go slowly, and be sure to check back in and see if you are still using as little effort as possible. This allows you to use your deeper intrinsic muscles while you relax the larger muscles. *(Watch to see that the larger muscles of the shoulder are released. You can work individually with students by holding the wrist and asking them to let you hold up their arm. Once the muscles have released, ask if they feel a difference. You can also put one hand under the shoulder, and let them relax down into your hand. This allows you to feel if they have relaxed or may still be holding tension there.) (Fig. 10.9c.)*
- Once you've drawn a few of your biggest circles, start to make them smaller, smaller, and smaller, until you find you are making just a small circle on the ceiling again. Keep making your circle smaller until your arm is resting in the center.
- Relax your arm back down, this time first letting the fingers relax, and then the wrist, the elbow, and the shoulder, until your arm is lying by your side.

- Take a moment to feel that arm and shoulder. What do you notice? Feel both of your arms now. What do you notice? Take a moment to feel both sides of your body. What do you feel? *(You can invite students to stand at this point to experience any changes as well, or just continue to the next side.)*

Repeat the directions for the other side.

Variation

Students can perform the arm circles while lying on one side, which provides for a fuller range of motion of the scapula and engages more of the muscles of the back. You can begin with the original Circles exploration and then repeat it using this variation on another day.

Discussion

- What did you feel? Did you notice any difference between the side that you moved and the side that you didn't? If so, why do you think that was? (*Refer to the skeleton to discuss the relationship between the shoulder girdle and the arms.)*
- What did you notice as you did your circles? Did the circle feel smooth, or did you feel any jerking or "rough spots" as you traced your circle?
- Was it hard to use less effort? What else did you experience? Did anyone experience anything different?

You can repeat this exploration again on a subsequent day after having reviewed the specific anatomy to clarify the shape and articulation of the shoulder joint.

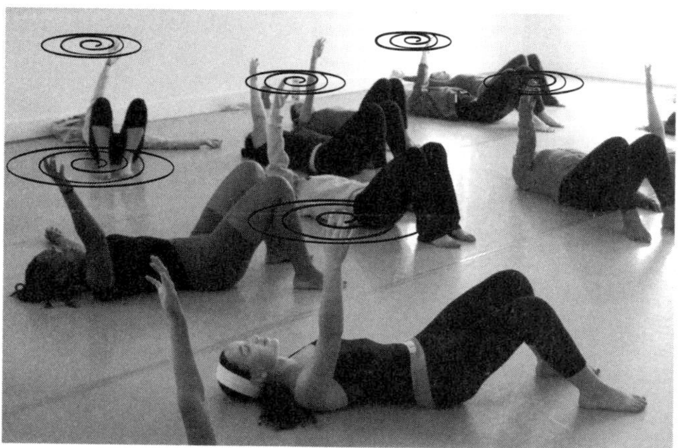

Fig. 10.8. The circling activity helps students understand how their habitual patterns may affect or limit their movement. As they discover, learning to reduce their muscular effort often increases both their flexibility and their actual range of motion, essential aspects of moving with ease and avoiding injury.

Tips for Teachers

- The type of jerking movements mentioned in the discussion will often occur as the more extrinsic muscles are releasing and students are getting used to a new way of using just the deeper, more intrinsic, muscles at the joints. Those who experience this are generally able to circle the arm more smoothly after a few minutes, especially if guided to slow down the movement.
- If students continue to have difficulty, suggest that they stop and rest, and then continue this at another time. This likely indicates a previous shoulder injury or more tension in the shoulders. Students can also be guided to reflect on this to see if they discover any correlations. For example, many students find that they carry more tension in one shoulder than the other, only to realize that this is the side on which they carry a heavy bag or backpack throughout the week! Making such discoveries can inspire them to make further adjustments in their lives that support the health of their bodies.
- When students first try this activity, you may find that some students extend fully through the arm and hand, but not through the fingers. You can assist those students through touch by gently extending their fingers for them with your own hands, as you follow along with the circling motion. To initiate this, ask the student first if you can help them by touching their hand. This is important in touch-based interventions in general, but especially in a case such as this, in which they will likely have their eyes closed when you approach them. Also tell them that you will be following their movement, rather than directing it, so that they will keep initiating the movement on their own. This intervention helps bring heightened proprioceptive awareness to the hands and particularly to the fingers *(Fig. 10.9d)*.

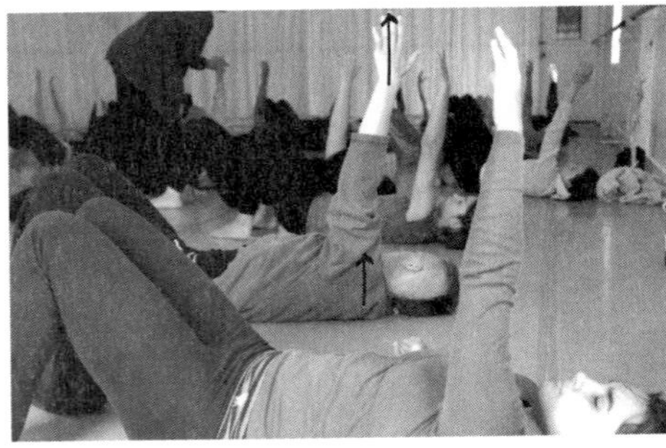
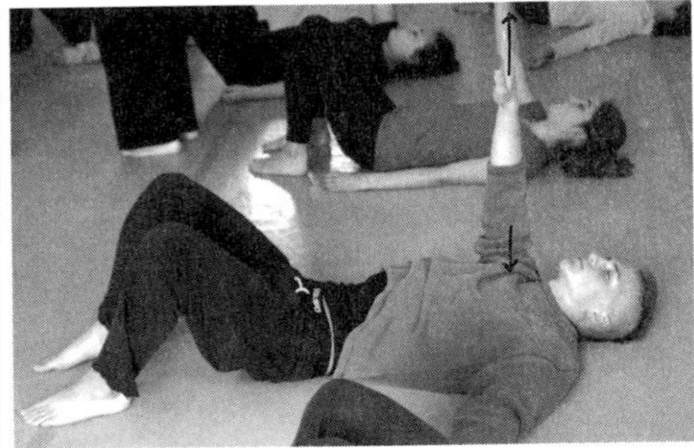

Fig. 10.9a, b. In the arm circles exploration, students first reach their arm up and lift the shoulder off the ground (a), and then allow it to drop back down to the floor to help relax the shoulder (b), before circling the arm on their own timing.

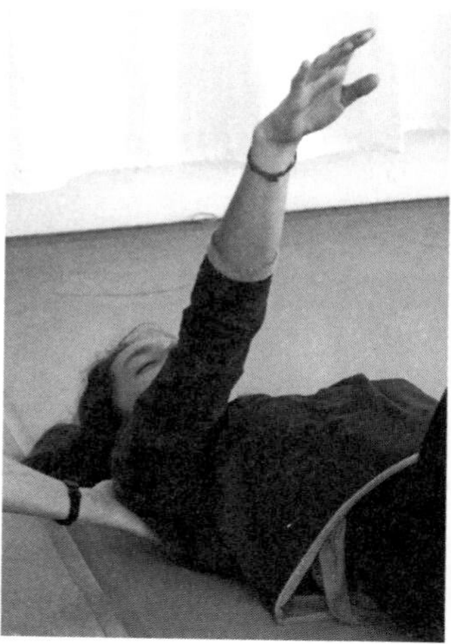
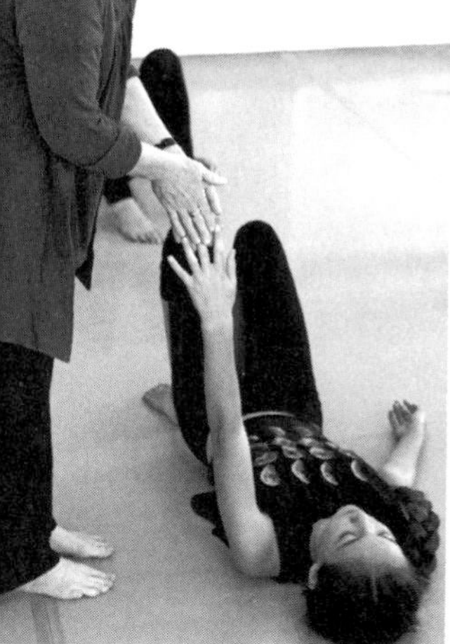

Fig. 10.9c, d. You can also assist students to feel the release of the shoulder by placing your hand under the shoulder and prompting them to drop their weight into your hand (c). You can also assist them in lengthening through the full length of the arm, hand, and fingers by gently extending the fingers with your hands (d).

Exploration: Circles—Legs and Hips

(20 minutes)

PURPOSE. To balance the use of muscles around your joints; to focus your mind through imagery and spatial intent; to recognize the amount of muscular effort being expended in your movement; to learn to regulate your muscular effort; to experience using only the muscular effort needed to produce easy, efficient movement in your hips.

Activity

This activity is done in Constructive Rest.

- Rest here and let your body be supported by the earth.
- Now gently lift one leg up toward your chest, so it is perpendicular to the floor. Keep your knee, lower leg, and foot relaxed.
- Using the center of your knee, "draw" a tiny circle on the ceiling, the way you did with your fingers when moving your arm. You can tap the spot at the center of your knee to feel it more distinctly if you like. Be sure that the opposite leg

stays still while you move the other side. Let your foot and leg help to stabilize the supporting side while you draw your circle. Move very slowly while drawing your circles. *(Fig. 10.10.)*

- See if you can make your circle without also letting your hips move. *(Watch to see that the leg is moving separately from the pelvic girdle.)* Then allow your circle to get a little bigger and bigger as you go. Still go slowly.
- Begin to make your circle smaller and smaller again, as you did with your arm circles, until your leg is resting back in the center.
- Place that leg down again, so you are resting in Constructive Rest again. Bring your attention to the leg and hip on that side. What do you notice? Feel both legs, both sides of your body. What do you experience? Is this the same on each side, or different?

Repeat the directions for the opposite side.

End with students standing to do their body scan.

Discussion

- What did you feel? Did you notice any difference between the side that you moved and the side that you didn't? If so, why do you think that was? *(Refer to the skeleton to discuss the relationship between the femur and the pelvis.)*

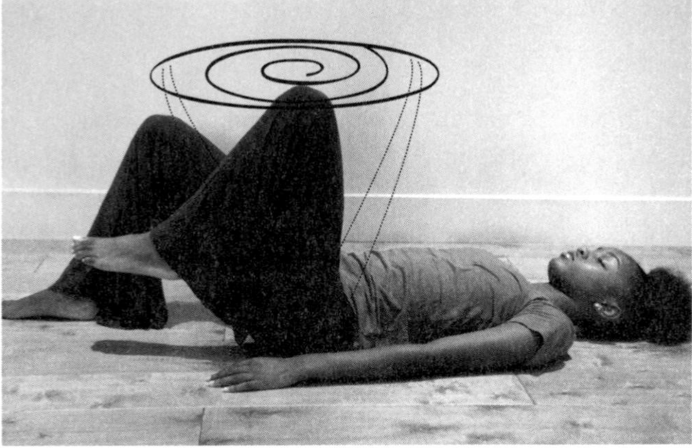

Fig. 10.10. In the Leg circles exploration, students can begin to release excess tension in the hips and release the femur into the acetabulum. When standing after this activity, students often express feeling more "grounded," as they begin to feel more weight in their feet. They also find it easier to balance, such as when standing on one leg or the other, as well.

- What did you notice as you made your circles? Did the circle feel smooth, or did you feel any jerking or "rough spots" as you traced your circle?
- Was it hard to use less effort? What else did you experience? Did anyone experience anything different?
- Was it easier to make these circles with your arms? Or with your legs? What did you notice? How was it the same or different?

You can repeat this exploration again on a subsequent day after having reviewed the specific anatomy to clarify the shape and articulation of the hip joint.

Variations

If students are having difficulty isolating the leg (femur) from the hip (pelvis) in this activity, you can have them explore the difference between moving the femur on its own, or allowing the pelvic halves to respond. This can be done sitting or standing. In sitting with legs outstretched, the pelvis will be stabilized, and students can just explore the rotation of the leg in the hip socket; in standing, both the leg and pelvis can move.

Students can try balancing on one leg and then the other both before and after doing this activity, and then compare the two experiences. Often they find that it is much easier to balance after engaging in this activity, as it heightens their proprioceptive awareness in the hip joints.

Tips for Teachers

- Many students have excess tension in their hips, which restricts movement of the legs and pelvis. With this activity, then, it is quite common for them to experience jerky movements in the hips as the bigger muscles let go and the head of the femur settles into the hip socket or acetabulum. The variation above can help them experience this deep release, so you may even introduce it as a precursor to the previous exploration of circling the leg.
- Ideally students can wear loose-fitting long pants like sweatpants for these activities. Otherwise, if they are wearing tight pants, like jeans, it can be difficult to explore a full range of movement at the hip socket. Conversely, if they are wearing revealing clothing, like loose-fitting shorts or a skirt, they may feel self-conscious doing this, particularly when lying down and circling their legs. Advise students to dress comfortably and appropriately for somatic work.

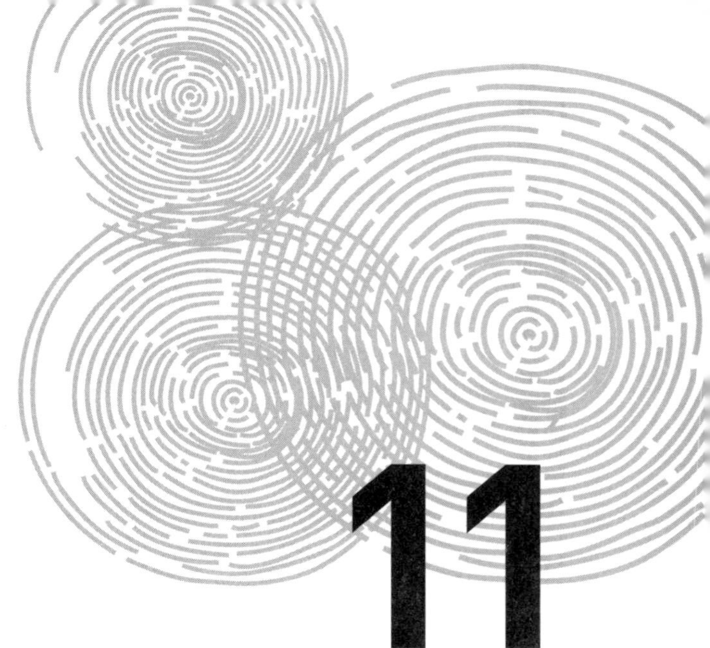

11

Organs

While the explorations presented so far have primarily focused on the musculoskeletal system, these next activities begin to help students differentiate the skeleton from the organs, as well as to integrate them. The skeletal system provides support for our bodies in gravity and also protects the internal organs. We could consider the skeletal structure to be our "container," while seeing the organs as the "contents." The organs also serve as support for the skeleton, with their soft resilience serving as a counterforce to our structure.[1] Exploring through movement, we can feel the weight and fullness of our organs—gaining vitality, stability, and fluid, three-dimensional support.

Whether consciously or unconsciously, we also associate the organs with our inner lives and emotions, as our language often reveals. For instance, we search for the essence of something to "get at the heart of the matter," or express our difficulty accepting a situation that we "can't stomach," or refer to someone who acts boldly as having "a lot of guts." In this sense, our organs represent our deepest core and authenticity; accessing our organ presence puts us more in touch with ourselves and can evoke confidence from feeling the sensation of inner support. On the other hand, we may feel embarrassed if our stomach gurgles when we are hungry or have indigestion, for instance, or try not to burp in public; we often restrict our organs to satisfy social conventions. Especially in adolescence, the need to conform makes the ramifications of any missteps feel even greater. This is compounded by a multilayered relationship with sexuality, as teens struggle to relate to both inner experience and outer social, cultural, and religious norms.

With time and structured guidance to focus on the internal organs and the emotional centers of the body, students have an opportunity to develop self-awareness and come into a healthier relationship with themselves.

Vitality and Rest

As students discovered in their study of joints, we *feel* our position in space through an intricate system of sensory nerves called proprioceptors. These specialized nerve cells help us to register our body position and move with awareness. Your internal organs provide another level of awareness—along with the inner vitality necessary for survival, through processes such as digestion, circulation, and breathing. For instance, notice how you are feeling right now. What comes to your awareness? Are you tired? Thirsty? Hungry? Agitated? Calm? What about your breathing … is it shallow? Or deep? Noticing your internal sensations with a level of specificity is related to another set of sensory nerves, your interoceptors, located in your internal organs—such as in the circulatory, respiratory, and digestive systems. These specialized nerves help you to regulate your body's homeostasis and relate to your sense of well-being.

Together, your proprioceptors and interoceptors contribute to a sense of full body awareness. Yet just as tension in your muscles can limit your proprioceptive awareness, you can develop related tensions that limit your *interoceptive* awareness as well. For example, a pattern of holding in your abdominal muscles causes tension in the intestines that then affects your digestion. Various postural holdings may restrict other internal organs: tension in your upper chest or back can restrict your lungs, while tension in your lower back can compress your kidneys. As you learn to allow your organs (contents) to rest within your bony cavities (container), you begin to release excess muscular tension and allow your body to *soften.* Beginning to rest and feel the weight of your organs can be a first step to rejuvenating them.

In the first exploration, students are guided to lie on the floor and rest their organs—such as relaxing the lungs and heart in the rib cage, the digestive organs in the abdomen, and even the brain in the skull. Resting the organs is important to experience in all four dimensions—on your front, your back, and both sides of your body. Initially, some people find it easiest to feel their organs when resting on the belly or ventral side, where you can more directly feel the soft front surface of your body against the floor. After lying down like this for some time, and then coming back up to stand and walk around the room, students are often surprised at how different they feel! Experiencing the weight of the organs helps them to slow down and gives them a more grounded and full-bodied sense of themselves.

When you have this kind of internal support from the organs, less muscular effort is also needed to support yourself upright in gravity. Although primarily the bones of the skeletal system should bear the majority of the weight as it passes through your body, in healthy embodiment the organs also provide internal support, like a balloon expanding outward. In fact, in addition to having our "skeletal alignment," we also have our "bellital alignment," a concept coined by somatic educator Caryn McHose to refer to the three-dimensional presence of the organs.[2]

How do you gain this internal support of your bellital alignment? One way is through bringing tone to the organs, which is developed through compression. In the same way that you gain proprioceptive awareness through compression of your joints—so that the nerve cells "register" each other, helping you to feel your position in space—you gain interoceptive awareness from the pressure exerted on your organs through gravity. Yet if you are always in the same relationship to gravity, your organs bear weight in an uneven way, such that the *base* of the organ is always compressed by supporting your weight.[3] By changing your position in gravity, you shift the weight-bearing side of the organ, which helps to strengthen its tone.[4] With today's more sedentary lifestyle, you may find that you are most often in an upright position, such as when standing, sitting, and driving. Students have this same problem from hours of sitting at desks and computers.

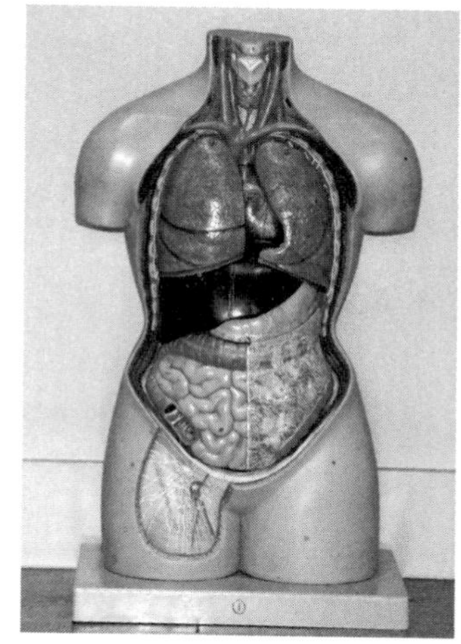

Fig. 11.1. Organ model.

To counteract this tendency and revitalize the organs, these activities serve to "mix things up a bit" by providing a more rich and varied relationship with gravity, such as in a next activity that involves simply rolling along the floor. In this exploration, students first rest with a sense of the weight of the bones, and then roll across the floor letting the bones guide them. This provides a familiar starting point for them, since many of the activities have focused on the bones. Then they are guided to pause, bring their awareness to the weight of their organs, and then begin rolling again. Afterward, they can stand, move, and then see how they feel.

Another image that may be useful for students in this activity is to have them imagine that they are a single cell and are "pouring" their body weight as they roll, as described by Caryn McHose and Kevin Frank in an activity they call "Rolling and Pouring the Cell."[5] In this version, you imagine your body as a weighted, fluid-filled container, and notice the contact with the floor of each part of this outer container as you roll the fluid within. Here the emphasis is on the head, torso and pelvis, with the limbs of the arms and legs coming along for the ride as you roll and pour your body weight. This activity also encourages the establishment of a boundary between self and other, establishing your location in space, both physically and emotionally.[6]

All of these initial activities awaken a more full-bodied sense of the weight and presence of the organs. They can also provide a context for students to learn about specific organs in the upper torso and abdominal cavity, after gaining an initial experiential sense of them, through further discussion and by looking at organ models or anatomy plates.

Exploration: Resting the Organs

(20–30 minutes)

PURPOSE. To release excess muscular tension by resting the organs; to gain a fuller perception of your body to include your organs; to experience the organ support of your "bellital alignment" along with your skeletal alignment.

Activity

Begin with students standing and doing a body scan; then progress to lying in Constructive Rest and lead a shortened version of body scanning that focuses on feeling the support and weight of the skeletal system. Then continue:

- Now as you rest here, begin to bring your awareness to your organs, inside of your skeletal container, and allow these to be supported by the earth as well. Relax your lungs and heart in your rib cage, and your digestive organs in belly and abdomen. Rest your brain inside your skull. Your eyes can also rest in their bony sockets, like pools of water.
- Feel your whole body relaxed and supported by the earth. *(Pause here for a minute or so.)*
- Now let your knees drop to one side or the other, and then gently roll onto your right side. Feel your bones and organs resting in this new position.
- When you are ready, roll over onto your belly. Adjust your head so you are comfortable, and rest in this new position. Take a few deep breaths in … and out … and let all your organs soften into the earth. *(You can suggest that students can add any sound on the exhale, such as a sigh as described previously, if that has worked well with your group.)*
- Now you can just rest here for a few minutes. *(Pause for 3–5 minutes; it's best if you don't talk during this time.)*
- Take another deep breath, in and out, and when you are ready you can roll to your left side now, and rest there for a moment. *(Pause.)* Keeping your eyes closed,

take your time to come up to sitting and then into a crouched position, and then slowly push back onto your feet and pause there a moment.

- Then slowly roll back up to standing, still keeping your eyes closed. Just notice how this feels. *(Alternately, you can specifically guide students to feel their skeletal alignment and also feel their organs as they roll back up, naming this as their "bellital alignment." Or you can save naming that for the discussion.)*
- When you come to standing, take a few moments to do your body scan again, and see what you experience. Does this feel the same as or different from when you stood at the beginning before lying down?
- When you are ready, open your eyes and take a walk around, or move in any way you would like. How does this feel?

Variation

Students can also then engage in other movement practices, such as practicing the Sun Salutation in chapter 8, with an added focus on organ support.

Discussion

- How do you feel? What did you experience when doing your body scan at the end? *(Often students will notice a wide variety of changes, from feeling more grounded and heavy to feeling taller and stronger.)* Did anyone have a different experience?

You can then discuss the difference between skeletal and bellital alignment, using any supplemental materials that may be helpful. Students can also learn about specific organs and name them, by referring to the skeletal and organ models or the anatomy coloring plates—first by sharing what they know—and then with you adding any further information.

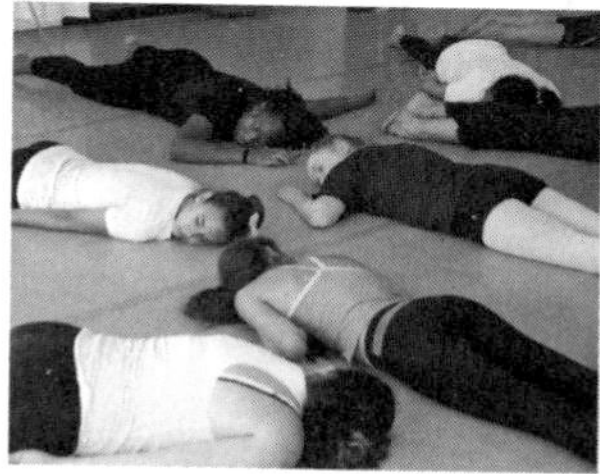
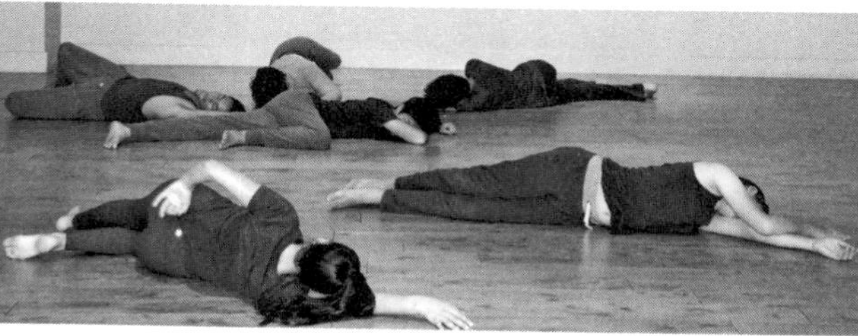

Fig. 11.2a, b. Resting the organs: Resting on the belly, or ventral side, can help bring awareness to the organs through the soft surface of the body (a). It's also helpful to rest in all four dimensions—on the front, back, and both sides of your body—as students change their position as well (b).

Tips for Teachers

- The first time you lead this activity, you can use the general suggestion to "rest your organs." Later on, after students have looked at the organ model or colored related anatomy plates, you can repeat the activity and include more specificity. For instance, you can suggest that they rest their brain in the skull; the lungs and heart in the upper torso; the stomach, liver, gallbladder, pancreas, kidneys, spleen, and small and large intestines in the mid-abdomen; and the reproductive organs, bladder, and part of the large intestines in the pelvic bowl. This serves as both a good cognitive review and a method of bringing more focused attention to particular organs.
- Making sound can also be a fun way to enliven your organ presence. Encouraging sound in this activity can help students to relax further, while the vibration of the sound itself helps to awaken the organ tissue. As another way to explore this, you can even try singing a song together, and have students notice how they feel beforehand and then afterward!
- Though as a starting point students can rest on their belly side for 3–5 minutes, you can gradually increase the time when repeating the activity, extending it to 10–20 minutes. You can encourage them to shift their positions as needed, or to rest on their belly the entire time if preferred. We often underestimate the benefits of deep relaxation. Contacting the organs often initiates deep layers of release in the body, so more time here may be necessary and beneficial.

HOME PROJECTS

- Students can color anatomy plates related to specific organs; they can also research particular systems, such as the digestive or circulatory systems, in relation to their interests.

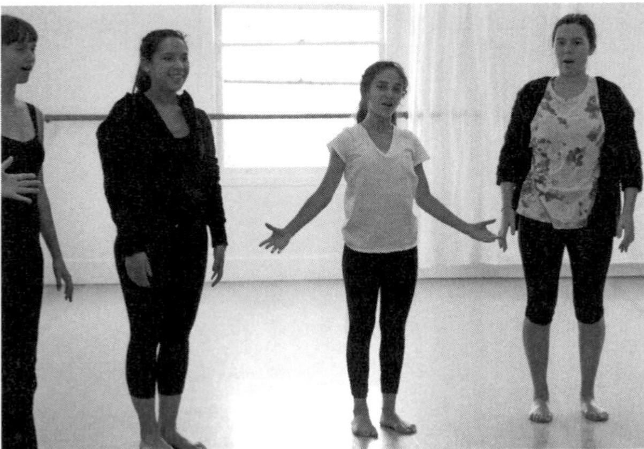

Fig. 11.3. Teens experiment with making sound, which helps to vitalize full-bodied organ presence as the tones vibrate within the body.

Exploration: Rolling from the Organs

(20 minutes)

PURPOSE. To differentiate between skeletal system initiation ('container') and organ initiation ('contents'); to awaken interoceptive awareness of our organs; to encourage an increased range of movement through the internal viscera (internal organs and fascia).

Activity

Students can begin standing and do their body scan, then come into Constructive Rest. They should have enough space between them to be able to roll several feet in either direction.

- Take a moment to feel yourself resting here, letting yourself relax and be supported by the earth. Take a few breaths, in and out.
- Now begin to bring awareness to the bones in your body, your full skeleton resting on the earth. Feel where you are taking your weight. Which parts of your body are heaviest, which are lighter?
- Now begin to stretch out so your legs are long and your arms are up over your head, but still resting on the floor. Feel the length of the bones of your arms, legs, and torso.
- Begin to roll along the floor, feeling your bones as you roll. *(Leave a few minutes for them to explore this.)*
- The next time you roll to your belly, rest there a moment. Take a few breaths in and out.
- Now bring your awareness to your organs, the contents within the container of your bones. Feel your lungs and heart, nestled inside your rib cage; your intestines and organs of your abdomen, in your belly and pelvis; your brain inside your skull.
- Let all of these organs rest, your organs resting on the earth. Take a breath in, and out.
- Rest here, feel your organs being supported by the earth. *(Pause for a minute.)*
- Begin to roll again, but this time as you roll, let your organs lead the way. Can you feel your organs as you roll on the earth?
- Rest again and see how you feel. What do you notice? Come back to Constructive Rest again now, and rest here. Does this feel the same or different, from when you were lying in this position earlier?
- When you are ready, take your time to push up to one side, and sit for a bit, still with your eyes closed. Then find your way back up to standing in whatever way you like.

- How does it feel to be standing now? What do you notice? Take a moment with your eyes closed to do your body scan again and see how that feels.
- When you are ready, open your eyes and take a walk around. How do you feel? What do you notice?

Students can then share their experience in partners or small groups.

Variations

Students can come to one side of the room and take turns rolling across the room. Have one line of students lie down and go first, and then when there is ample free space, the next group can lie down and begin to roll as well. In this variation, they can all roll across the room first from the bones, and then do this a second time with a focus on rolling from the organs. Alternately, you can have them roll halfway across the room with one focus, and then switch to the other mode when they get to the middle of the room as they roll the rest of the way.

Students can, of course, also just roll freely through the space and explore these variations on their own, but then keep in mind that they may also gently collide with each other! This can bring a fun and spontaneous quality to the activity. In other instances, it may create unnecessary problems, so you can assess what is best in each situation.

Discussion

- What did you experience? What did you notice? How did you feel when walking around after doing this activity?
- What changed as you switched your focus from your bones to your organs? *(Often students will find they move more slowly and with more weightedness when initiating from the organs.)* What did you feel? What did you prefer? Why?
- What did you learn? Were there any surprises?

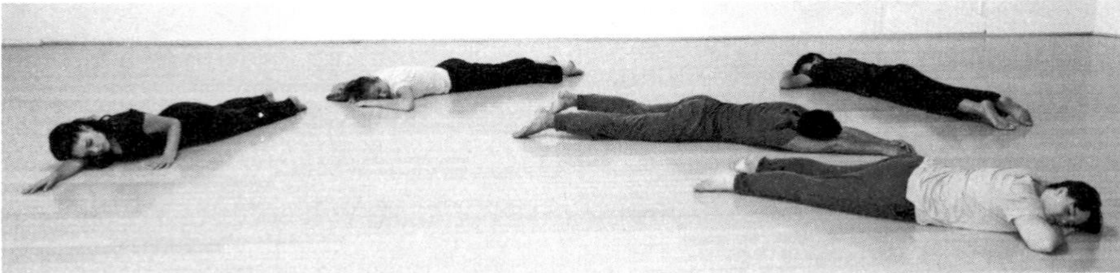

Fig. 11.4. Teens rest on their ventral side before beginning to roll from the organs; for many of us, rolling on the floor can be a novel orientation to moving and relating with gravity that helps us to slow down and enlivens our interoceptive and proprioceptive awareness alike.

Moving with Three-Dimensional Support

As explored in the previous activity, you can learn to shift your attention from one body system to another—from the bones to the organs, for instance—as a means of changing the initiation and quality of your movement.[7] This is another way to experience the three-dimensional fullness and support of the organs. In a next activity, students learn to differentiate between moving from the rib cage (the container) and moving from their internal organs within the rib cage, the heart and lungs (the contents). A variation of this activity focuses on the lower body as well, by lying in Constructive Rest and experiencing the pelvic bowl (the container) and moving from the internal organs of the intestines (the contents).

Another variation includes using warm-water-filled balloons to represent the organs. Students can first hold them to evoke the weight and soft malleable tone of the organs. They can also place them on the torso and move with them, imagining the organs inside, which encourages softening in the musculature. This also provides a fun and tactile way to invite a deeper source of movement initiation. In another example, as they sense the fullness of the organs in the lower abdomen and pelvis and their connection to the legs and feet, they may feel more grounded. Another way to explore the organs is to feel their buoyancy and lightness, such as the lungs as they support your rib cage; in this case you can use air-filled balloons. These activities encourage an enlivened interoceptive awareness of the organs to expand students' movement and expression.[8]

While we generally think of the neuromuscular system as being responsible for initiating movement, all of our body systems are engaged when we move. Movement that is initiated from the organs can also help to stimulate new proprioceptive and interoceptive pathways. This is important because, as Bonnie Bainbridge Cohen has noted, many injuries occur from moving without internal organ support, such that the muscles and joints are strained beyond their range.[9] This can occur in sports, dance, yoga, or a variety of daily movement activities such as housecleaning or lifting heavy items, or in recreational activities like swimming, skiing, kayaking, or playing volleyball. As we learn to access organ support when moving, we help protect ourselves from injury. Health and vitality depend on fully developed proprioceptive and interoceptive sensory awareness—with movement as the key to this inner body intelligence.

Organs also represent our deepest reserve and vital life-force, and can be a storehouse for many other emotions, beyond a sense of confidence already discussed. Both positive and negative feelings can emerge, even in something as simple as rolling on the floor, or initiating movement from the organs of your torso or pelvis. For instance, here is what one student had to say in her journal about doing the activity of holding the rib cage and moving from the organs of the lungs and heart:

> *It was a moving experience to "hold" and become aware of my bellowing lungs and pumping heart. I began to feel vulnerable and was glad to later experience the protection of lying on my stomach. Exposing the skin is one kind of vulnerability, exposing the organs is another.*

To help students process their emotions, another activity draws on free-association journaling to give them a chance to express themselves, privately first, and then by sharing with others. The conversation that ensues from these journal entries can take many forms, from discussing the general "hush" we have in society about our internal organs and their functioning, to a recognition that we do have certain parts of our bodies that are more private and not to be openly shared. Students may become aware of feeling a hesitancy or fear of moving in certain ways, or a feeling of joy and freedom in moving in other ways. As students share their perceptions and open up to others' points of view, they begin to reflect on the many ways they experience movement, as well as how they perceive and are perceived by others.

Exploration: Moving from the Bones, Moving from the Organs[10]

(20 minutes)

PURPOSE. To differentiate between the skeletal system (the "container") and the internal organs (the "contents"); to experience initiating movement from both the contents and the container; to encourage moving from a fuller perception of your body to include the organs.

Activity

Have your students practice this exploration in either a seated or standing position.

- ❍ Place your hands on your rib cage in the front. Close your eyes. Feel the bones of your hands resting on the bones of your ribs. Now move your rib cage by moving your ribs, so you are turning to your right and to your left. Can you feel how your ribs lever into your spine, so that your spine rotates also as you turn from your ribs, so that you turn side to side? *(Pause while they explore this.)*
- ❍ Rest a moment.

- Now place your hands on your rib cage again, this time a little more to your sides. Close your eyes. Imagine what is inside your rib cage.... What do you see? Breathe. What do you feel? Let's consider your rib cage a container for all that is inside. The organs inside your rib cage are the contents. Let your hands "hold" the contents. What are you holding? What organs are in your rib cage? Now move your "contents" inside the rib cage, turning to each side again, and feel them move as you turn side to side. *(Fig. 11.5.)* Rest a moment.
- Now let that movement move the ribs; the contents move the container.
- Now let the ribs move the organs; the container moves the contents.
- Do this again, but this time try to feel both the movement of the rib cage and of the internal organs.
- Now move around just as you want. *(Pause as students explore this.)* Are you moving from the contents or the container? Can you tell?
- Take a minute to walk around the room or move in any way you want. What do you feel as you move? What do you notice?

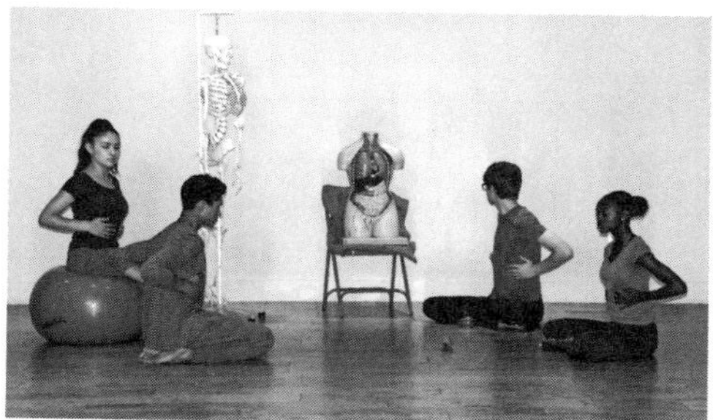

Fig. 11.5. Students rest the hands on the ribs (the container) and feel the organs within (the contents) to initiate movement from within.

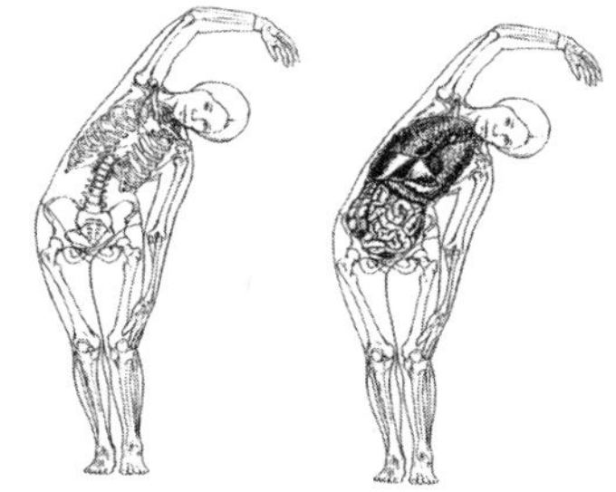

Fig. 11.6. Moving from the container (bones of the skeleton) versus the contents (the organs); actively engaging our organs helps us to move with more internal support.

Variations

Lower Body: In study of the abdominal cavity and pelvis the initial activity can be repeated while lying in Constructive Rest, first moving from the big bones of the ilium, sacrum, and ischium, and then from the organs of the pelvic girdle. You can then similarly use the organ model or drawings to discuss the specific organs in this region.

Water Balloons: Before beginning this exploration, you can also use small warm-water-filled balloons for students to hold to get a physical sense of the weight and movement of the organs. I prefer to prepare these in advance and keep them hidden until I will be using them. You can gather students in a circle and have them close their eyes and put out their hands, and then you can give the balloons out one by one. *(Fig. 11.7.)*

You can guide students in exploring this process in several ways. You might first invite them to, with eyes closed, just feel and experience the weight and temperature of the balloons in their hands, and then begin to move them gently *(Fig. 11.8a)*. They can also then place them on their torsos, at the chest or belly, as they move their spine in various ways, such as they have just done in this activity *(Fig. 11.8b)*. Or when lying in Constructive Rest, they can rest the warm balloons on their bodies *(Fig. 11.8c)*; they can also open their eyes and roll the balloons gently along the floor to visually see the outer balloon (container) and inner water (contents) both moving. They can also just move on their own with the intention of initiating and supporting their movement from within. *(Fig. 11.9.)* There are many creative variations you can discover together—using a balance of directed guidance and more improvisational modes of exploring—as appropriate to the comfort level of your group.

Use your own discernment as to whether the group can handle this responsibly, and be sure they use caution so as not to break the balloons. Water balloons and regular air-filled balloons can also be used on separate days, or they can be used in conjunction to explore as a means of comparison.

Discussion

- What did you experience? Was it easier to initiate your movement from either the contents or the container for you? Why do you think that was? How does the quality of your movement change? What happened when you moved around without deciding which to focus on? Was the system you moved from then the same one you felt was easiest at the beginning of the exploration? What did you notice as you moved or walked around? Were you more aware of your "contents," i.e., your organs, than before? What organs were you aware of? How did you feel when doing this?
- *(For variation with balloons)* What was your experience from holding the balloon? What did you feel from moving with the balloon? Were there any surprises? Did anyone have a different experience?

Tips for Teachers

- When facilitating any of these explorations that explore the organs, students can also rest in what is called "child's pose" in yoga, so they are curled up and resting the chest on the legs, with the arms relaxed by the sides. This position is another way to feel the fullness of the organs more distinctly, while providing an integrative respite from the activities themselves as needed.

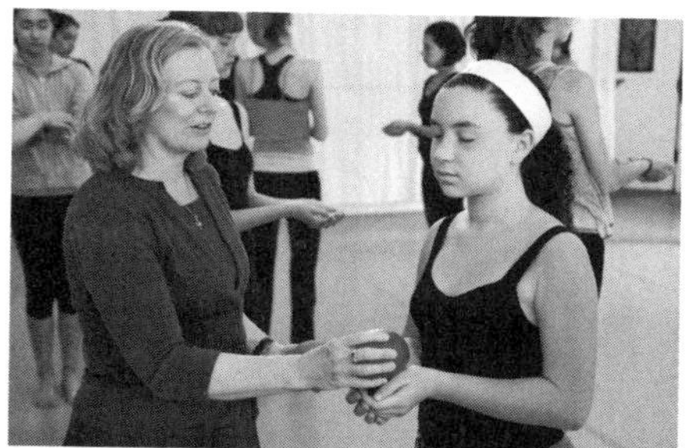

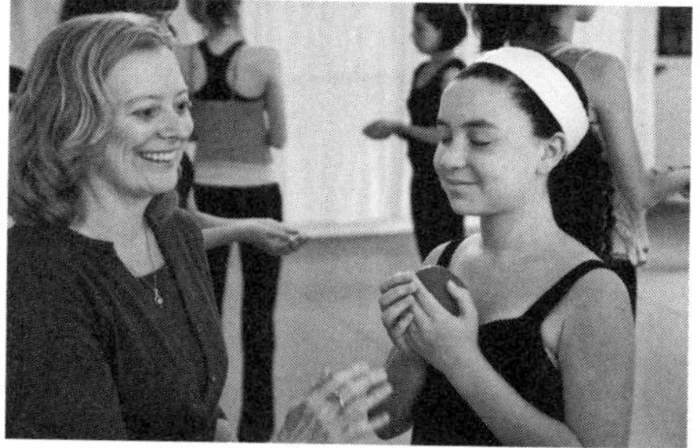

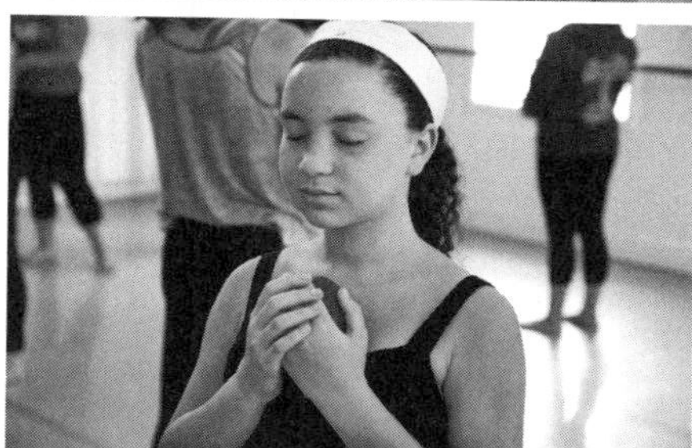

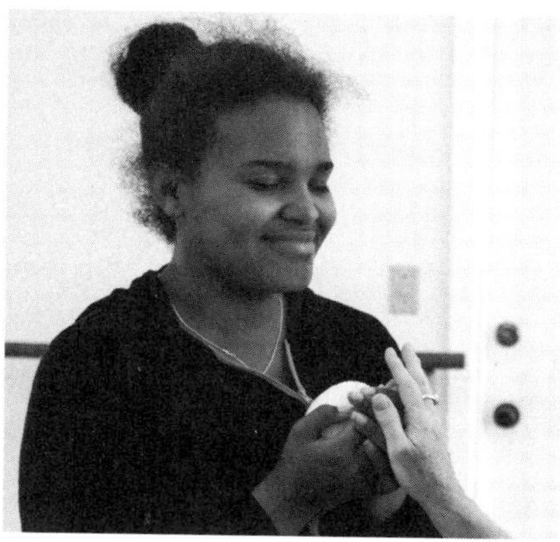

Fig. 11.7a, b, c, d. Variation: Handing out water balloons. Students close their eyes and are each given a warm water balloon to represent their organs. They then place them on their bodies to help them imagine and focus within on their organs.

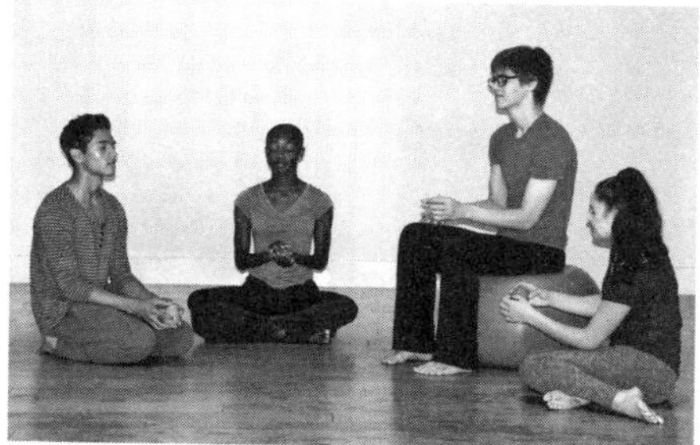

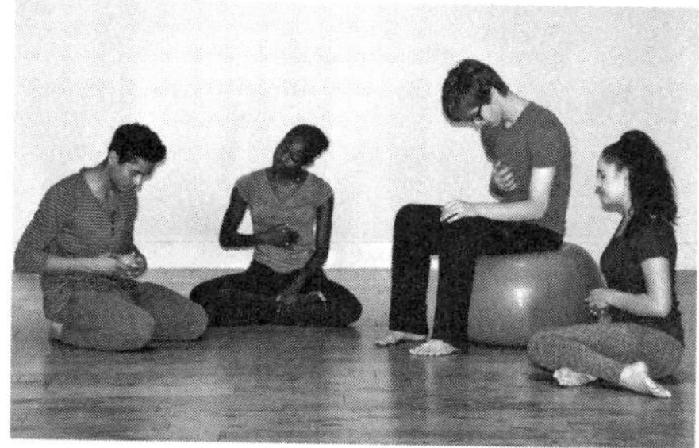

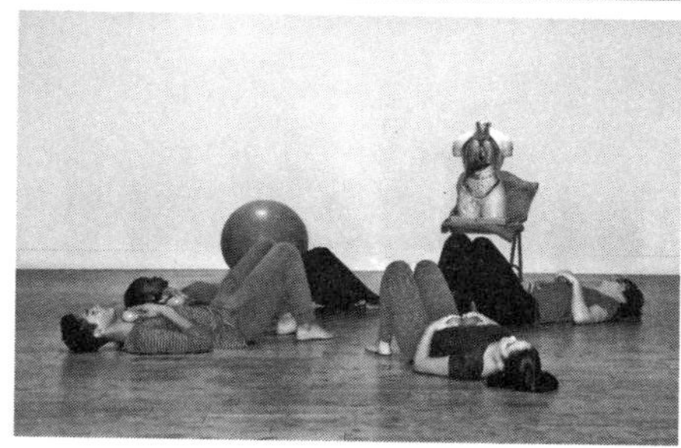

Fig. 11.8a, b, c. After holding the water balloons, students begin to slowly move with them; their body tone and posture inevitably soften in response. They can also just rest with the balloons on their bodies.

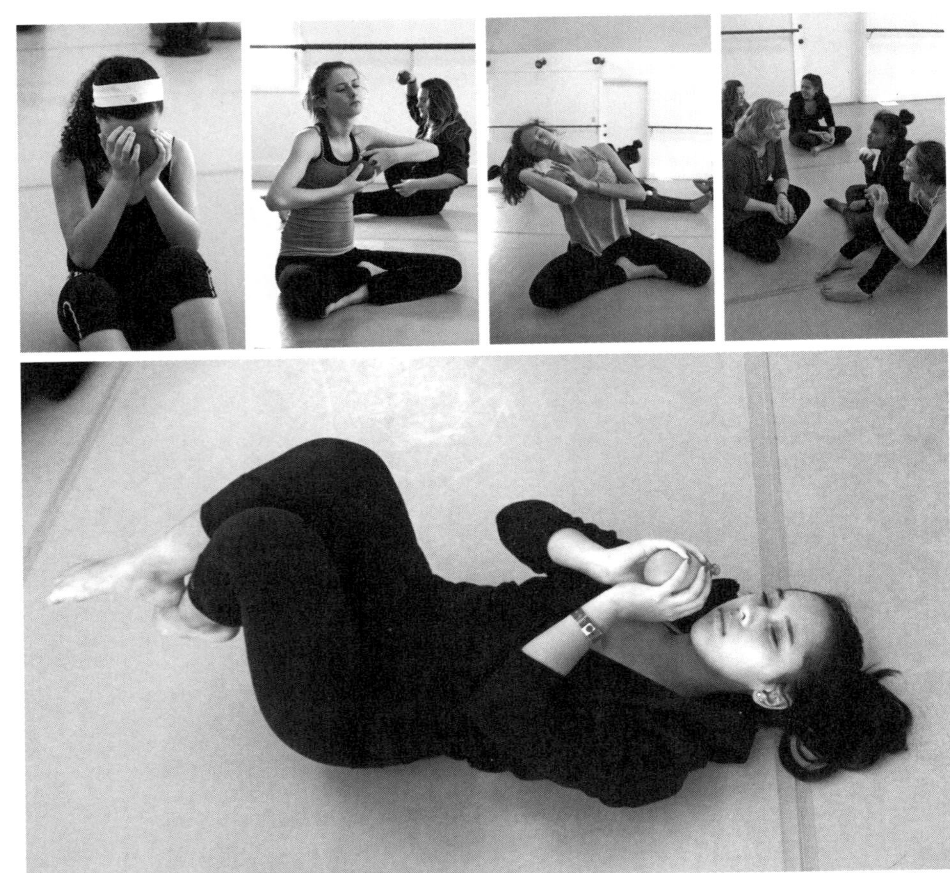

Fig. 11.9a, b, c, d, e. Teens begin to experiment with moving from the organs while holding the water balloons, and then sharing together about their experiences.

Exploration: Organs and Emotions (Journal Entry)

(20–35 minutes)

PURPOSE. To provide a container for your thoughts, feelings, and reflections related to previous activities focused on the organs; to have an opportunity to share these with others and discuss them as a community; to encourage empathy and listening skills; to support recognition of cultural influences and perceptions that impact your relationship with your body and your movement.

Activity

MATERIALS

- Writing paper or journal
- Pen and drawing supplies

This activity can be done after either of the previous explorations.

Have students write in their journals, giving them a certain time frame for responding. You can either suggest that they write about their experience in the activity, leaving it very open-ended, or you may want to ask them to respond to a specific prompt to guide their writing, such as to the title: My Organs. You might also use more specific prompts on certain days, like My Heart or My Lungs. Students can also be invited to draw, instead of or in addition to writing.

Discussion

Students can talk together in pairs or small groups, and then write a brief list of main topics that came up in their group. This provides them with a way to later offer their comments more anonymously in the full group conversation if they choose. You can also have each group of students write their thoughts on big pieces of paper that they can then present to the full group in turn, or use the scribe method instead to record topics and themes as they emerge.

These are just some initial questions that can serve to get the conversation going, though you may prefer to improvise your own.

- What are some of the things that you wrote about? Did some themes also come up from your drawings? Were there some things you had in common? Or other things you experienced very differently? Why do you think that was? Did anyone have a different experience they want to share?

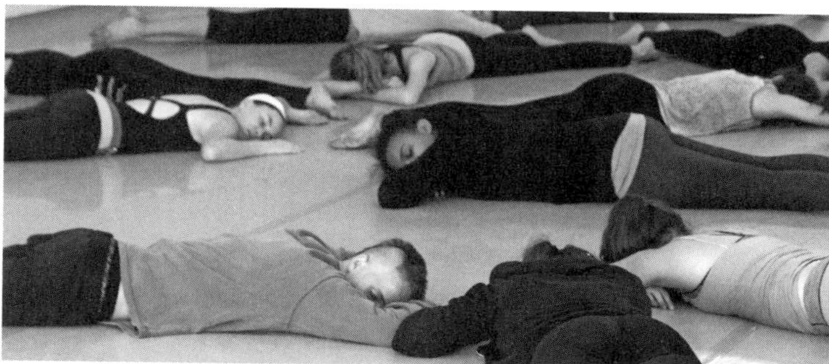

Fig. 11.10. Even resting on one's belly or being guided to focus on the organs can evoke deep feelings and associations; journal entries allow students to reflect on their various responses.

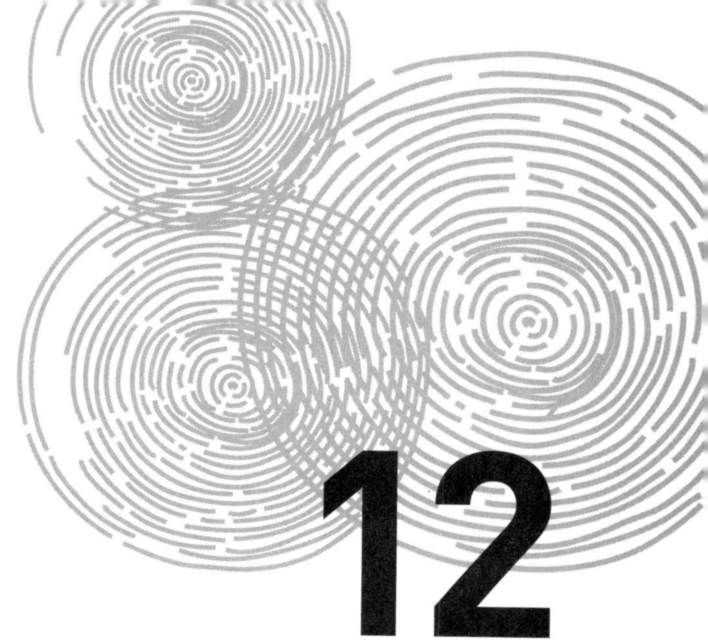

12

Fascia and Movement Qualities

Throughout the body there are many different types of tissues. Fascia is a type of connective tissue—a thin, viscous, continuous sheath throughout the body spanning all layers of your body—from skin, to muscles, to bones, to organs. Depending upon where it is located, fascia serves to support, separate, and provide ease of movement between muscle groups. For example, superficial fascia is located just under the skin and serves as a container and support for the whole body. The periosteum is a connective tissue on the outer layer of bone tissue to which tendons and ligaments attach. Muscles are encased in fascia that both separates specific muscle groups and permits their smooth passage over each other in muscular contractions. This fascia extends into the muscle mass as deep fascia that encases individual muscle fibers as well. Deep fascia also surrounds and supports all your blood vessels and vital organs.

Learning about and focusing on these deeper tissue layers, such as fascia and the internal organs, students enhance their body awareness and gain dynamic support in their movement.

Layers of Tissue

Initial explorations in this section help students use touch and movement as a means to learn about the various layers of tissue in the body. First through self-touch, students learn to differentiate among the skin, fascia, muscles, bones, and joints in their own arm.[1] Discovering and learning to differentiate these various layers of tissue enhances students' understanding of the complex interconnection of the body systems, while relieving tension and increasing their movement potential.

How is this possible that a simple activity of touching your arm can relieve tension? Since fascia interfaces throughout your body, restriction in one area will create a certain level of restriction throughout your entire body. Imagine, for example, pulling on one thread of a thick knitted sweater. Although only a small portion of the sweater's threads appear to tighten in response, the shape of the entire sweater is affected.[2] Likewise, release of tension in any area will begin to provide a certain level of increased ease throughout the body as well. Students experience this simple method of self-touch in the following exploration to distinguish between the levels of skin, fascia, muscle tissue, and bone in the body, and then notice the effect of their own touch on their body sensations and their movement.

Exploration: Variations in the Use of Touch

(10–15 minutes)

PURPOSE. To use varied methods of touch to distinguish between the levels of skin, fascia, muscle tissue, and bone; to physicalize the previous experiences of visualizing the body systems; to experience the use of self-touch for relief of tension and increased ease of movement.

Activity

Note: This activity builds on the exploration called Bone Touch from chapter 9, and assumes previous experience with that activity.

- Place your hand on your arm, in the middle of your forearm. Move your hand back and forth very lightly. What are you feeling? *(This is the skin on your arm.)* Feel how the skin slides from side to side? The layer just beneath the skin is your fascia.
- What is fascia—does anyone know? Where is it located in your body? *(You can add to what students say.)*
- Fascia is a continuous sheath of moist connective tissue in our bodies that surrounds all our muscles, encasing them and allowing them to glide over one another. You might picture something like slippery Saran Wrap! *(You can ask students if they've ever eaten cooked chicken—or seen raw chicken meat—and noticed the slippery covering along the length of the meat, which is the*

fascia. While some students may find this reference a bit "gross," they will often immediately get the idea from this image.)

- ❍ Now keep your hand in one place and use a little more pressure. Now what are you feeling? *(This is the muscle tissue.)*
- ❍ Lift your hand and repeat this in several different places on your arm. What differences do you feel? Now press a bit deeper until you get to a solid feeling under your fingers. What is this? *(This is bone. At the forearm, touching the sides of the arm helps to find the bone.)*
- ❍ You can imagine that you are going through sand, and letting it "ease" out of the way as you press more deeply to feel the bone.
- ❍ Keep your pressure firm and become aware of the bones in your fingers touching the bone of your arm. Move the bone of your arm with the bones of your hands.
- ❍ Lighten the pressure a bit and again you will be feeling the muscle. Become aware of the muscles of your fingers touching the muscles of your arm.
- ❍ Lighten your pressure again until you are again feeling the layer of the skin. Feel the skin of your fingers touching the skin of your arm.
- ❍ Now move the arm you were touching. Move both arms and notice any differences you feel. What do you notice?

Have students repeat this activity with the other arm.

Variation

This can also be done in partners, with one student finding the layers in the other student's arm. This would take longer to facilitate, and should be done only once students have some previous experience with self-touch and partner touch.

Discussion

- What did you notice? Could you feel the difference between your skin, fascia, muscle tissue, and bone? What did you feel when you moved both arms after having only touched one arm? Or once you had touched each arm? Was there any difference?
- Did anyone have a different experience?

Discuss the various layers of fascia, such as superficial fascia, periosteum, and deep fascia, adding any relevant information and referring to related plates from *The Anatomy Coloring Book*.

Types of Tissue, Movement Qualities, and Emotions

Our language demonstrates our intuitive understanding of the inherent connection between body, mind, and emotions. We use phrases that refer to states of being and associated psychophysical states all the time: such as "uptight" (a tense attitude or restricted expression), "laid-back" (an ease of character and relaxed body tone), or "cold-hearted" (not expressive or "heartfelt"). Body movement is an expression of the mind or our state of consciousness at the time. Likewise, movement can be a way to observe the expressions of the mind through the body—as well as a means to effect changes in the body-mind relationship.

All of the individual layers of tissue—like fascia, muscles, bones, and joints, for example—also relate to various modes of expression and vitality. In the following explorations, students move with a partner to explore moving from the joints, bones, muscles, and fascia. As students explore this they begin to discover the intimate body-mind connection. This process also allows them to expand their range of expressive movement qualities while discovering their own preferences. For instance, moving from the joints and synovial fluid often initiates laughter, while moving from the muscles initiates a sense of power and strength, or even feelings of resistance; moving from the bones elicits clarity and directness; and moving from the fascia often brings a sense of ease and interconnection.

These activities help students learn about themselves as well as gain tools to impact and change their physical and emotional state. By experiencing and discussing these variations, they begin to gain resources for continued self-care as they recognize the relationship between the quality of their movement and their expression and emotions. For example, if they are feeling tense and anxious, they might try sitting on a physioball and bouncing on it, which initiates easy movement in the joints and can bring back a sense of ease and playfulness that is recuperative. On the other hand, if they feel a bit scattered and distracted, they might try to move their arms with a sense of the bones, or move into a few yoga poses with a focus on supporting the movements through their bones: this initiates a state of mind that is direct and clear. Or if they are feeling lethargic or foggy, such as from sitting at the computer studying for a long period of time, they can take a brisk walk to get their body moving, which gets the blood moving and can initiate a feeling of greater vitality, warmth, and connection with life.

By simply changing our movement, we can change our mind, our mood, and our perceptions. These variations are explored in this next exploration. Students often feel enlivened from engaging in this activity, as it activates many qualities of movement and expression and invites a sense of self-empowerment and play.

Exploration: Moving from the Bones, Joints, Muscles, and Fascia[3]

(20–25 minutes)

PURPOSE. To differentiate initiation of movement of the joints, bones, muscles, and fascia; to use your focus to change the quality of our movement; to recognize your preferences for movement initiation, and any associated physical or emotional states.

Activity

Have your students work together in partners. (Journals may also be used; see variations.)

- *Movement from the joints:* Stand across from your partner and hold hands. Keep your arms out straight in front of you. Now release your wrists and shake them out. Let the shaking travel up to your elbows, and up to your shoulder girdle. Try to relax your muscles and let the shaking move you. Let it travel to your head and into your spine from your neck down to your sacrum, down into your pelvis to your legs, all the way down to your feet *(Fig. 12.1a).*
- Now let go of your partner's hands and stand with your eyes closed for a moment. How do you feel? What do you notice?

Students can take a moment to share their perceptions. Qualities and states of mind associated with movement in the joints are lightness and playfulness.

- *Movement from the bones:* Stand and close your eyes again. Slowly bring your weight forward over your toes and then back again to center. Now bring your weight back over your heels, and again back to center.
- Join hands with your partner again, this time so your palms are touching, and then close your eyes. Again bring your weight slowly over your feet, until you balance with your partner. Let your weight be supported by your partner through your hands. Try to release your muscles and let the bones support the weight, like you felt when lying in Constructive Rest. *(Fig. 12.1b.)*
- Now come back to standing in your own center, rather than leaning forward toward your partner, while still keeping your palms together. Begin to move your arms, using the bones as levers to move the bones of your partner. Can you do this with ease, or are you still holding extra tension somewhere in your body? Your shoulders? Neck? Hips? Legs? See if you can move with ease.

Take a moment to share perceptions. Qualities and states of mind associated with the movement from the bones are clarity and effortlessness.

- *Movement from the muscles:* Come back to a standing, centered position again. Place your palms together and drop your weight forward toward your partner again.

Now place one foot back a bit, as you begin to push with one arm and then the other. How does this feel? Plant your feet down and really push as hard as you can now. *(Fig. 12.1c.)*

- Now stop pushing, and come back to center. Close your eyes again. How does this feel?

Students can again share their perceptions. Qualities and states of mind associated with movement from the muscles are vitality, power, and resistance.

- Now stand again and shake out through all your joints again and release your muscles. *(This joint movement is done first here as recuperation from the previous pushing movement.)*
- *Movement from the fascia:* Step forward, so you are a bit closer to your partner now, and hold your partner by the wrists. Lean back, but keep your spine in alignment and feel the stretch through your arm muscles. Now bend your knees and let your head and back release forward as you pull away. Pull gently with one arm and then the other as you feel the muscles through the back and arms. Add to this the awareness of your fascia, feel the stretch extending through this continuous sheath in your entire body. As you move with your partner, stretch gently through the fascia throughout your whole body. *(Fig. 12.1d.)*

Have the students again share their perceptions. Qualities and states of mind associated with movement from the fascia are ease and smoothness.

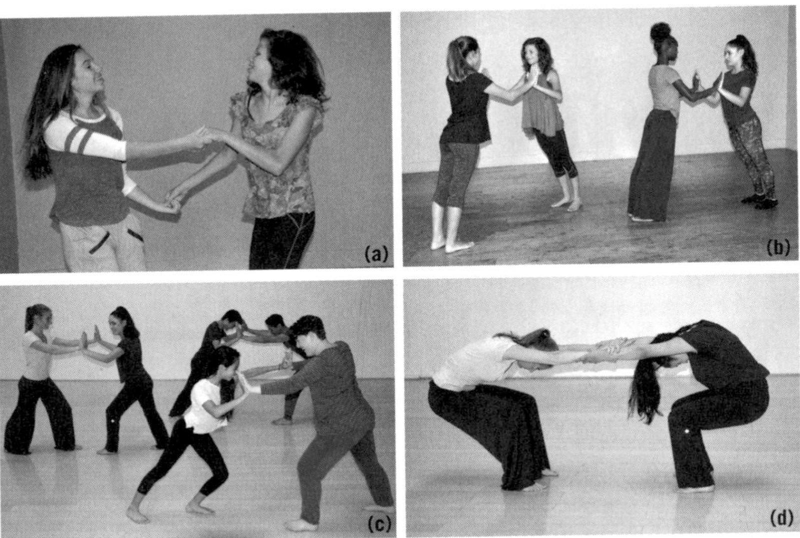

Fig. 12.1a, b, c, d. Teens experimenting with moving from the joints (a), balancing with the bones (b), pushing from the muscles (c), and stretching through the fascia (d).

Variations

You can guide students in exploring each of these types of movement initiation on their own first while standing in a circle, so they can get a sense of the different types of movement before getting into partners. *(Fig. 12.4.)*

In Partners: In the section in which students support weight through the bones by joining palm to palm, they can also explore balancing head to head, shoulder to shoulder, or back to back. You may want to demonstrate this first.

With Journals: Students can write in their body journals about their experience, noting the specific tissue types and their associated experience with moving from each one.

Discussion

- What did you experience? Which of these variations felt most comfortable to you? Which did you enjoy most? What system were you focused on at that time? What were the qualities that you enjoyed most? What was most difficult or the most uncomfortable for you? Why do you think that was true for you? What feelings did that experience evoke?
- Did anyone have a different experience?

Variation with Journals

- What words or phrases did you use to describe your experience of each of these ways of moving?
- How do you feel now? What did you learn about yourself from this experience? How might you apply this in your daily life?

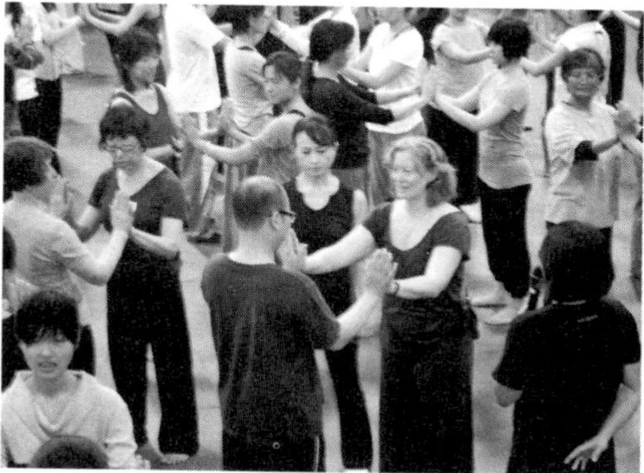

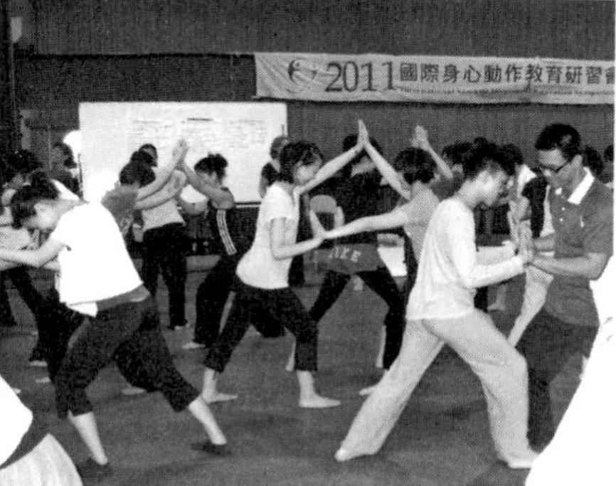

Fig. 12.2a, b. Adults exploring connecting with one another through bone touch versus through pushing from the muscles. (Photos courtesy of Somatic Education Society of Taiwan.)

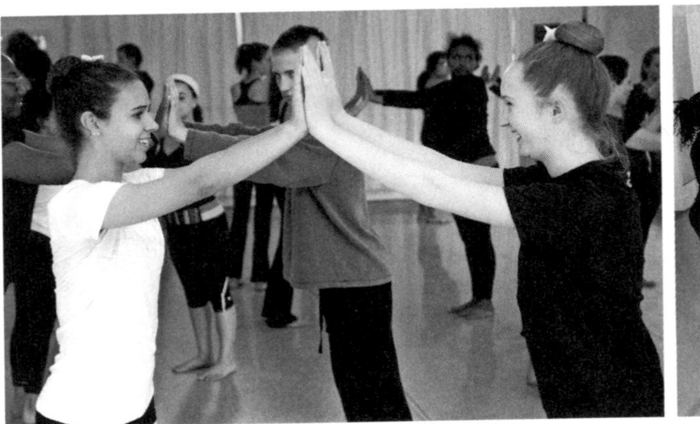
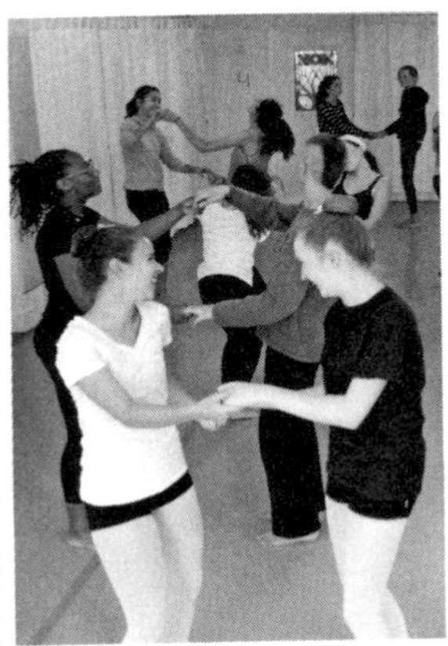

Fig. 12.3a, b. Teens exploring the difference between the solid clarity of bone support and the easy fluidity of synovial movement.

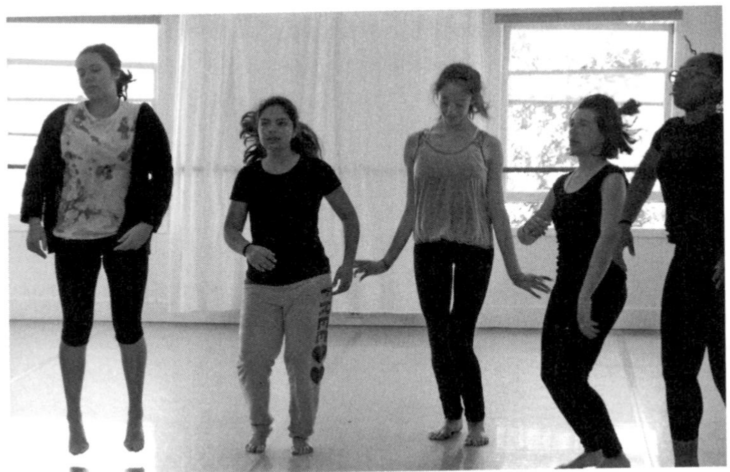
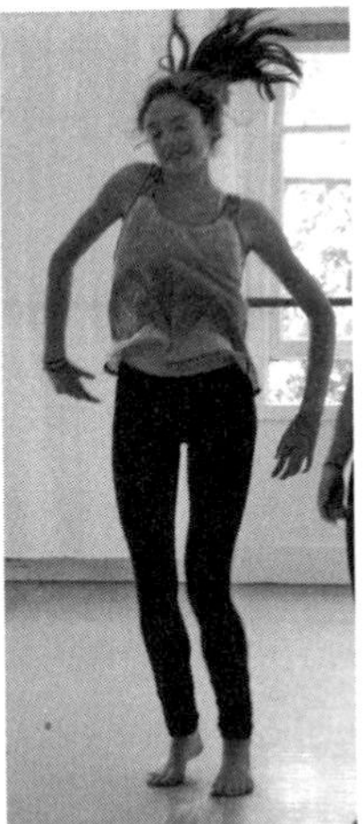

Fig. 12.4a, b. Students can also explore each of the qualities on their own to get a feel for it before working in partners; here teenagers explore the "jovial synovial fluid," as it is sometimes referred to in Body-Mind Centering.

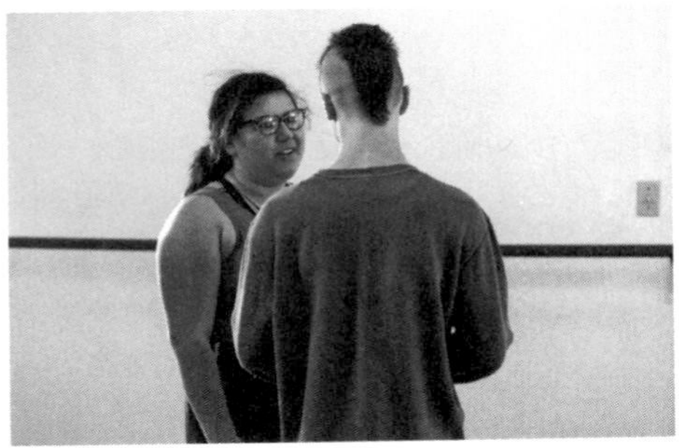
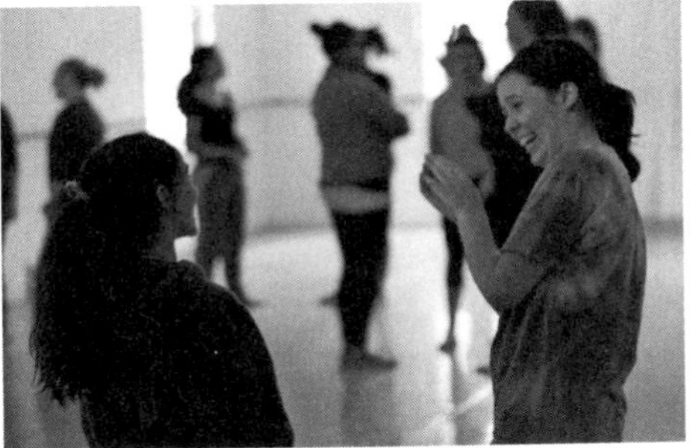

Fig. 12.5a, b. Students discussing their experiences in partners, as they discover the various feelings and associations they have with expressing a variety of different movement qualities.

ఌ

Having engaged in the previous explorations in this part of the curriculum, your students will likely have become more comfortable with themselves, their movement, and their own bodies. They will have also gained some basic knowledge of anatomy that, beyond being understood cognitively, will have begun to "make sense" to them in their own bodies. With these inner resources—of body listening, body scanning, and increased proprioceptive and interoceptive awareness—they are now more familiar with what it is to engage in a dialogue with their bodies through somatic practices.

Through an experiential study of the body systems, such as the bones, muscles, and organs—they've also had time to develop a more conscious awareness of some of the feelings and associations they have with certain qualities of movement, and been offered an opportunity to expand their comfort zone of expression—exploring the intimate interconnection between sensation and perception.

Building upon these Embodiment Basics that were covered in Level I of the curriculum, in the next section of the curriculum students apply this initial experiential learning to areas such as alignment, breathing, and warm-up. These next activities continue to inspire individual learning, while drawing upon the strong container of community that has generally become established among the group by now. Diving deeper into their bodies and being given time for personal reflections, students gain further confidence and self-understanding through these next activities—some of which challenge them to embody and reflect upon certain stereotypes (in an activity related to posture), consider how they relate to technology (related to care of the spine and morning habits), and gain a more personal understanding of their own breathing (in light of both internal and external factors that may inhibit them or free them to be themselves).

Sharing their insights also gives teens a chance to learn from one another; these conversations can take an additional level of maturity on the part of the students, to engage in the kind of self-reflection they require, so though I've presented a specific order of activities, you can be the best judge of when to introduce each of them with your particular group.

PART IV

A CURRICULUM IN SME: EMBODIED ANATOMY FOR TEENS

Embodiment Fundamentals–Level II

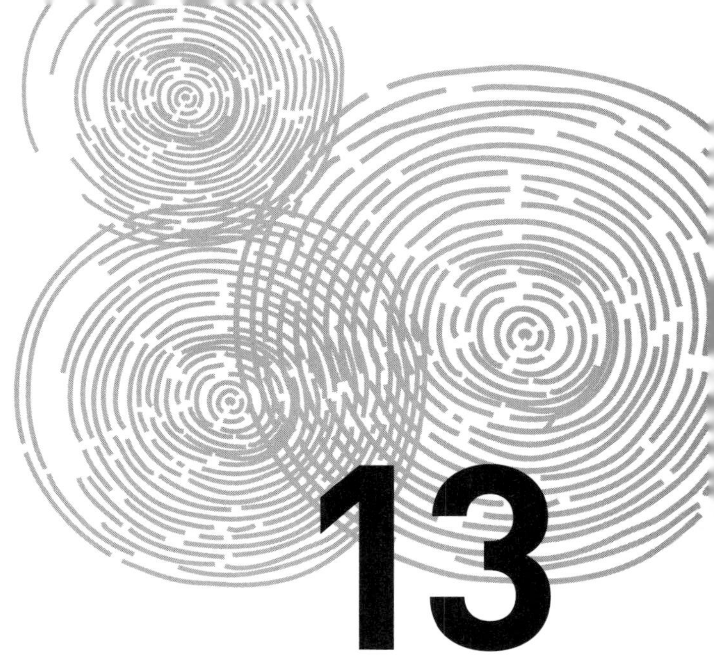

13

Structure and Posture

Structure is our physical form; posture is the way we live in and inhabit our body. Throughout life our bodies change in response to many factors, including diet, physical activity, emotions, and habitual ways of moving. The choices we make affect both the structure and functioning of our body and our sense of self. Many of these choices, however (such as how we sit, the positions in which we sleep, even the food we eat) are habitual; we may or may not be conscious of them. Underneath these habits are the feelings, attitudes, and beliefs that continuously influence our behavior. Initial explorations in this section are geared toward increasing students' awareness of their habitual behavior, as well as their cultural assumptions, which directly affect their bodies and their perceptions of themselves and others.

Perceptions of Posture

Because body image and self-image are so intertwined, the topic of posture can be a complex and sensitive one to address with teens. During adolescence, students' bodies can feel like a battleground for independence as parents and schools try to dictate how to look and behave. In studying posture, students are first guided to become aware of their present posture and to reflect on the many factors that influence their movement and attitudes. This serves as a means to bring more conscious awareness to their bodies and movement patterns, as well as to their cultural conditioning. Further activities in this section of the curriculum are designed to help students experience a more balanced and efficient alignment for better health, rather than to dictate that they adopt a particular physical aesthetic. This is an important distinction to communicate to students so that they feel supported rather than controlled.

Through the previous explorations in class, many students start to notice benefits of their improved alignment and become motivated to experience further change. Some students notice having more ease in dance or athletics as they gain more kinesthetic ability. Others find that chronic strains, such as lower back problems or recurring sprained ankles, are reduced. Many others notice they feel more relaxed and better able to concentrate after our class. Many find their self-esteem—as well as their grades—are improving as well. By the time they explore the topic of posture, students have often experienced some of these changes for themselves and can easily understand the benefits of these activities.

To begin to explore the topic of posture, you can lead a discussion of the concepts of structure and posture that includes such questions as "What is skeletal balance?" and "What is posture?" and "If we can define balanced alignment, why don't we all have it?" This helps students to reflect on the complex interrelationship of the body structure and the *soma*, the lived body. Then in the next exploration, Identifying Postural Tendencies, students change certain elements of their posture and reflect on their experience. After noticing the relative positions of each of the three body weights—head, torso, and pelvis—they then experiment with shifting each of them forward and back from center and observe their responses.

For example, as students shift the rib cage or torso forward, various reactions occur. In one class, a student who habitually stands with his chest forward of center expressed feeling a sense of pride and confidence in this position; another student who stands with her torso shifted back of center expressed feeling embarrassed and overly aggressive in this position. Another student agreed, saying that people who stand with their chests forward are often stubborn and bossy. These types of reactions are not uncommon, and often reveal certain stereotypes based on gender and other factors. As students begin to recognize their own postural tendencies, you can guide them to see how they interpret these tendencies in themselves and others.

The "What's My Line?" exploration takes this a step further by encouraging students to embody and reflect upon the stereotypical physical stances of particular groups of people. For instance, as they examine postures of various athletes, such as weight lifters, swimmers, and football players, they find that the movement required for each physical activity influences the skeletal muscular development of that athlete. Similarly, just as certain training in a particular sport can affect the body, practicing a particular postural stance over time will also influence the structure of the body. A person in the military, for example, may have been encouraged to adopt a posture meant to project a culturally recognized image of power, dignity, and strength, while a female ballet dancer may have developed a posture that reflects a certain cultural perception of femininity, characterized by lightness and grace. In many ways our present perceptions are influenced by ingrained cultural beliefs.

By examining such examples, students also discover that our underlying perceptions can influence our bodies and our movement throughout our lives. The person in the military, for example, will not necessarily be able to "drop" that physical stance upon returning home; the ballerina will not carry herself differently once her career has ended. The movement experiences you choose impact your body and your sense of self. Conversely, your sense of self may also affect your choices—such as whether to engage or not in certain types of movement. You may choose those that feel familiar based on your past experiences, and avoid other movement practices that fall outside of your current comfort zone.

As pioneering dance therapist Mary Whitehouse observes, "Any change has to come through consciousness, awareness, first of one's actual condition, and second, of the possible meaning of that condition."[1] By identifying some of the associations they have with particular postures, students begin to recognize factors that affect how they move, perceive, and are perceived. They discover that many of these body postures and body prejudices are often adapted quite unconsciously, based on stereotypical assumptions related to factors such as gender, class, ethnicity, or profession, which are also explored in the What's My Line? Exploration.

Through this process, students develop awareness as they acknowledge their own judgments—and the impact these judgments may have on themselves and others. Such predetermined perceptions can have huge ramifications, both personally and collectively, especially when we act upon our biased impressions of others. Evidence of this is ever-prevalent in our schools and in our society at large in the oppression of particular segments of the population based on skin color, gender, profession, nationality, and sexual orientation. As teens gain awareness and understanding of their present perceptions and related habits, they gain compassion, and also begin to have more *choice*—about how they live and move, how they perceive themselves, and how they act toward others. This helps students become less judgmental of themselves, as well as less reactive and more accepting of those around them.

To facilitate this process, during discussions following each of these explorations students talk about their own feelings associated with posture; they gain insight when given time to reflect on their experience. Rather than creating further expectations of what they should look like or who they should be, the facilitator supports students' ability to make conscious choices—serving as an *ally* who offers them tools to discover and decide who they are for themselves.

Exploration: What Is Structure? What Is Posture?

(20 minutes)

PURPOSE. To discuss the concepts of structure and posture and reflect on the interrelationship of these concepts; to understand alignment related to posture.

Activity/Discussion

- What is structure? What is skeletal balance? *(Discuss skeletal balance in terms of the three body weights [head, torso, and pelvis] and the structure and function of bone, muscle, tendons, and ligaments.)*
- What factors influence body structure? *(Factors include heredity, genetics, gender, race, use, injury, alignment, and diet.)*
- What is posture? *(Posture is the way we use our bodies; this will be examined further in chapter 14, "The Dynamics of Balance.")*
- If we can define balanced alignment, why don't we all have it? Why don't all bodies have the same alignment? What factors influence posture? *(Factors may include physical activity, emotional state, injury, cultural perceptions, media images, role models, and such.)*

Exploration: Identifying Postural Tendencies

(20–30 minutes; 45 minutes with variation)

PURPOSE. To discover your postural tendencies by shifting each of the three body weights (head, torso, and pelvis); to reflect, individually and collectively, on our associations with certain postures.

Activity

Begin this activity with everyone standing.

❍ Close your eyes. Take a minute to do a body scan, starting with your feet and progressing to the top of your head. Just observe how you are standing. Notice the weight of your head. Does it feel centered? Or do you notice the weight falling more forward or backward? To one side or the other? Don't try to change it; just notice it.

❍ Now let the weight of your head come slightly forward by lowering your chin toward your chest. Notice how that feels. How does it affect the rest of your body? How does it affect your spine? Shoulders? Pelvis? Knees? The balance of weight on your feet? Now come back to what feels like a more centered and balanced position of your head.

- Now let the weight of your head fall slightly back of center. How does this feel? Again notice how this affects your spine, shoulders, pelvis, knees, the weight on your feet.
- Notice what feels familiar, what feels strange or new, or what tendencies you have ... what images or feelings you become aware of.

Repeat the directions with shifting the torso forward and back of center.

Repeat the directions with shifting the pelvis forward and back of center.

- Now relax and stand in any way you like. Take a breath, in and out. Stretch or move as you need to now, and open your eyes when you are ready.

Variation

Ask students to hold the position they have arrived in, and then open their eyes and walk through the room in this new posture. For example, after shifting the head forward of center, students walk around with their heads down, looking at the floor, and notice what they experience walking in this way. Then they come back to standing still, close their eyes, and realign into what feels like a more balanced relationship of the three body weights of head, torso, and pelvis, before taking on the next postural variation, and then walking again *(Fig. 13.1a, b)*. You may also ask students to notice each other as they are walking, or perhaps stop and have a conversation with someone else while embodying each new posture *(Fig. 13.1c)*. After exploring all the variations, ask students to embody the position that felt most familiar to them *(Fig.13.2)*, and walk again; they can then go back to the posture that felt most unusual or uncharacteristic of them. As they do this, you can remind students to notice any differences in how it may feel to move in each case, as well as to be seen by others when embodying these various stances.

Teens and adults alike really enjoy this activity—especially this variation of walking through the room—as it can be fun to "try on" various personas and to perceive themselves and others in a new way. This invites humor and spontaneity while building a sense of community, as students' own attitudes and prejudices inevitably emerge and they begin to recognize them. These more unconscious attitudes will be explored briefly in the discussion section that follows, and then examined further in the next exploration, What's My Line?

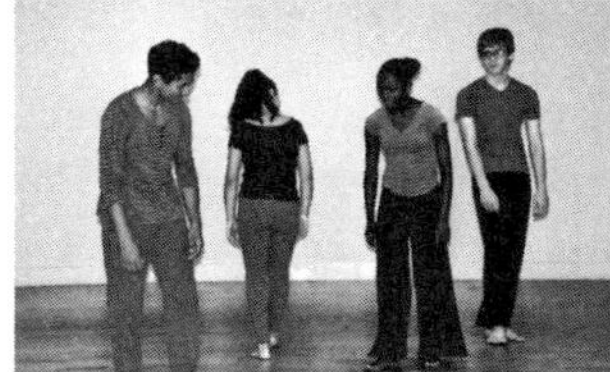
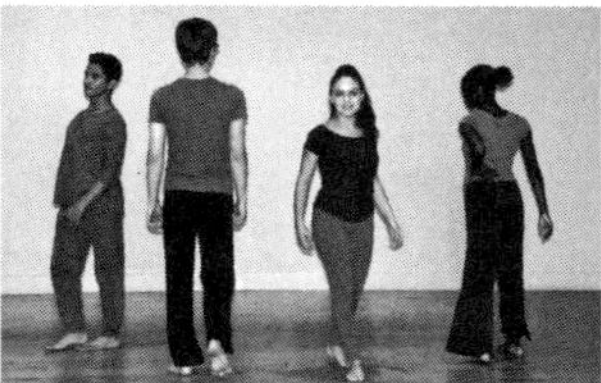
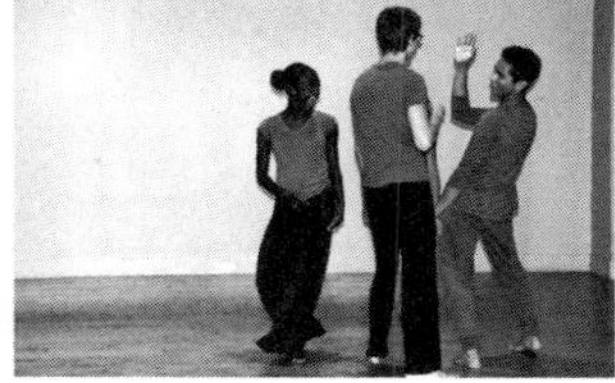

Fig. 13.1a, b, c. Identifying Postural Tendencies, Variation. Students shift their three body weights (head, torso, and pelvis) one at a time to explore various postures while walking among themselves. This provides a fun in-road to exploring the complex topic of posture and perception.

Discussion

Students can first discuss their experience in partners.

- *(In large group)* What did you experience? Were there any positions we explored that felt familiar? Why do you think that was? Were there any that made you uncomfortable? Why do you think that was? Were there some positions that brought to mind certain people? Or an aspect of yourself?
- Were there some things we did that made you laugh? What was so funny?

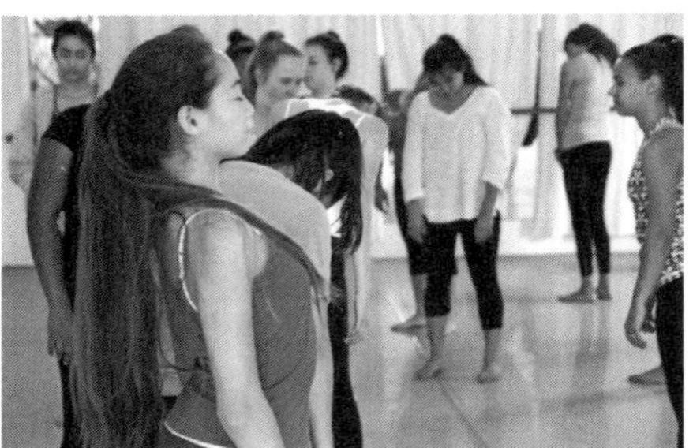

Fig. 13.2. Students explore the posture that feels most familiar to them, and later compare that with a position that feels most unfamiliar.

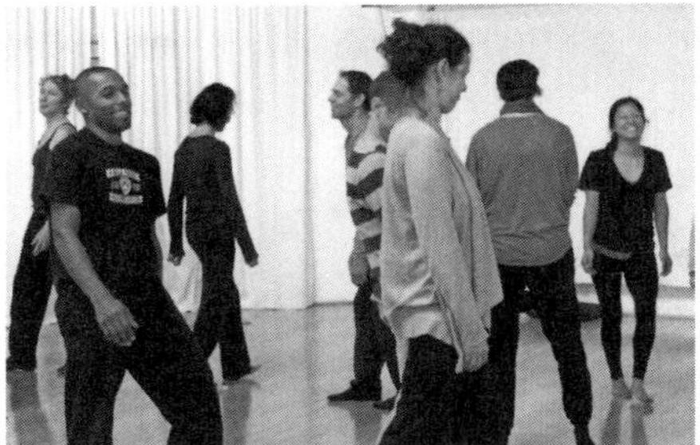

Fig. 13.3. Participants in the Embodiment in Education training have fun trying on different postural "personas" while participating in the exploration Identifying Postural Tendencies.

Exploration: What's My Line?

(50–60 minutes)

PURPOSE. To discover and discuss stereotypes related to posture and body image; to gain an understanding of ways that specific *body use* affects body structure over time, such as training in specific movement forms; to reflect further on your associations with certain postures as a means to discover our individual and collective cultural assumptions and body prejudices.

Activity

Have students write down on separate pieces of paper specific types of people they identify as having a particular postural stance. Categories might include someone who is depressed, shy, or confident; a particular type of athlete, such as a weight lifter or gymnast; or a particular media image or stereotype, such as a fashion model. They then give them to you. Read each one as it is submitted, and choose the ones that seem most appropriate to the context of your class; you can also add a few of your own if you like.

Divide the class into two groups. Each group takes turns picking a piece of paper and doing their best to demonstrate the posture of that type of person. The other group tries to guess who they are. Facilitate this by having the group that will be guessing close their eyes while the students in the other group choose a particular posture. Those who will be demonstrating the posture can also close their eyes, so that they each come up with their own version rather than referencing each other's positions. Then they all open their eyes and the guessers try to determine who they are portraying. Once the group has guessed, the full group discusses how they came up with their perceptions, as in the following sample discussion.

Discussion

- *(Directed to group guessing)* How did you guess who they were? How did you know? What particulars about their posture did you notice? What corresponding association do you have with that? Why do you think you have that perception? How did you interpret what you noticed? Where does that association come from? Why do you think most of you thought that? [or] Why do you think your perception differed from that of others in the group?
- *(Directed to group demonstrating)* How did you choose what to do to show who you were portraying? Did you all do the same thing? Why do you think you had similar (or different) perspectives? How did it feel to move or stand like that? How did it feel to be seen in that way? Why do you think that was? Did anyone have a different experience?

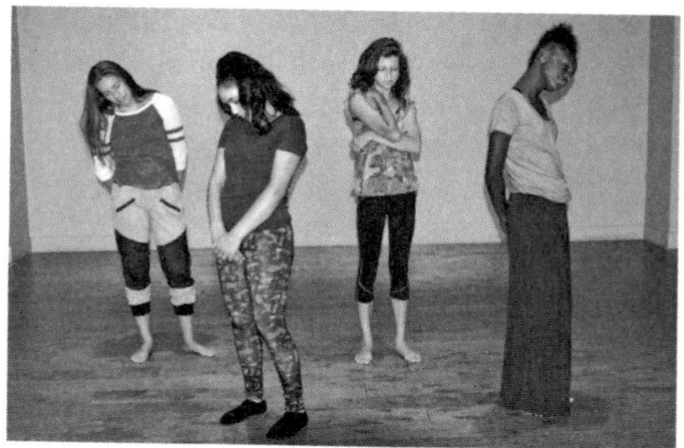

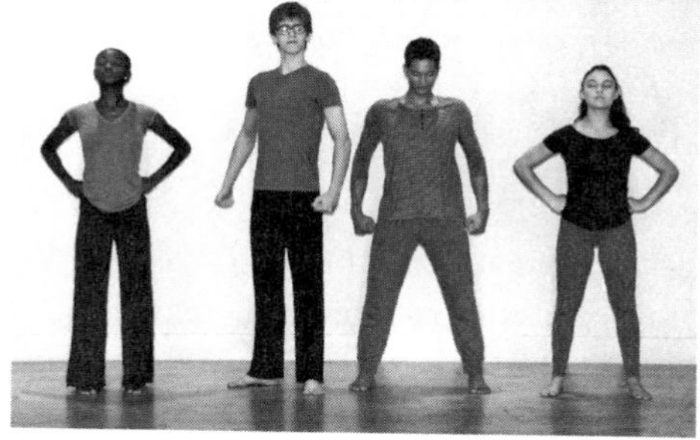

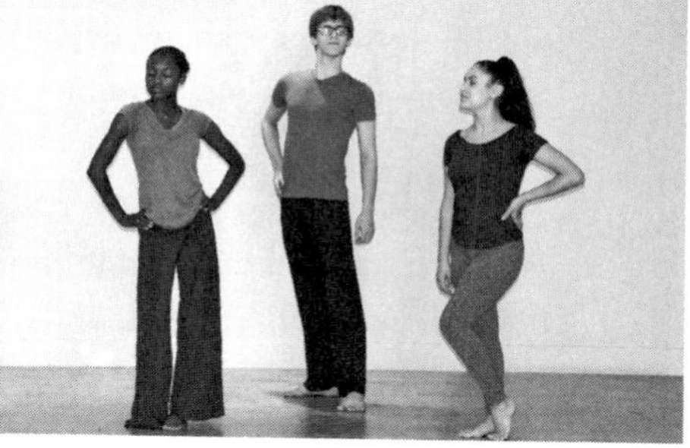

Fig. 13.4a, b, c. Teens participating in What's My Line? as they explore stereotypical postures: someone who is shy (a), a body builder (b), a fashion model (c).

Tips for Teachers

- By specifically focusing on stereotypes and encouraging an open discussion, we are inevitably stepping into sensitive and potentially controversial territory. In choosing which student topics to accept, you define your own comfort zone, likely based on both your own attitudes and your confidence in facilitating such a discussion. Yet also be aware that even if you have "edited out" certain topics, they may still emerge in the students' responses during the activity or the discussion! You may want to try facilitating this activity with a group of peers first, to experience various ways in which this conversation might unfold.
- In facilitating the discussions, include all student perceptions as valid, and then inquire deeper into them. For example, a student may say that someone's posture looks "retarded." Rather than impulsively objecting to the use of such a derogatory term, guide the group to look objectively at what they saw that evoked that perception. You might respond by saying, "that's an interesting observation." Then you might ask, "Did anyone else have that perception? What about their bodies or movements gave you that impression? Why do you think that is associated with being "———"? (retarded, gay, depressed, arrogant, sexy, or whatever stereotypical assumption has been identified). You might also ask the students who were demonstrating, "how did it feel to be associated with being "—-" based on how you were standing/moving?" You can also directly discuss the use of such terms as being offensive or oppressive to some people, if that is the case, and the reasons for this—and in fact I have found that students will often take the role of advocate and bring this up themselves.
- These types of conversations can be especially helpful in addressing various social issues, like racism, sexism, and homophobia, for instance, that inevitably emerge. This activity can also be applied in instances of bullying that may have occurred in school to help students gain greater insight into their own judgments. In addressing specific situations, you may also want to coordinate this activity with other supportive methods, such as counseling or restorative justice meetings. It is challenging to skillfully facilitate these types of conversation, but when done well they have the potential to foster greater awareness, compassion, and sensitivity in the school community.

HOME PROJECTS

- Follow-up projects can include research on posture and body image as represented in media, advertising, films, and so on, such as making collages or photo exhibits; related topics such as body image related to gender, class, ethnicity, and other stereotypes can also be explored.

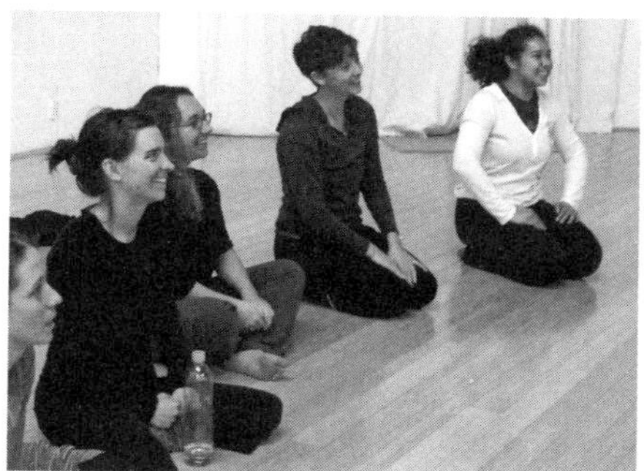

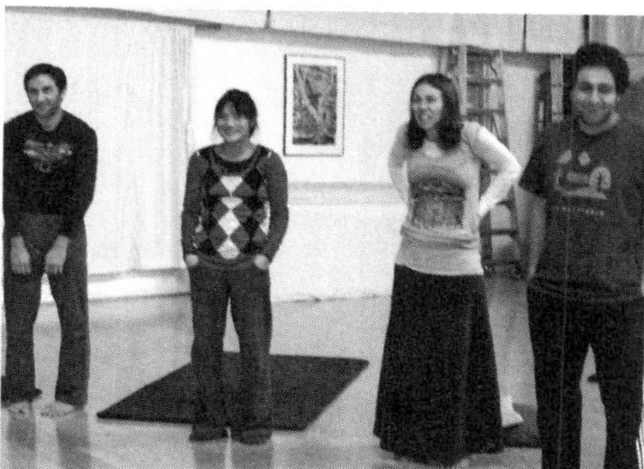

Fig. 13.5a, b. Participants in the Embodiment in Education training participate in What's My Line?, with one group acting out the stereotype and the other group guessing who they might be portraying based on their body posture.

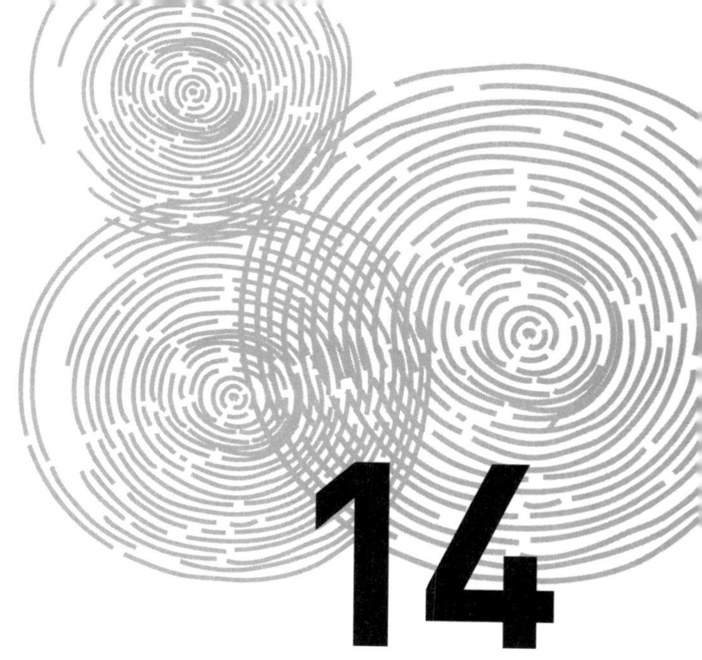

14

The Dynamics of Balance

Teens generally assume there is such a thing as a "correct posture" that must uniformly be achieved. At the mere mention of the word *posture,* some students throw their shoulders back and lift their chins, others press their shoulders down and tuck their chins, others lift their shoulders up and push their chests forward—all to match an image of what they have come to perceive as ideal posture. Yet although people often think of posture as a fixed position in space, posture is actually more of an *activity* related to maintaining balance within the body, rather than a position. Redefining posture as relationships within the body is a first step in unraveling neuromuscular patterns that may be inhibiting our movements, and even our lives—as is evident in the following story of a former student of mine.

Perceptions of Alignment

As we began to study the spine, one young girl in the class named Karla told us, "The spine is like a pole that has to stay lined up." She added, "My dance teacher told me that." She eagerly showed us her drawing to illustrate this fact. Indeed, she held her spine rigidly, with her chin tucked in firmly to keep "the pole" in line—a position she had spent hours perfecting at her dance studio. Although she was proud of her accomplished posture, Karla often experienced muscle spasms in her neck when under emotional stress, sometimes to the point that she couldn't even turn her head! At those times, she would stay home from school, which only added to her distress as she fell further behind in her schoolwork. Although the pole was just an *image in her mind,* the neuromuscular adjustments she made in response to this image were affecting her movement, her health, her self-esteem, and the quality of her life.

Although Karla may be an extreme example, many people have images of the spine as being straight and solid from being told to "sit up straight" or to "stand tall" or to "not slouch." They also often imagine their spine to run along the surface of their backs. When they are asked to draw a side view of the head and spine, students often draw this "straight pole in the back" image. In attempting to achieve a better posture, then, students readjust and attempt to hold a position that appears straighter.

Alignment, however, is a *dynamic balance* within the body. It is a felt sense, an *experience,* rather than a position. An exercise called the Small Dance, developed by Contact Improvisation founder Steve Paxton, encourages an awareness of the fact that even within stillness, there are very subtle postural shiftings that happen as the intrinsic muscles, tendons and ligaments, especially in the joints of the feet and legs, adjust to hold the body up in gravity.[1] The exploration called "What Is Balance? The Small Dance," derived from Paxton's exercise, helps introduce students to this new way of experiencing and perceiving posture.

Exploration: What Is Balance? The Small Dance

(10 minutes)

PURPOSE. To feel the postural shifts that occur in balancing your structure in the force of gravity; to encourage an expansion of the term *balance* to include movement.

Activity

Have students stand in a circle.

- We are going to try an experiment! I'm going to invite you to close your eyes and stand as still as you can. I'll be timing this for exactly one minute. Let's see how still you can be.
- OK, now close your eyes. Feel what happens as you try to stand perfectly still. And begin. *(Begin to time one minute.)* Stay as still as you can! *(At the end of one minute)* OK, relax, but keep your eyes closed.

Variation

You can end with the previous activity and move to the discussion, or proceed to this variation, which adds an amusing additional element of comparison.

- ❍ Now we're going to do this again, but this time, I want you to exaggerate whatever you just experienced in your body as you tried to stay still. For instance, if we imagine that what you just experienced was at "volume 1," now you are going to repeat that but at "volume 10"! I'll be timing this again for one minute.
- ❍ Close your eyes again. Ready, go. *(Students often begin to sway, or exaggerate holding their breath, or tighten their shoulders or legs, and so on. After thirty seconds or so of this, add this new directive.)* Keep going with what you're doing, but gradually open your eyes so you can also see what others are doing.
- ❍ *(At the end of one minute)* OK, relax.

Discussion

- What did you notice as you tried to stand as still as you could? Could you stand absolutely still? What did you experience? Did anyone have a different experience? What does balance mean? *(Discuss this in terms of skeletal balance and the subtle postural shifts made to stay balanced in gravity, as described previously in the introductory text in this chapter.)*

Anatomy of the Spine

Once students have experienced this more dynamic notion of posture, they can begin to learn about the actual physical structures in the body that provide us with such amazing resilience against the forces of gravity. Rather than being a rigid column, the spine consists of the four curves of the cervical, thoracic, lumbar, and sacrum-coccyx regions.[2] In addition to absorbing shock, the curves of the spine serve to counterbalance the three major body weights: the head, torso, and pelvis. The spine, actually a series of joints, is made up of vertebrae and the cartilaginous discs between them, which provide mobility of the spine.

Although people often perceive the spine as the column of bones they feel in their backs, what you are actually able to touch along your back are the posterior spinous processes, the bony projections on the back of each vertebra. The weight-bearing part

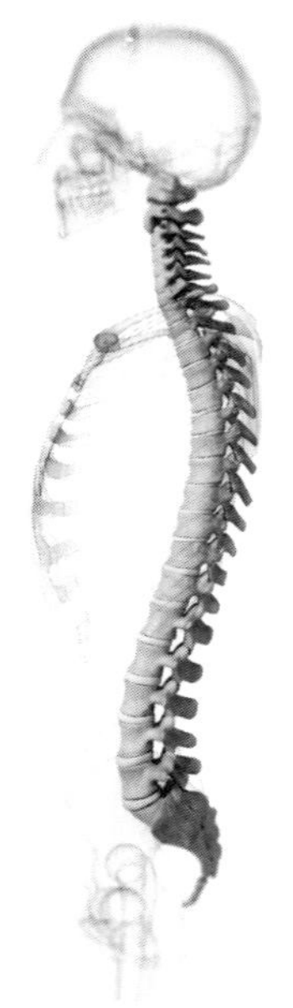
Fig.14.1. Side view of the spine.

of the vertebrae, called the "bodies," actually project a third to halfway into the thoracic cavity and are more in the center of the body.

Rather than connecting at the very back of the skull, the spine actually balances the skull at its center, on the first cervical vertebra called the atlas. Because the spinal column houses the spinal cord, alignment of the skull on the spine is important for the healthy functioning of the nervous system. Skeletal alignment refers to the balance of the three major body weights (head, torso, and pelvis) along the central vertical axis, or plumb line, of the body. The term *plumb line* refers to a string suspended overhead with a small weight attached at the bottom end, and is a term often used when assessing standing alignment in reference to the positioning of the head, upper torso, pelvis, legs, and feet.

Benefits of Skeletal Alignment

In using the body efficiently, weight is transferred through the skeleton along this vertical axis, with the connective tissues of tendons, ligaments, and fascia supporting and stabilizing the joints. If the three body weights are not in alignment, strain is placed on these supportive tissues. As you approach a more vertical alignment, less muscular effort is needed in standing, so you feel less strain. More muscular energy is also available to accomplish movement.

A more balanced alignment allows all the body systems to function more freely: the spinal cord and peripheral nerves receive less compression, the organs of the thoracic and pelvic cavities are able to function with minimal compression or restriction, and the major vessels can provide for unimpeded circulation of the blood. Improved alignment can lead to a reduction of chronic strains and stress, greater physical vitality, and an enhanced sense of well-being. When students understand the complex relationship between skeletal alignment and health, they become more motivated to improve their alignment. As they study the specifics of alignment, students refer to their own bodies, their original drawings of the skeleton, and the skeletal model to gain a more accurate image of their structure, which also affects their *movement.*

For instance, as Karla examined the structure of the spine more closely, she was able to relate her image of the pole to the actual structure of her own body and gain a new image, one that supported her to develop a healthier, more fluid way of moving. First, as she learned about the curves of the spine and could feel her skull balanced on the first cervical vertebra, she could relax the muscles of her neck and allow the curve of the cervical vertebrae to exist, without feeling wrong. By learning that her spine projects deeply into the center of her body rather than at the back, she could also begin to feel her balance through her vertical axis. Over time this allowed her to begin to release the extra tension in the larger muscles of her back, which she had thought she needed "to hold up the pole."

Once she gained a more anatomically accurate experience of her spine, *her new image was supportive of her body's structure, rather than fighting it.* Although it takes time to change the body's structure, this experience positively affected her self-perception, her movement, and her health. Through the study of alignment and the anatomy of the vertebrae and spinal column, students begin to gain a more realistic understanding of posture as a dynamic, living process. In the explorations in this section, students work in partners to feel the curves of the spine, and further experiment with shifting the three body weights to help them internalize their understanding.

Other activities encourage care of the spine, first by exploring the relationship of the pelvis and spine in sitting. No doubt, many teachers and parents alike have dealt with the issue of trying to get teens not to "slump." When sitting in a slumped position we are actually sitting on the base of the spine—the sacrum—rather than on the base of the *pelvis,* which puts strain on the lower back. Rather than "correcting" this tendency, in this activity students try both ways of sitting and compare the two. You may find that students report they still prefer the "slumped" position and wonder what to do! Rather than feeling discouraged, you can see this as a wonderful launching point for an important discussion about body use, habitual patterns, and health.

For many people our habitual pattern just *feels* right, even if it is not most aligned or efficient. Yet as we develop new patterns, the musculature can change such that the new pattern begins to feel more familiar and supported from within. Discussing body learning objectively like this gives students more information about their bodies—as well as more choice in how to respond. From the many other activities done already, students often find they can sit and stand upright without as much strain in any case, as their three body weights are more aligned and they've become more flexible, so that balanced alignment becomes easier. If some students are still having difficulty sitting upright, it may mean that their hamstring muscles are particularly tight, in which case they can practice exercises to lengthen these muscles, or try sitting on a cushion to raise up the pelvis to help them to sit more comfortably. The sitting exploration presented here may be helpful to do early on in the class, so that students can sit comfortably and with less strain when doing further activities that involve sitting on the floor.

An additional exploration encourages students to become aware of specific movement habits, such as observing their posture when texting on a cell phone, to experience how this can affect both posture and health. For example, if we habitually bend forward for long periods of time, such as by texting on our phone, reading a book, or working on a computer, we put strain on our cervical spine while compressing the organs in our thoracic cavity—our lungs and heart. This impedes our respiration and circulation, all necessary for full vitality.

Learning about the relationship of their upper body—head, spine, lungs, and heart—to their health brings teens' awareness to the need for alignment and ease of movement in this area. Instead of teaching them a "correct" way to organize their bodies, in this exploration students are again given an opportunity to experience their habitual pattern first, and then to experiment with other modes and compare them for themselves to discover what feels best in their own body, and then to discuss this together.

Exploration: Spine and Pelvis—Sitting

(15–20 minutes)

PURPOSE. To understand the relationship of your pelvis and spine in sitting; to encourage sitting on the base of your pelvis rather than on your sacrum; to encourage an understanding of the relationship between body use and both care of the spine and full breathing.

Activity

With the group sitting on the floor in a circle, ask students to freeze, close their eyes, and notice the position they are in.

- How are you sitting? What part of your body are you sitting on? Which part of your skeletal system is supporting your weight in this position? Can you tell? How does this feel? *(Fig. 14.2a.)*
- Now open your eyes and sit with your feet on the floor or with your legs crossed. Hold onto your knees and allow your weight to rock slightly backward. What are you sitting on? *(This is the sacrum.) (Fig. 14.2b.)*
- What part of the body are you sitting on? *(The sacrum is part of the spine.)*
- Close your eyes and see how this feels in the rest of your body. What do you notice?
- Shift your weight forward until you feel two bony projections, one on either side. What are you sitting on? *(These are the sitz bones, or ischial tuberosities.)* What part of the body is this? *(This is the pelvis.) (Fig. 14.2c.)*
- Notice how this feels in the rest of your body. What do you experience?

- OK, open your eyes. Let's take a walk on our sitz bones, moving forward with first one and then the other. Now let's walk backward the same way. *(Fig. 14.3.)*
- Stay seated on your sitz bones, and gently lengthen your spine by reaching the top of your head upward. Take a minute to close your eyes and notice how this feels.
- What happens in your rib cage as you do this? Go back to sitting on your sacrum. What happens in your rib cage now?

Discussion

- How were you sitting when I asked you to freeze? Was this similar to what you consider to be your "normal," or habitual, way of sitting?
- Which was more comfortable for you: sitting on the sacrum or on the sitz bones? Why do you think that is? *(Look at the skeleton and discuss sitting on the pelvis versus on the sacrum or lumbar spine in relation to the health of the spine.)*
- How did lengthening your spine affect your sitting? Did it make it easier to sit on the sitz bones? Why might that be?
- How did your rib cage change as you lengthened your spine? How would that affect your breathing? Did you notice anything else?

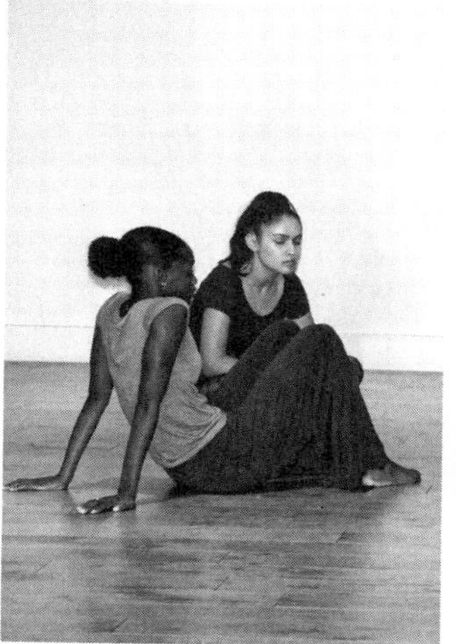
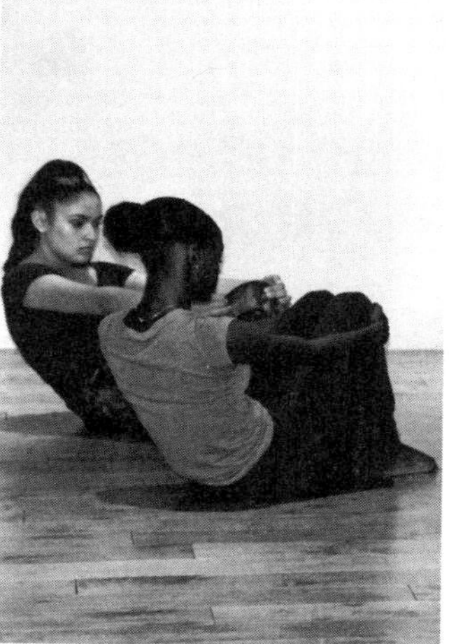
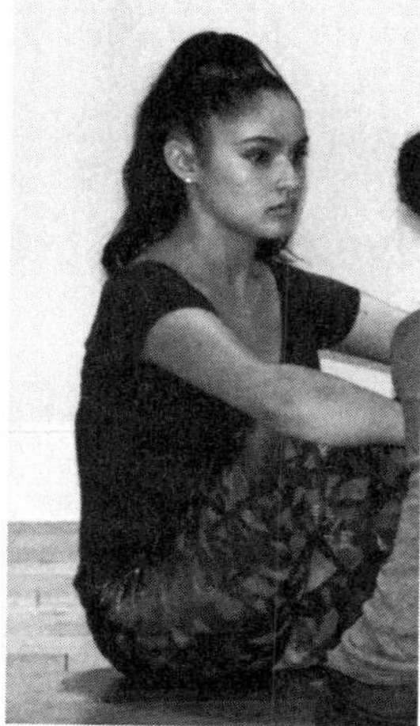

Fig. 14.2a, b, c. Sitting on the sacrum puts strain on the spine, while sitting on the sitz bones (or ischial tuberosities) allows the pelvis, rather than the spine, to take the weight. Students are asked to freeze in whatever position they are in and notice what part of their bodies they are sitting on (a); they then experiment with shifting back to their sacrum (b), and then to shift forward onto the sitz bones of the pelvis to experience the difference (c).

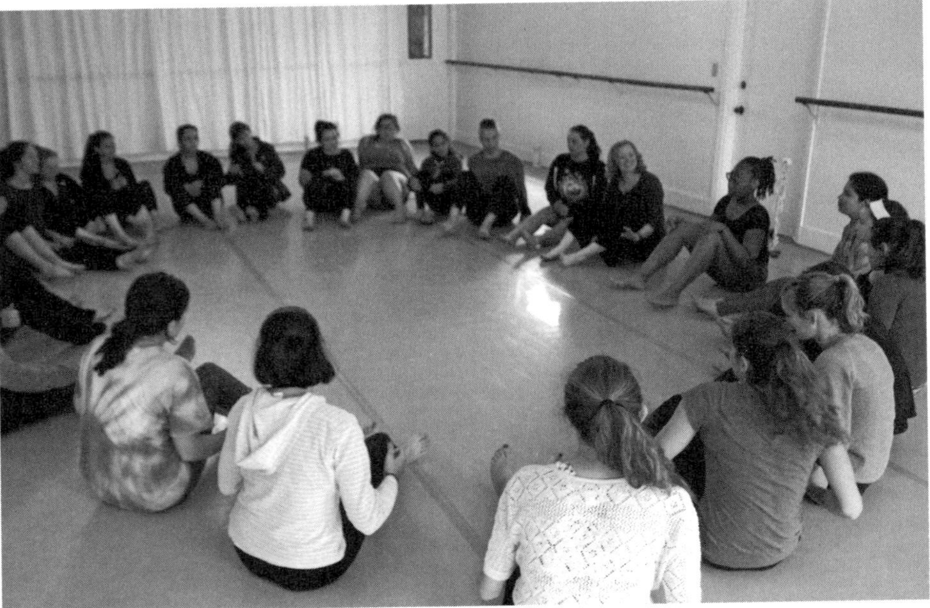

Fig. 14.3. After experimenting with feeling the difference between supporting weight on the sacrum versus the pelvis, students can "take a walk" on their sitz bones, moving forward and then back, to help to locate them and enhance the proprioceptive awareness of the bony base of the pelvis.

Exploration: Curves of the Spine

(20 minutes)

PURPOSE. To identify and feel the cervical, thoracic, and lumbar curves of the spine; to feel the spinous processes of the spine; to gain a cognitive and proprioceptive understanding of the location of your spine.

Activity

Have your students do this activity in partners with one partner seated behind the other.

Before facilitating this activity, be sure to see notes about facilitating touch in chapter 6. Take a few minutes to demonstrate this activity first by showing the method of touch with a volunteer partner while the group observes. Then when students get in partners remind them to check to be sure they are sitting on the pelvis (sitz bones) rather than on the spine (sacrum), as in the previous exploration.

- *(To the person touching)* Feel the spinal curves along your partner's back, starting from the cervical vertebrae and working down to the lumbar vertebrae. Use a flat hand so you can trace the length of the spine and feel the curves. Do this a few times. Notice the direction of the curve as well as the projection of the back surface of each vertebra. How close to the skin do you feel the bony processes? *(Refer to the skeleton to clarify the structure of the spine.)*
- *(To the person being touched)* Feel the spinal curves along your back as your partner traces them. You may want to close your eyes to focus on this sensation. What do you notice as your partner traces your spine? Talk to your partner if anything is uncomfortable, for example, if the touch feels too soft or too hard. Ask your partner to make any changes that you need.
- Now stand up and take a walk. Notice what you feel. Move around in any way that you like, and see what you experience in your spine, or in the rest of your body.

Partners can take a few moments to share their respective experiences.

- Switch roles with your partner.

Repeat this activity, guiding it verbally again with partners in their new roles.

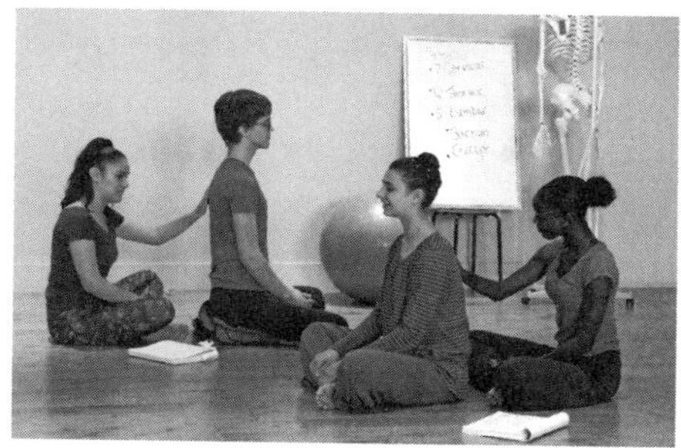

Fig. 14.4. Students learn about the curves of the spine by working in partners to trace the spinal curves through touch.

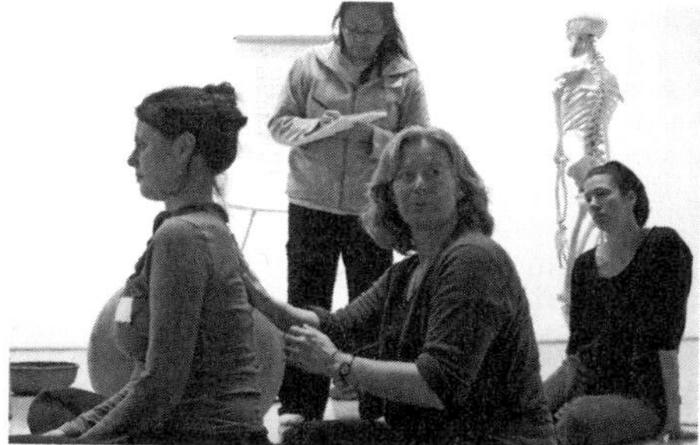

Fig. 14.5. Adult educators learning how to facilitate the Curves of the Spine exploration.

Discussion

- What did you feel when touching your partner's back? Could you feel the curves of the spine? Was this what you expected to feel? What did you feel as your partner touched your back? Was this what you expected to feel? *(Refer to students' drawings of the skeleton and a skeletal model if possible to discuss the location of the spine in the body.)*

- How does your drawing compare with what you felt in your own or your partner's back?
- What did you notice as you walked and moved after the activity? Was there a change in your perception of your spine? In your movement? Anywhere else in your body? What did you learn?

After this activity, students can be invited to redo their drawings of the side view of the spine and head (see the activity Drawing the Skeleton, p. 155); this may take an additional 10 to 15 minutes in class, or they can do this activity on their own.

Exploration: Alignment of the Three Body Weights

(15–20 minutes)

PURPOSE. To experience postural alignment; to activate imagery in your body related to weight and space; to use imagery to activate postural tone and vibrancy in your body.

Activity

This activity revisits material from the Shifting Perceptions exploration in chapter 7, with a more specific focus here on how imagery affects alignment. It also assumes experience with the Identifying Postural Tendencies exploration done previously in chapter 13.

- ❍ Stand and take a moment to close your eyes and do your body scan. Just notice what you become aware of.
- ❍ Bring your awareness to each of your three body weights: your head, torso, and pelvis. Don't try to change anything; just notice the relationship of these three places in your body. Is your head forward or back of center? Your torso? Your pelvis?
- ❍ Now feel yourself standing just as you are. Imagine standing in soft, warm sand, letting your weight be taken through your feet and into the earth.

- Now use your finger to tap the center of the top of your head, and then relax your arm back down.
- Feel the spot you have tapped, and lengthen up from that spot, up and up toward the ceiling or the sky. *(You can also introduce any imagery that has been helpful here.)*
- Now see if you can keep this feeling of lifting, and relax your muscles. Perhaps you have lifted your shoulders along with the top of your head, or lifted your chin, or tightened your knees.... Let all that release, and still feel the lift through your spine and up through the top of your head.
- Bring your awareness again to each of your three body weights: head, torso, and pelvis. Don't try to change anything; just notice the relationship of these three places in your body. Is your head forward or back of center? Your torso? Your pelvis? Is this the same as or different from what you felt before?
- Open your eyes. Take a walk around the room, trying to keep this awareness of the warm sand under your feet and the length of your spine. How do you feel as you walk now?

Alignment of Three Body Weights

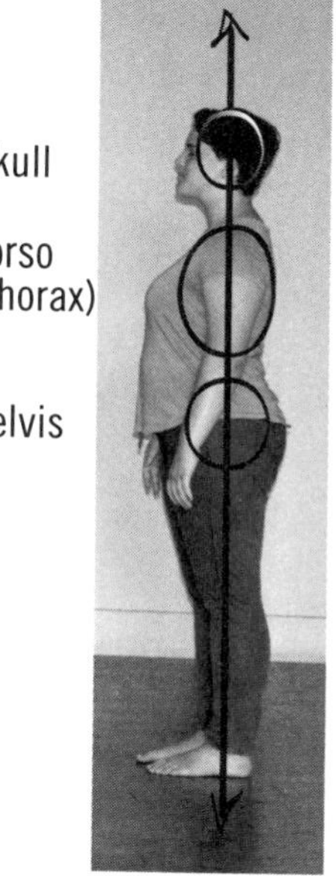

Fig. 14.6. Extending your energy in two opposite directions at once helps to lengthen the spine and align the three body weights.

Discussion

- What did you notice in this activity? How did the imagery affect your alignment? How did it feel to walk while using these images?
- How did it affect the alignment of your three body weights? What did you experience? Did anyone have a different experience? What did you learn?

Exploration: Care of the Spine—Using Technology

(15–20 minutes)

PURPOSE. To experiment with postural alignment; to recognize habitual tendencies related to using technology, such as cell phones and computers; to notice the effect of your habitual postures on your body and your health; to explore alternative dynamic relationships (such as the relationship between the head, spine, and arms when texting or reading); to invite choice in how you move and relate to your devices.

Activity

MATERIALS

- Students' personal cell phones; students can also pretend to use them
- Alternate: books for students to hold, if you feel some students may not have phones and you don't want to bring attention to this fact, as this activity easily also relates to how we use our bodies when reading

Have students spread out in the room and take a minute to check out something on their phones. They may do this activity standing or sitting, or you can have them try it both ways.

There are two ways to facilitate this activity. Students can pretend they are holding their cell phones and looking at a text; or they can use their actual phone and try this.

If they will be using their phones, note that as part of the activity you may be taking the phone from each of them, so they can stay in the exact same posture and see how it feels in their bodies. Tell them this ahead of time, and assure them that they will be getting their phones back in a few moments! Alternately, you can just have them do the full activity while holding the phone, and adapt the directions accordingly.

- ❍ Take a moment to look at your phone as you normally do. *(Figs. 14.7a and 14.8a.)*
- ❍ Now keep this same position in your body, and I'm going to come around and take the phone from you. When I've taken the phone, you can close your eyes, stay in this same position, and take a moment to do your body scan. How do you feel in this position? What do you notice? *(Figs. 14.7b and 14.8b.)*
- ❍ Now align your three body weights of the head, torso, and pelvis, but keep your arms in the same position as when you were holding the phone.

You can then give each of them back their phone.

- ❍ Now once you have your phone back, open your eyes. What would you have to do to still see the screen and yet stay in this new aligned position? Try this. *(Likely this means they will have to lift their arms to hold the phone up slightly higher than they had done before, so as to avoid bending forward as much in the cervical and thoracic areas of the spine.) (Figs. 14.7c and 14.8c.)*

- ❍ Now how does this feel? Open your eyes, and take a minute to use your phone, but in this new position. What do you notice? How is this the same or different than before?
- ❍ Now experiment with a few different positions. Hold your phone up very high, or much lower, and notice what happens in your body. Find a place that feels best. How can you tell? How does that feel?

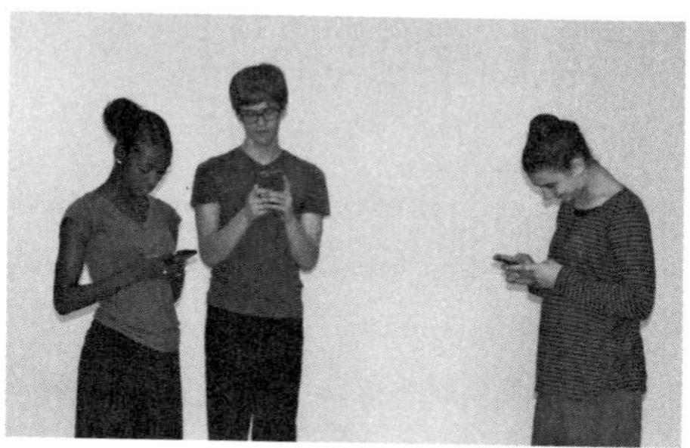

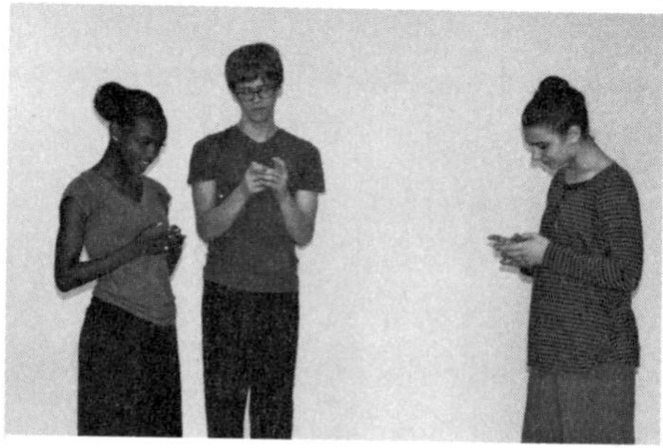

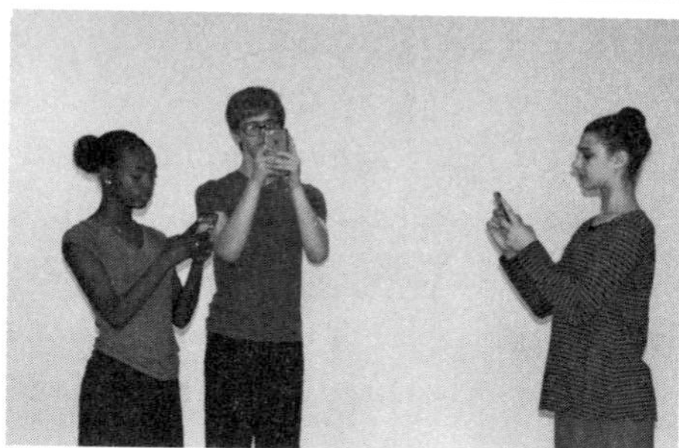

Fig. 14.7a, b, c. Care of the Spine—Using Technology (Standing). Teens can benefit from taking some time to consider their postural tendencies in daily life, such as when reading or using technology. Here they are guided to experiment with how they generally move and organize themselves—such as when using their cell phones—while exploring new options as a means to discover what may feel best to them in their own bodies.

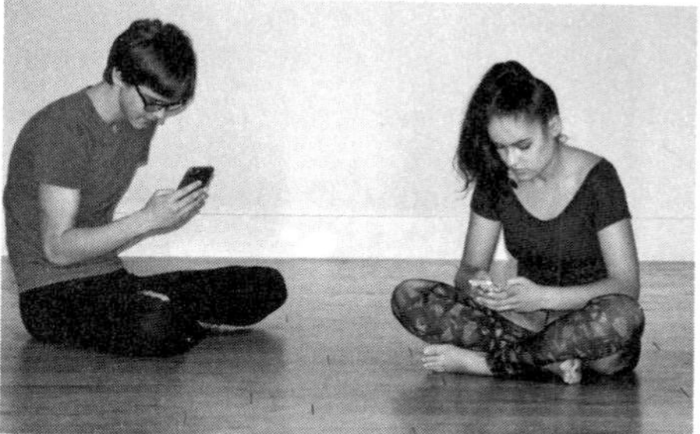

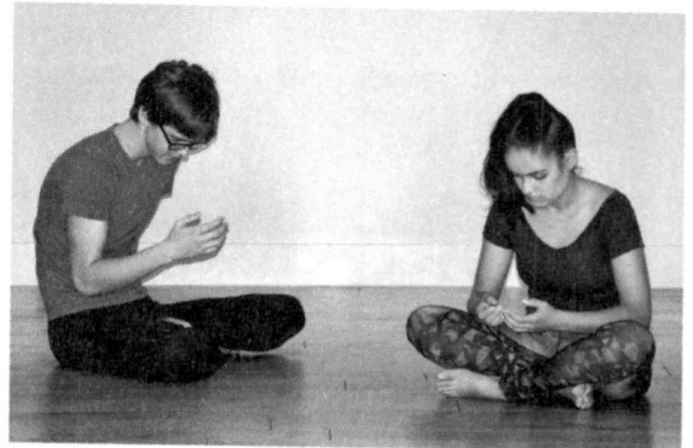

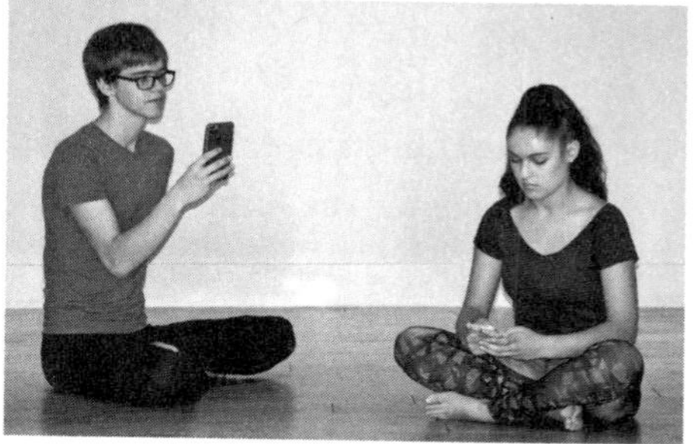

Fig. 14.8a, b, c. Care of the Spine—Using Technology (Sitting). Students can also explore this same activity when sitting. Here they notice the relationship of the pelvis, spine, neck, and head, and experiment with various ways of sitting when using their phones. With awareness comes choice.

Discussion

- What did you notice about your posture when you were using your phone? What did you experience? What has changed in your sternum? In your rib cage? How does that affect your lungs? Your heart? What do you notice? Did it affect your breathing? How?
- How often are you on your phone? For how long at a time? How else might you hold your phone?
- What happened when you aligned the three body weights and then tried to use your phone? What changes did you have to make? How did that feel?
- What kind of devices do you use? Do you have a similar posture when you use them, or is it different? How? How often do you use your other devices? For how long at a time? How else might you use it?
- What did you experience from doing this? What did you learn? Did anyone have a different experience?

Movement of the Spine

The spine has a wide range of movement potential, defined as flexion (forward bend), extension (backward bend), lateral flexion (side-to-side bend), and rotation (turning around the central axis), with combinations of these basic actions providing for even more mobility. Many people hold tension in the larger muscles of the back, as well as in the deep postural muscles of support that run along the spine, which can limit their full range of movement. The force of gravity also inevitably works to compress your body, particularly at the central axis of the spinal column. In fact, you continuously work to maintain an upright position—such that of your hundred billion neural cells, 90 percent of them are engaged in keeping your body functioning in gravity! Through the proprioceptive feedback of touch and movement, you can regain much of your full potential for movement in the spine. This helps you to relax the larger muscles of the back, while activating the core, intrinsic muscles of support along the spine.

To explore movement of the spine, students first work in partners to distinguish movement of the vertebrae in the cervical, thoracic, and lumbar regions. In the first exploration, students sit together, one behind the other, as one partner curls forward while the other person touches each vertebra along the spine in the back. This helps both partners feel the location of each vertebra, and also helps the person receiving touch to articulate each one *separately,* rather than moving whole sections of the spine as one "block." This movement activity also helps create space between the vertebrae, such that the intervertebral discs can decompress and the spine is able to lengthen. Although in certain areas of the spine it can be more difficult to feel the spinous processes, such as in the lumbar region where the vertebrae are deeper in the body, the proprioceptive feedback this activity provides is nevertheless helpful in increasing awareness and movement potential.

Students may have some difficulty with this activity at first, so it can be helpful to repeat it several times over a period of weeks so they have a chance to become familiar enough with it that it gets easier. In a subsequent class I will often ask students if they want to repeat the activity again or move on to something else, and find that they often choose to repeat it. As they become more comfortable with this activity, they often even request it, asking that we do that "getting taller" activity again!

Further explorations in this section help students discover the various movement possibilities of the spine. In a duet movement practice called Dance of the Spine, students sit back to back and explore movement potential in their spines and learn to integrate movement of the head and spine. In another exploration, based on an activity developed by Caryn McHose that she calls Fish Swish,[3] students pull each other gently across the floor to feel lateral (side to side) shifting of the spine. These activities provide creative, interactive modes of experiencing and learning about the movement of the spine.

Exploration: Movement of the Spine—Forward Curl

(40–50 minutes)

PURPOSE. To articulate your vertebrae and lengthen your spine; to integrate the intervertebral discs into your cognitive and proprioceptive perception of your spine; to use touch to activate increased proprioceptive awareness of your spine; to begin to release the larger muscles of your back and activate the core intrinsic muscles of support along your spine.

Activity

Note: This particular activity is best facilitated only once the group has previous experience with the simpler touch-based activities, and only when there is sufficient trust among students in the group.

One partner is seated behind the other partner; the mover sits in front and the facilitator/observer sits behind the mover.

Demonstrate this first by working with a volunteer partner as the facilitator/observer, with the rest of the group watching. Also discuss that you will be using the "bone touch" practiced previously in chapter 9, and review this briefly with them.

- *(To all students, once they are sitting in partners)* As you begin, take a minute to organize your sitting posture. Are you sitting on your sacrum, or your sitz bones? Do you need a cushion or mat, or can you sit comfortably as you are? Can you lengthen through your spine and still stay relaxed?
- *(To facilitator/observer)* Take a moment to tap the top of your partner's head, to help them to lengthen up from that spot and be sure they are beginning from a lengthened position before rolling forward. *(Fig. 14.9.)* Then relax your arm back down.

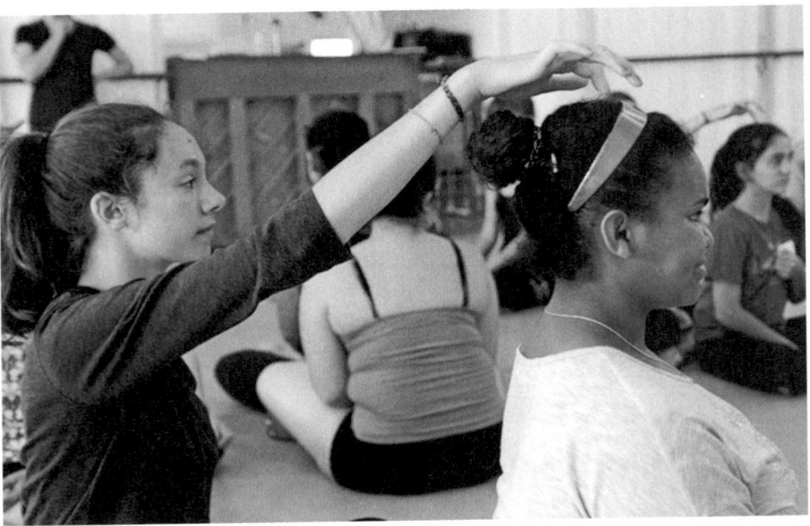

Fig. 14.9. Students learn to gently tap the top of the head to help provide proprioceptive feedback for their partners.

- *(To mover)* As your partner touches the spinous processes along your back, you will be "rolling down" your spine by letting the weight of your head come forward toward your chest and then curling forward. Close your eyes, and feel each vertebra releasing forward into gravity as the weight of your head pulls you gently forward. Try to move only the spot where your partner is touching, and let the rest of your spine relax.
- *(To facilitator/observer)* Place one finger on the spinous process of each vertebra, starting with the cervical vertebrae. As your partner curls forward, you can trace

the pathway of the movement by moving your finger down to each vertebra, one at a time. Feel the movement of the spine as your partner allows each vertebra to move forward with the weight of gravity. *(Move from the cervical to thoracic to lumbar vertebrae.)*

- Notice the difference between the bony projections and the flatter spaces between them as you go. If you can't be sure you are touching the next vertebra, move down about an inch and do your best to feel each one. This is the first time you have done this, and it can be difficult at first to locate each vertebrae. The touch will help your partners feel their spine, even if you aren't 100 percent accurate.
- *(To both partners)* Are you holding your breath? Sometimes we do that in a new experience like this. Bring your awareness to your breath, and allow your breathing to help you to relax and focus.
- *(To facilitator/observer)* Continue to feel each vertebra as your partner rolls back up, starting with the lumbar vertebrae. *(Reverse the order.)*
- *(To mover)* As you roll back up, be sure to allow space for the intervertebral discs, letting each vertebrae release back up into alignment over this soft cushioning.

This next section serves as a transition to change roles. *(Fig. 14.12.)*

- *(To the mover)* Take a minute to close your eyes and notice how you feel. Then open your eyes, stand, and walk around the room. What do you notice?
- *(To the facilitator/observer)* Watch your partner walk. What do you notice? *(Students will often observe that a partner looks taller, more lifted, or lighter on his or her feet.)* Take a minute to sit and close your eyes. While you wait for your partner to return, do a body scan and see your spine in your mind's eye. Has what you feel or visualize in your body now changed from touching your partner's back? How has that changed your perception?

Partners can take a few minutes to talk together. Then repeat the activity with the same partners switching roles.

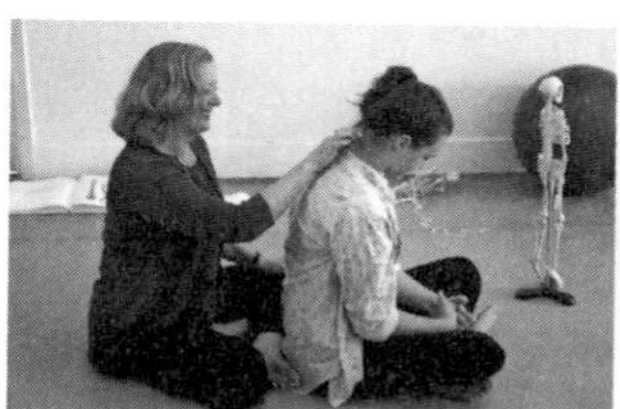
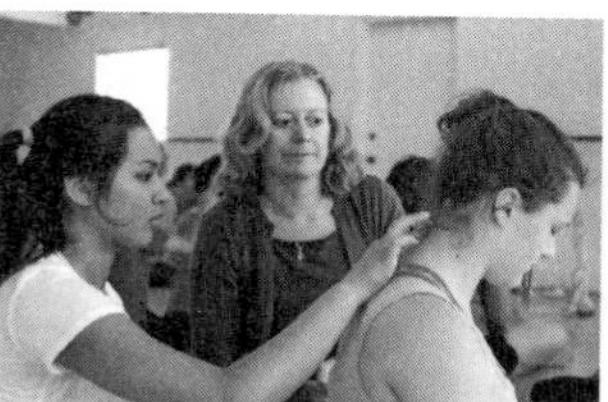
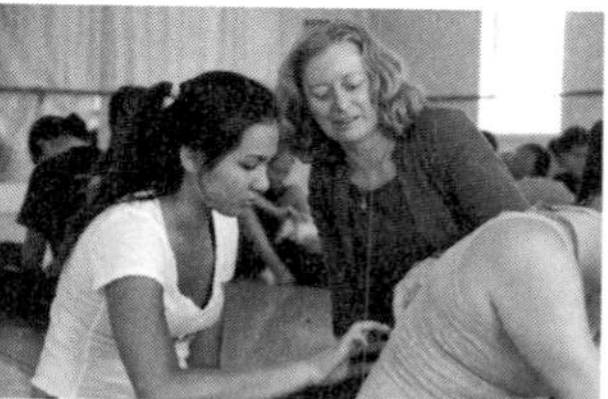

Fig. 14.10a, b, c. To best facilitate this exploration, demonstrate it first with a student (a). You may also need to help students to locate the individual vertebrae and touch the spinous processes (b and c).

Discussion

- What did you learn from doing this? What did you feel or observe from touching your partner along the spine?
- What did you notice as your partner walked?
- What did you feel or observe from curling forward?
- Did the touch from your partner affect your experience? How? Did you notice any difference as you walked? Did anyone have a different experience?

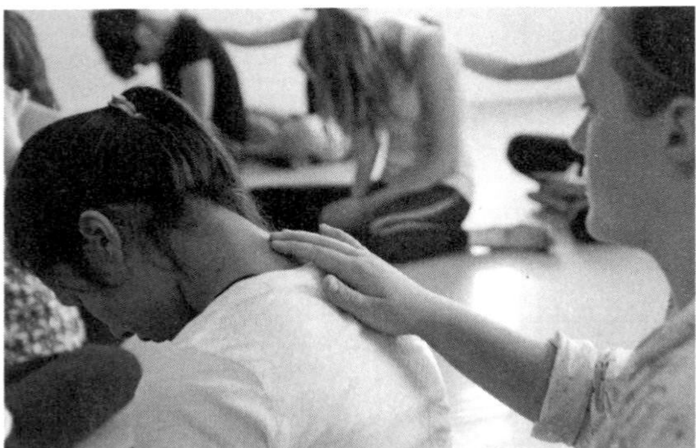

Fig. 14.11. Teens learning through movement and touch: the one being touched gains increased proprioceptive awareness at the point of touch, and the one touching learns to feel the location of the vertebrae.

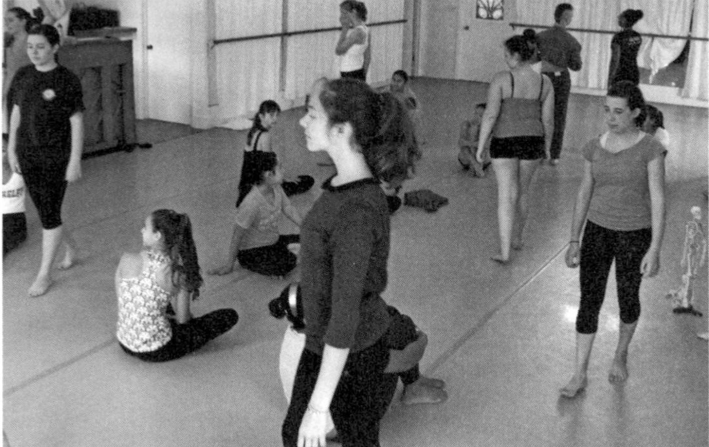

Fig. 14.12. Before changing roles, the person who has received touch along their spine can take a walk to notice how they feel, while their partner observes any changes they perceive. Students often find they feel more lengthened through their spine—and often look taller as well.

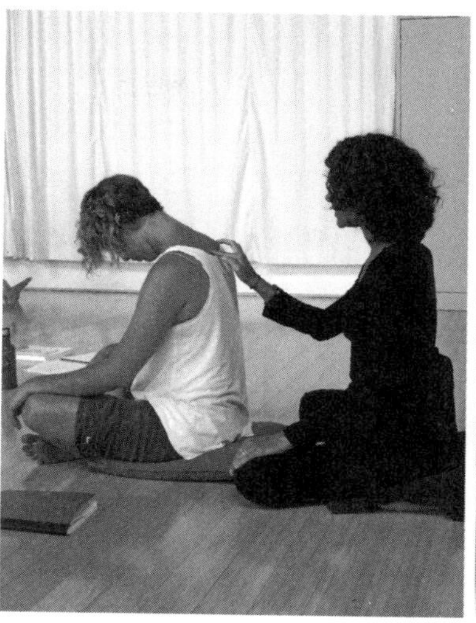

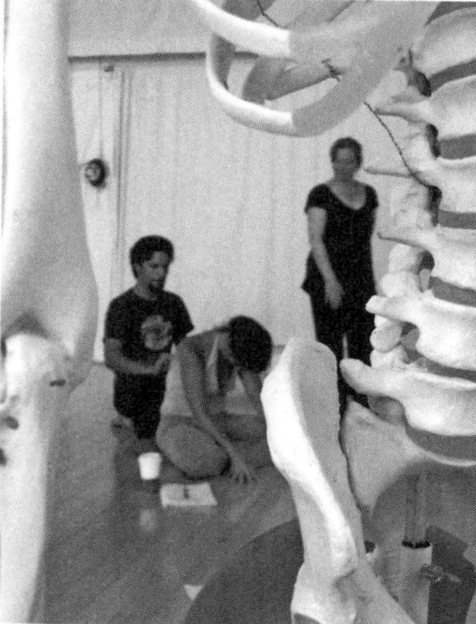

Fig. 14.13a, b. Educators in the Embodiment in Education training learning to do the Forward Curl activity. For both the person being touched and the one touching, it is important to organize your own body so you are supported and lengthened through your own spine so you can touch and move with ease.

Variation

Before or after this exploration, you can help students to understand the structure and function of the intervertebral discs with this fun demonstration: Have one student sit on top of a large physioball; then have them move slightly forward so as to sit more to one side of it. As they will notice, the side they are sitting on will compress, making the back side expand a bit more. This is equivalent to what happens in the discs in spinal flexion, if you imagine that the side you are sitting on is the ventral (front) side *(Fig. 14.15a, b)*. They can then reverse this, sitting on the other side, and imagine this as spinal extension, when the dorsal side would become compressed and the ventral side would expand *(Fig.14.15c, d)*. You can also have another student stand up behind them and demonstrate spinal flexion and extension simultaneously so they get the idea. *(See Fig. 14.15.)* This helps them understand more specifically how the cushioning role of the intervertebral discs actually works.

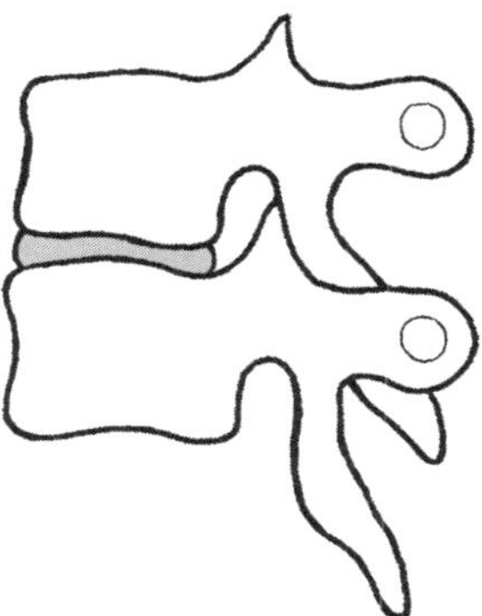

Fig. 14.14. In an aligned position, the intervertebral discs have relatively equal amounts of compression on the front (ventral) and back (dorsal) sides.

Alternately, you can also demonstrate this yourself, with a student as your partner *(Fig. 14.16)*.

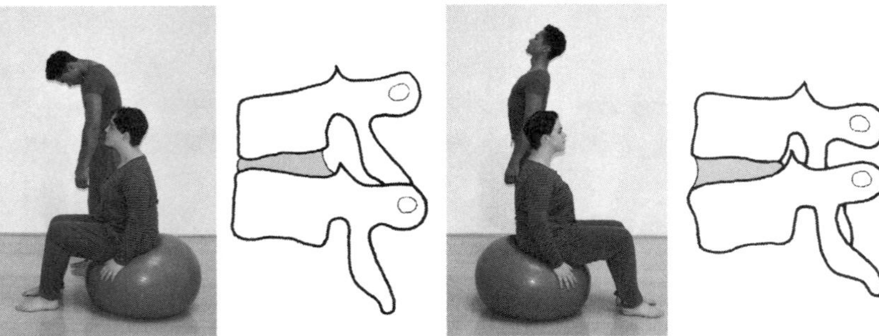

Fig. 14.15a, b, c, d. Variation with physioball: in flexion of the spine, the ventral side of the disc is more compressed, while the dorsal area expands (a and b). In extension, the dorsal side compresses, while the ventral side expands (c and d).

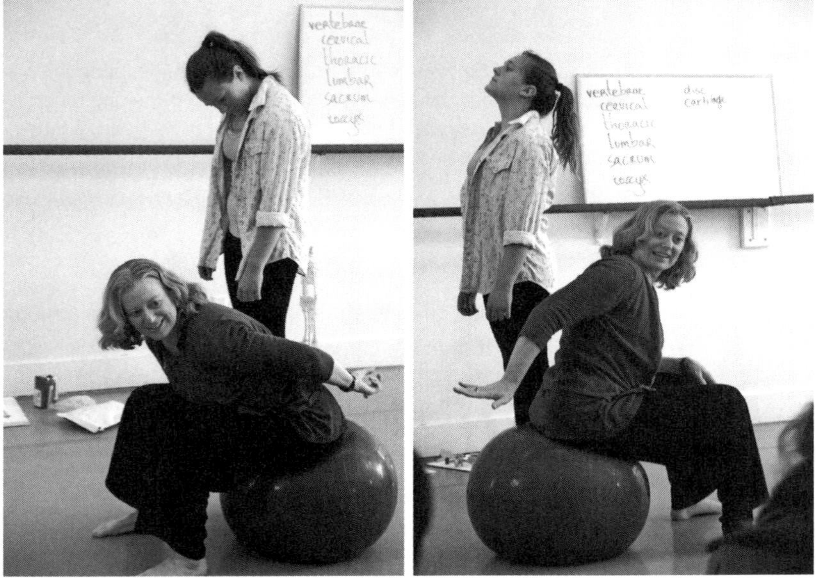

Fig. 14.16a, b. Variation with physioball: you can demonstrate this variation with a student, or have students demonstrate it together as in Fig.14.15.

Tips for Teachers

- You can also facilitate this exploration by guiding the touch more directly—counting each vertebra out loud for the group as they trace the spine. Begin with the cervical vertebrae, often referred to as *C*, followed by the number of the vertebra, so that the first cervical vertebra would be *C1*. Count *C1* and then *C2, C3, C4, C5, C6,* and *C7*. Then the twelve thoracic vertebrae: *T1, T2, T3,* and so forth, all the way down to the five lumbar vertebrae and the sacrum. When tracing back up the spine, begin with the lumbar, counting *L5, L4, L3,* and so on.

- Students find this guided counting very helpful in building group concentration and focus, especially the first time doing the activity. Be sure to let students know that your counting is to be used as a guide, so they are free to go slower or more quickly than your directions if needed.
- Tell students that it is fine to estimate and do their best, rather than needing to be precisely accurate on a first attempt. If you repeat the activity, with practice it gets easier for students to feel comfortable with the process and become more specific in their use of touch.

Exploration: Dance of the Spine—Back to Back

(20–25 minutes)

PURPOSE. To explore the movement potential of your spine; to play with various movements of your spine in a duet movement practice; to encourage responsiveness of your spine and head.

Activity

MATERIALS

- Journal or paper and writing supplies (optional; can be used at the end of the activity)

Have your students do this activity sitting and working with a partner.

❍ Sit back to back with your partner. Take a minute first to breathe, to take a few big, full breaths. Take another deep breath in, and exhale with any sound. *(Do this with them.)* And again, inhale, and exhale with any sound, as you relax back into your partner.

- ❍ As you rest into your partner's back, begin to feel your partner's breathing through your back surface. As you bring your awareness to your breathing, you may notice that you begin to synchronize your breathing with your partner ... breathing at the same time, inhaling and exhaling in the same rhythm.
- ❍ Now together you can begin to explore all the ways your spine can move. Move slowly at first so you can stay together. Just see what evolves as you begin to move, leading or following along. *(Pause to allow students a few moments to explore this.)*
- ❍ Notice if your head is moving as well, or are you holding your head upright? Can you allow your head to respond to the movements of the spine as you move? Continue to move without talking with your partner about what you are doing or what you will do next.
- ❍ How else can your spine move ... what else can you do?
- ❍ Now begin to let your arms respond as well as you move. Did you explore all the possibilities for movement? Can you try something new? Or see what evolves as you follow your partner?
- ❍ Now begin to find a way to end. *(Pause.)* When you are done, just rest again with your partner.
- ❍ Move away by peeling your back away from your partner, turning to one side or the other, and thank your partner.
- ❍ Now close your eyes again, and take a few moments to try some of these variations on your own. *(Pause.)* Do you have a favorite way of moving that you explored? Or one that felt strange or uncomfortable? See if you can let your spine move in whatever way feels best. Is your head responding as well? Try this while standing as well if you like.

Students can talk in partners to share their respective experiences. You can also ask them to write down some words they would use to describe the movements of the spine that they experienced.

Discussion

- What did you experience? Were you able to communicate with your partner without talking?
- Was it different to do this while sitting than it was while standing? How?
- Were you able to let your head respond to the movements? Or did you find yourself holding your head upright? Why do you think that was?

- What did you notice about how you moved? About how your partner moved? Did your partner get you to try anything that felt new to you? Were there any surprises?
- How does your spine move? What did you discover? What words did you write down?

Use the student scribe method to record the various words and phrases. These might include words like "slithering," "snake-like," and "rocking," or phrases like "waves rolling," "stretching up," or "curling over." Students may also offer some of the more anatomical words, such as "flexion" or "extension" as well.

Once the list is complete, distinguish between words that are more descriptive and the anatomical words generally used. Together you can then relate the descriptive phrases they generated to the anatomical terms. For instance, a "wave-like motion" might be a combination of flexion and extension in various parts of the spine at once, while a "turning and arching back" motion would be anatomically defined as a combination of rotation and extension of the spine.

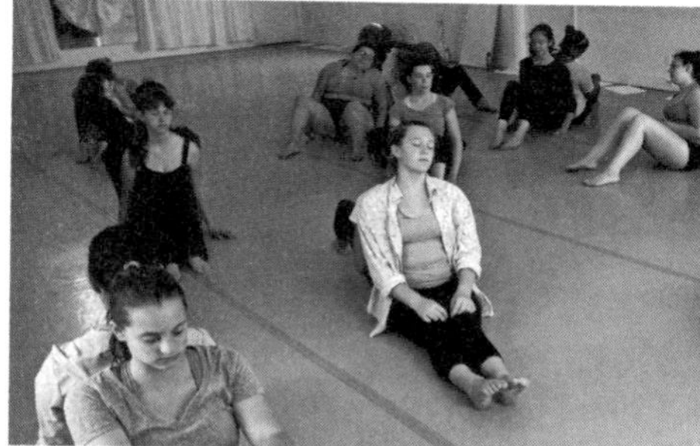
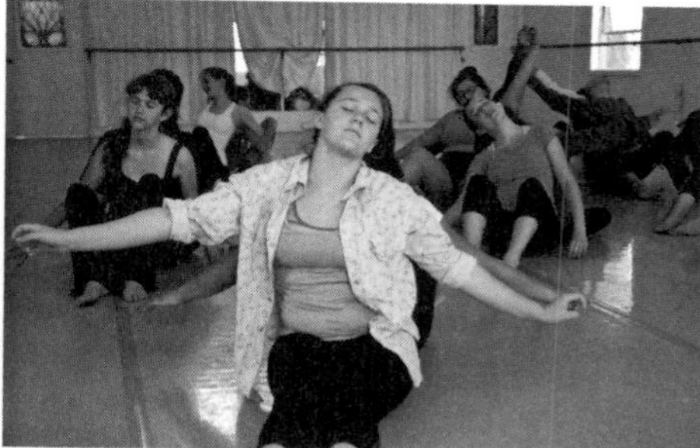

Fig. 14.17a, b. In the Dance of the Spine exploration, students first sit back to back, which increases the proprioceptive awareness of the back surface of their bodies as they lean back into their partner (a). They then explore through movement to discover all the possible ways the spine can move (b). This activity also encourages mutual cooperation and kindness to emerge naturally between them.

Tips for Teachers

- You can also add music to accompany this activity. Music often frees teens to respond more spontaneously. If you choose to use music, add it in part-way into the activity, only once you see that students have made an initial connection with their partners, such as that their breathing has become synchronized and they are moving slowly and in a responsive manner. Otherwise, they may resort to "moving to the music" rather than paying closer attention to their own bodies and their partner's body. You may find it best to use melodic music without words, with a variety of rhythmic pieces to encourage a variety of movement qualities to emerge.

Exploration: Movement of the Spine—Side to Side

(20–30 minutes)

PURPOSE. To experience the interconnection of your head, neck, and spine; to experience lateral flexion of your spine and the easy response of your pelvis, rib cage, and head; to practice organizing your body for lifting.

Activity

This activity is done in partners; demonstrate this first.

One partner lies on the back (supine); the other partner stands and will be gently pulling the partner across the floor by holding the partner's ankles, slightly elevating the legs while moving them side to side. Be sure the partner who is doing the pulling is bending at the hip sockets to support the weight, rather than bending forward at the back, which may strain the lumbar spine. Demonstrate these two ways of bending first, and have students practice this, as indicated below, before working in partners.

❍ *(To the standing partner)* Stand by your partner's feet. Close your eyes and focus on your own body first. Take a moment to do your body scan. Feel your weight being supported through your feet and the full length of your spine reaching up toward the sky.

❍ Now open your eyes, and begin to bend forward as we practiced, by softening and bending first at your ankles, then your knees, and then your hips, still keeping your spine long as you bend forward. Reach your sitz bones back and down, while reaching the top of your head forward and up.

❍ Now reach down and hold your partner's ankles, and lift them up just slightly off the floor. Walk backward, pulling your partner as you move their legs gently from side to side as you move back. *(This works best by shifting side to side fairly quickly, and within a small range of movement, so it initiates a gentle "jiggle" side to side like a fish uses to swim.)* Watch the spine respond as your partner glides along the floor. Notice what happens in his or her body while moving from side to side. How does the spine move?

❍ *(To the lying-down partner)* Relax your head and neck as you are pulled by your partner. Feel this swishing movement travel through your spine. Does your spine move easily? Is there anywhere you feel it gets "stuck" or tense? Can you feel the "contents" moving as well as the "container"?

Switch roles and repeat.

Variation

Students can recreate this lateral swishing of their spine individually while in various positions, such as lying down, sitting, or standing.

Discussion

- What did you notice about your partner's movement? What did you experience as you were being pulled? What about the structure of the spine allows for this type of movement? What animals move like this?
- How did your other three body weights of the head, torso, and pelvis move in response to your spine? What did that feel like?
- Could you feel the "contents" moving as well as the "container"?

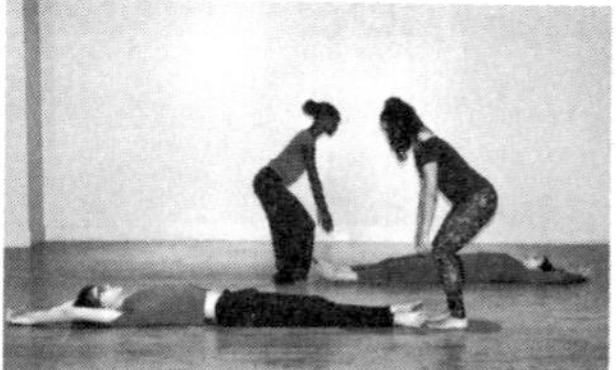
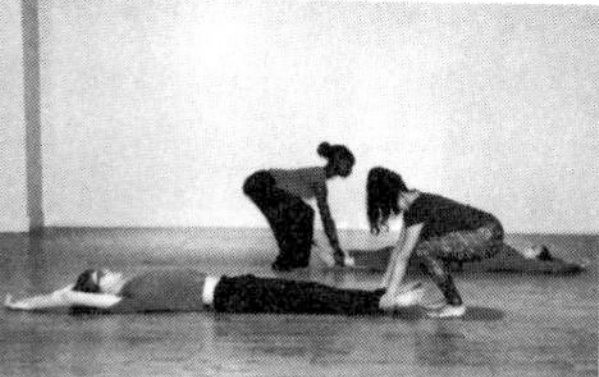
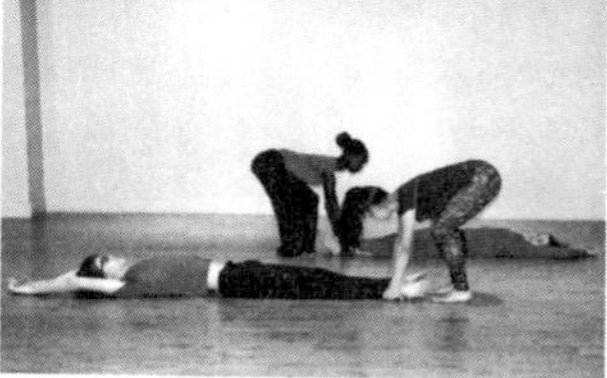

Fig. 14.18a, b, c. In this Movement of the Spine exploration, students play with gently pulling each other across the floor to feel the side-to-side movement (lateral flexion) that gets initiated in the spine. (Before beginning the process, it is important to let them practice organizing their own bodies first—so they can pull their partners without straining their lower backs.)

Tips for Teachers

- While it can be fun to have spontaneous play as part of the class, it's important to be clear with students when that is being invited, or when a more directed focus is needed for all to feel safe. When you teach this activity, be sure to go slowly and methodically, since it involves students moving each other's bodies and necessitates a high level of trust. By giving clear directives and an opportunity to practice each one—individually first and then when working with their partners—students gain a sense of security and trust. The students who are guiding the movement feel confident in knowing what they are doing, and the ones who are being moved can trust that they won't just be pulled about wildly in an unstructured way. Once students have learned how to do the activity with your guidance, they enjoy exploring it on their own, taking turns pulling each other. As they get a better sense of how to do it, this activity inevitably evokes a fun and playful tone among them.

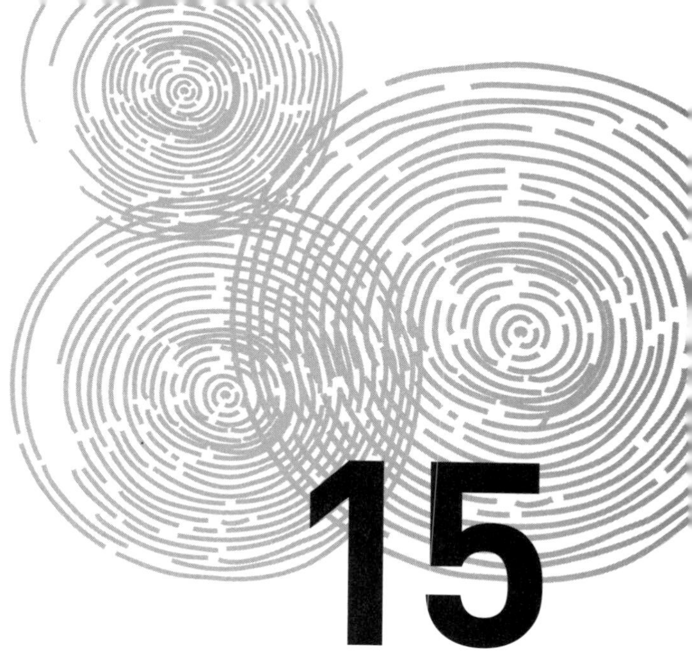

15

Breathing Basics

"How's the concert coming?" I asked a colleague.

"Oh, in a few weeks when more of the details are taken care of, I should be able to take a deep breath."

"Hear from that college yet?" one student asked another.

"No, but I'm not holding my breath. That's my long-shot anyway."

"When is that vacation coming up? I sure could use a breather!"

Anticipation, pressure, fear—all are internal emotional states, which, literally and figuratively, cause us to hold our breath. Our language reveals that we imagine we can postpone breathing until convenient times when we can let down and relax. Yet this pattern likely will take its toll on us—in our bodies and in many aspects of our lives.

Perceptions of Breathing

Breathing is a natural process that occurs without conscious effort. We can, however, alter our breathing by directing our awareness to it. By using conscious control over breathing to reduce chronic tension, students learn to reverse the shallow breathing often caused by emotional stress and to play an active role in maintaining their health. Taking a deep breath, sighing, and laughing create fuller breathing and a sense of ease that helps to restore our physical and emotional health. Breathing can teach us to slow down and to learn not to put the body "on hold" while we push ahead through our lives. In a healthy lifestyle, work, rest, and play are balanced. One of my college students named Calleja had come to realize this on her own, as expressed in her weekly journal:

> *Both the way I grew up within my family and early dance training methods emphasized the value of continuous hard work. There is something to be said for that, but at certain points, without rest, the approach can actually backfire. Instead of running towards a goal, I might run myself into the ground. Thus, I have slowly been learning the value of rest.*

With a balanced lifestyle, we find it easier to relax; otherwise, our level of stress increases. As we experience stress, we become constricted in many areas of our bodies. Just as emotional stress can cause us to tighten the muscles of our shoulders, for instance, we may also tighten the muscles of the ribs, belly, and back, leading to shallow breathing. By restricting our breathing and decreasing the flow of oxygen to our bodies, we decrease our vitality. We may also be making other changes in our lifestyle that further deplete our energy, such as sleeping less, eating quickly, or neglecting to get outdoors or exercise. As we find we have less energy to meet the many demands that made us feel overloaded to begin with, our anxiety increases. Teenagers experience this same pressure from the demands of their academic and personal lives from school, parents, peers, and a dynamically changing body in adolescence—and could benefit from learning to "take a breath" once in awhile.

To begin to focus on breathing, students are first guided to explore ways that sound and movement affect their breathing. These movement activities inevitably evoke discussion of topics such as the difference between full and shallow breathing, the relationship of heartbeat (circulatory system) and breath (respiratory system), and perceptions and feelings we may have about expressing through sound and movement. Students then create journal entries through a free-writing process by responding to the prompt, "I can't breathe when …" and then to the prompt, "I can breathe when …" These writings put them in touch with situations, thoughts, and feelings that may restrict their breathing, as well as those that support them to breathe more fully.

Sharing their responses also allows them to discover common experiences that have emerged from the group community as a whole. Teenagers find these discussions especially engaging, as they give them a chance to give voice to their many experiences—visceral and emotional—related to feelings of being either restricted and repressed, or free to be themselves.

Here are a few examples of the kinds of responses students have had to this journal writing activity. One student wrote:

> *I can't breathe when I am nervous. I can't breathe when I am crying. I can't breathe when I am overthinking things. I can't breathe when I am watching something scary. I can't breathe when I'm trying really hard to fall asleep. I can't breathe when I see something beautiful.*

And then:

> *I can breathe when I feel comfortable. I can breathe when I am outside and under the sun. I can breathe when I dance. I can breathe when I am moving. I can breathe when I am confident. I can breathe when I am with my friends.*

Here is how another student expressed herself in her response:

> *I can't breathe when I try too hard, when I'm worried if I will be good enough. Or when I* know *I am not good enough. Then the life force is gone. Fear is at the heart of it. I'm afraid I'll fail, and I forget to breathe.*

And then:

> *I can breathe when I stand at the edge of the ocean and look out at the expanse of the sea. I can breathe in the fresh spring air with my arms wide open, ready to receive. I could breathe when I used to run through the hot Houston streets. I can breathe when I find a good beat in the song to tap my feet to.*

And finally, here is another response from a student who later wrote in her journal about this free-response writing activity she had done in class:

> *When responding to the prompt, "I can't breathe when," I was instantly taken deep into memories or images that were dark and discomforting. I said I couldn't breathe when I think about what life would be like without God, or when I think about my best friend dying, or times when she has been hurt in life. I also started thinking in more literal terms, like if I imagine myself underwater, or emotionally like when there is a heavy weight on my shoulders. But when I wrote about the*

"I can breathe when" one, I started to think about places where I feel connected to the creator of my breath, like standing on top of a mountain, or sitting on the beach watching the waves. The way the ocean stirs in and out, crashes and calms is the same as my steady breath, moving in and out.

Interestingly, the student who had been her partner in the activity when they shared their writings together afterward also wrote about this experience in *her* journal. Here is an excerpt of her response:

When we shared our experiences, my partner shared that she can't breathe when she thinks about the bad things that happened to her best friend. I thought that was incredibly selfless for her to not be able to breathe, which is such a personal and vital thing to do for yourself, because of another person. This got me really thinking. How does the outside world affect our internal experience, such as breathing?

As these reflections all reveal, students learn from their own insights when given time to reflect on their experiences and share them with each other.

Exploration: Breathing and Sound

(10–15 minutes)

PURPOSE. To practice using breathing and sound to release tension and increase physical vitality; to notice the effect of breathing and sound; to identify ways in which fuller breathing can be integrated into your daily life.

Activity

This activity is done in Constructive Rest.

- Take a few deep breaths and allow your body to relax. In your mind's eye, see if you can imagine breathing into any areas of your body that feel tense.
- Now, as you exhale, let the air seep out gently through your teeth, making a hissing sound. *(This can also be done with an "ahhh" sound.)*[1] Imagine this sound filling through your spine, allowing it to lengthen. Send this sound to any place in your body that feels tense.
- Now, as you exhale, let out any sound that comes out. It might be a big, quick sigh, a rolling lingering sigh, a laugh ... just see what happens. Allow this sound to evolve as you exhale, letting the sound vibrate in your body. Send this sound to any place in your body that needs this inner massage of vibration.

- ❍ Take a few deep breaths again, breathing in ... and out. Do you notice any differences in your body from when we began this activity? Any places that feel more open or relaxed?

Discussion

- What did you notice from doing this activity? What helped you to release tension the most? How did you feel making sound? Could you let the sound come out as you exhaled? Could you feel it vibrate in your body? Where?
- What types of things affect how you breathe? *(Examples might be levels of physical activity, stress, and emotions.)* Can you think of any examples of when you spontaneously use sound to relieve tension? *(Examples might be yawning, groaning, or laughing.)*
- Can you think of ways you could use breathing in your daily life to help you relax or to focus? *(A few examples might be taking a few deep breaths before taking a test or having a difficult conversation, using the previous activity before going to bed at night, singing, or taking a brisk walk and breathing deeply.)*

Exploration: Breathing and Movement

(15–20 minutes)

PURPOSE. To explore the way various types of physical activities affect your breathing.

Activity

Lead students in a movement improvisation based on a variety of types of movement that vary in speed and energy such as running, moving in slow motion, and jumping. After each variation, ask them to pause, close their eyes, and notice how they feel in general, as well as how each activity affects their breathing.

Discussion

- What did you notice about your breathing from moving? When did your breathing speed up? Did you find you were ever holding your breath? What made you do that? What does that feel like? What happens in your body when you hold your breath? When you breathe fully?

Exploration: Breathing and Emotion (Journal Entry)

(40–50 minutes)

PURPOSE. To explore your associations with breathing; to notice elements such as situations, thoughts, or feelings that may restrict your breathing, as well as those that may support or nourish your ability to breathe fully; to share these perceptions as a group.

Activity

MATERIALS

- Writing paper or journal
- Pen and drawing supplies

This journal writing can be combined with either of the two previous explorations, in which case you can include the writing immediately after the activity, before the discussion section. When done as a separate activity, include a brief version of Constructive Rest as described below.

Part 1 (Constructive Rest)

Have students first place their journals somewhere to the side of the room, so they can easily come back to them later. Then have them get into Constructive Rest.

- Take a few deep breaths, in … and out. Take a moment to do your body scan in this position, noticing the weight on your feet, all the way up to your head. *(Leave a few minutes for this.)* Take another few deep breaths, in … and out.
- Place one hand on your belly, and one on your upper chest or sternum area, and just bring your awareness to your breathing. You don't have to try to change anything; just rest here and allow yourself to breathe however it feels natural to you. Rest here. *(Allow 2–3 minutes for this.)*
- What do you notice? What does it feel like to "breathe naturally"? What allows you to do that? What makes it harder to do?
- Take a last minute to do your body scan again, and see what you notice after having rested and focused on your breathing. Take a few deep breaths, in … and out.
- When you are ready, begin to transition out of Constructive Rest, by rolling on your side to come to sitting.
- Then go get your journal, and find a place to sit where you will be writing for a few minutes once we are all ready.

Part 2 (Journal Writing)

Explain that this is a free-response journal entry, in which students can write whatever comes to mind once they are given the prompt. Tell students they will have 2–3 minutes for each topic. Also explain that they can write complete sentences, just phrases or words, or even choose to draw as part of their response.

Also explain that after writing they will be sharing their responses with each other, but will be able to choose which parts to share from their writing, and will not need to hand it in to you.

- ❍ Here is your first prompt. "I can't breathe when ..."

After a few minutes, ask students to complete the sentence or thought they are writing before going on to the next prompt.

- ❍ Here is your second topic: "I can breathe when ..." *(After a few minutes, again ask them to complete their writing.)*
- ❍ *(Done in partners or groups of three.)* Take a few moments to share your responses. Start with one person sharing, and then switch to the next person. *(Alternately, you can time them and let them know when to switch to the next partner so there is equal time for each person in the group.)*

When done, end here or add this variation: Explain that they will next be taking a few minutes to gather the themes that were mentioned in their groups. For the purpose of this exercise, a theme will mean anything that was mentioned more than once, in other words by more than one person in the group. Ask them to each keep a list of the themes.

Discussion

- What did you learn? What types of things restrict your breathing? Why might that be? *(You can start with the first prompt, "I can't breathe when ..." and then move to the second topic, or just let them respond in general.)*
- *(Or with the variation of gathering themes)* What were some of the themes that emerged from your group? *(You can have students rotate in the role of the scribe to write all of the themes on a board or newsprint paper for the whole group to see together as the discussion unfolds.)*
- What types of things restrict your breathing? Why might that be? What types of things support breathing fully? Why might that be?
- Were all of your responses the same, or was there some variation? Why do you think that is? What has been most important to you about this discussion? What have you learned?
- What topic areas seem to affect our breathing in either case, positively or negatively? *(Discuss themes that appear on both lists, such as exercise/movement, emotions, and so on.)* Why might that be?

The Anatomy of Breathing

In one small group of teen girls I worked with, we were beginning to study about breathing. Each of the five students was asked to place their hands on their ribs, first in front and then in back, to breathe deeply and fully, and to notice what happened under their hands. What happens in the rib cage? All five said that the ribs move up and out on the inhale, down on the exhale. What happens in the back? Not much, they said.

Then, they were asked to place their hands on their belly, again to breathe deeply and to notice what they felt. What happens in the belly or abdomen? Three told me that their stomach moved in on the inhale and out on the exhale. One girl said that her stomach didn't move at all. The last girl seemed hesitant and said she didn't know. Finally, she admitted it seemed to her that her stomach moved out on the inhale and in on the exhale. She was the heaviest girl among them and seemed to think that was why. "Maybe it's because I'm fat," she said.

I asked them why they thought we had a discrepancy here. The other four girls each discussed how they learned to breathe like that from others—parents, siblings, and, in one case, a previous dance teacher—telling them to "keep their stomachs in." One girl confessed that she and her sister practiced together for hours and hours to get it right. The fifth girl, by now, was very discouraged. "No one told me how to breathe right," she complained.

"Let's not assume you are wrong," I reminded her. Ironically, she was the only one allowing the body its natural rhythm of inhaling and exhaling, expanding and releasing, in the dynamic flow of breathing.

In an attempt to conform to our culture's image of the ideal body, many students limit the fullness of their breathing to attain the "flat stomach." Although some people may naturally have a flat abdomen, others may not. Because the image of the flat stomach is proscribed as an ideal for both males and females through the media (in dance, aerobics, weight lifting, and modeling, to name a very few), students may hold their stomach muscles tightly to achieve this aesthetic. Moreover, this image encourages an experience of the abdomen as a region of muscle, rather than also as a container for the vital organs organs such as the stomach, liver, and intestines.

In full breathing, both the thoracic cavity and the abdominal cavity alternately change in volume, causing three-dimensional movement in both the rib cage and the belly. The diaphragm, the muscle responsible for 90 percent of our breathing, separates the thoracic and abdominal cavities. As the muscle of the diaphragm contracts, it moves downward toward its stable points on the ribs and spine, causing it to flatten. This shift increases the volume in the thoracic cavity, allowing for the inflow of oxygen as air rushes in to fill the lungs. As it flattens, the diaphragm also presses on the abdominal region and causes the contents to expand outward, often giving the appearance of a more rounded belly. Holding in the muscles of the abdomen inhibits this wave-like motion of the diaphragm and restricts the natural movement of the organs.

In the thoracic cavity, the ribs house the lobes of the lungs and the heart, nestled between the lobes. As the lungs fill with oxygen, they expand in six directions like a balloon—front, back, side to side, and up and down. Simultaneously, the rib cage expands when inhaling and contracts when exhaling, allowing the container (ribs) to be responsive to the contents (lungs). Holding tension in the intercostal muscles between the ribs or the more external muscles in the torso inhibits this rhythmic response of the ribs and limits the full expansion of the lungs. In unrestricted breathing, the ability of the lungs to completely fill and empty brings more oxygen into the circulatory system and enhances functioning of all the cells in the body.

Learning about the structures and dynamics of breathing—the actual anatomy and physiology—can help students to more readily identify and alleviate any holding patterns in the muscles of the rib cage and abdominal wall which may cause shallow breathing. The initial exploration called How Do We Breathe? is designed to provide a context for students to begin with what they each experience and know about breathing, by first observing their breathing and then discussing what they discover. They can then learn further information. As students recognize their own breathing patterns, further activities help them expand their perceptions and their movement.

Exploration: How Do We Breathe?

(30–45 minutes)

PURPOSE. To discover what you know about the process of breathing; to elicit questions about the process of breathing; to learn about the mechanics of breathing.

Activity

MATERIALS

- Blank paper (or students can use their own journals)
- Pencil or pen for each student

Part 1 (Done in Constructive Rest)

- ❍ Bring your awareness to your breathing, and take a few moments to see what you become aware of, what you feel.
- ❍ Why do you breathe? What is the purpose of breathing?

- Imagine inside of your body ... how does breathing take place? Take a minute to observe and to feel how this process occurs.
- What do you know? What is a *mystery*?...
- Place your hands first on your rib cage in front, take a few breaths, and notice what you feel under your hands.
- Feel your back against the floor as you breathe. What do you feel?
- Now place your hands on your belly, and take a few breaths again. What do you feel under your hands?
- Now keep one hand on your belly, and place the other hand on your upper chest or sternum. Notice what you feel under your hands now. *(Fig. 15.1.)*
- Relax your arms back down, and rest here as you breathe. What do you notice?
- When you are ready, roll to one side and come back up to a sitting position.

Part 2 (Journal Writing)

- What do you know about how you breathe? First, take some time to make some notes about what you felt or experienced in this activity. Then, make a list of everything you know about breathing. You can just jot down words or phrases if you like, or use some complete sentences. Include anything you know about breathing, like the purpose of breathing and the structures in the body responsible for breathing. You might want to also include any questions that you have. *(Leave 5–10 minutes for this journal-writing exercise. Students can discuss their experience in partners or small groups of three or four before proceeding to the group discussion.)*

Discussion

Students can alternate as scribes to record the information garnered by each group.

- What did you discover in your group? What questions did you have?

Other leading questions may include any of the following:

- Why do we breathe? What is the purpose of breathing?
- What did you experience happening under your hands in your upper torso or rib cage? What did you experience in your lower torso or belly?
- Did anyone have a different experience? Why do you think that is?
- How do we breathe? What happens in your body?

Add relevant anatomy/physiology information, such as tracing the flow of oxygen from the nose and mouth to the trachea and lungs, to the capillaries and blood to the cells. The additional explorations related to breathing can then also provide experiential learning to address questions that arise.

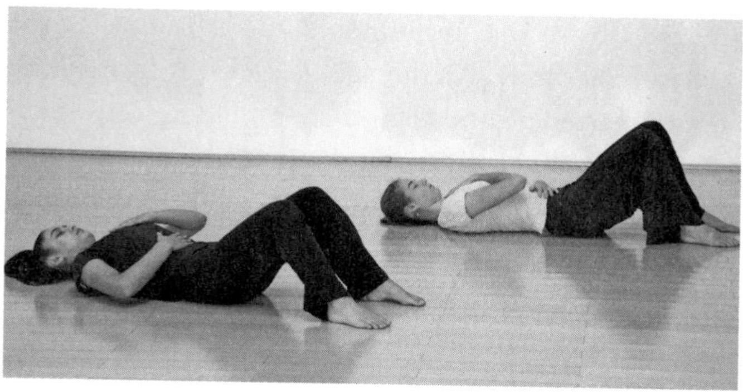

Fig. 15.1. In How Do We Breathe? students place their hands on their bodies to feel their breathing, as they discover both what they experience physically and consider what they know about the process of breathing.

Tips for Teachers

- The discussion of the anatomy/physiology of breathing can also be extended to include issues of health. Remind students of the need to fully exhale—releasing all the carbon dioxide—in order to bring fresh oxygen to the body when they inhale. You might also discuss the relationship of breathing and blood flow to overall health, such as feeling vital or depleted, or to disorders related to lack of oxygen, such as asthma or anemia.

HOME PRACTICE

- Students can write in their body journals to track their experiences during the week, expanding on the journal prompts related to what activities or situations impact their breathing.

Breathing and Movement

Breathing also affects our movement—inhibiting or freeing it; likewise our movement can inhibit or free our breathing. The lobes of the lungs, two on the left and three on the right, embrace the heart three-dimensionally and gently massage the heart as we breathe. Opening in the upper body allows for the full expansion of the lungs and healthy functioning of the heart—so that movement is free and unencumbered. The lungs also expand upward all the way beneath the clavicles, and can help to support movement of the arms and upper spine. The intercostal muscles between the ribs expand and contract the ribs, while the cartilaginous joints connecting the ribs to the sternum allow for this ease of movement in the front (ventral) side of the body. At the spine, each rib forms a hinge joint with two adjacent thoracic vertebrae and their disc, providing responsive movement at the back (dorsal) side as well. Healthy alignment allows our spine, rib cage, lungs, and heart to have ample space for full movement and functioning; otherwise, we restrict our potential.

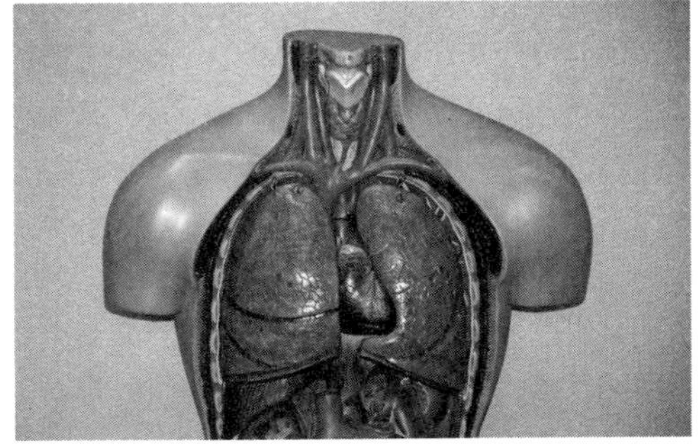

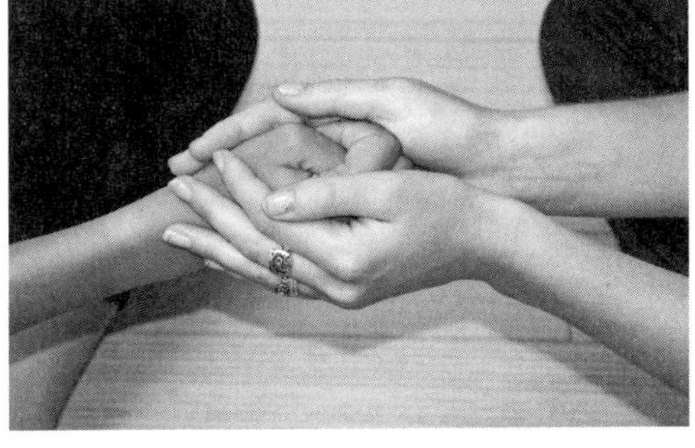

Once students understand the purpose and dynamics of the anatomy of breathing, they explore the many dimensions of their movement as they breathe: to feel the support of the internal organs of the lungs and heart (the "contents") within the rib cage (the "container") when moving; to visualize the relationship of the lungs and heart; to experience the movement of the rib cage in breathing; to feel the back surface of their bodies in breathing; and to feel the location and movement of the thoracic diaphragm; and finally, to integrate all of this awareness into full breathing. All of these activities provide more full-bodied breathing leading to increased vitality and health.

While most of these explorations are done individually, some include partner activities, like sitting back to back to feel the back surface of one's body respond when breathing, or variations with props, such as working in groups with a parachute to simulate the movement of the diaphragm when inhaling and exhaling. These interactive methods help bring the anatomy to life and create a fun and creative learning community. They also help students to personalize their learning, as noted in this journal response about the activity done in partners to experience the way the lungs "hug" the heart that was written by Lani:

> *A lasting thought for me was the image of one's hands cupped around another's closed fist. It reflects the very image of the heart encased by the lungs. Just as how the lungs shield the heart, so does the sternum and the ribs protect the lungs. Thinking about this just made me feel safe in my own body.*

Exploration: Contents and Container[2]

(10–15 minutes)

PURPOSE. To differentiate between the rib cage (the "container") and the internal organs of the lungs and heart (the "contents"); to expand the concept of breathing to include movement of the internal organs and ribs; to experience the movement of the rib cage and organs in breathing; to feel the support of the organs of the lungs and heart when moving.

Activity

This activity builds on the exploration Moving from the Bones, Moving from the Organs in chapter 11, and may be practiced sitting or standing.

- ❍ Place your hands on your rib cage in the front. Close your eyes. Feel the bones of your hands resting on the bones of your ribs. Now move your rib cage by moving your ribs. *(Fig. 15.2.)* Relax your hands and rest a moment.
- ❍ Next place your hands on your rib cage again, this time a little more to your sides. Close your eyes. Imagine that your hands are resting gently on your lungs. Feel the heart nestled between the lobes of the lungs, two on the left and three on the right. Now move your "contents" inside the rib cage; feel them move back and forth between your hands. Relax your hands and rest a moment.
- ❍ Let that movement move the ribs, the contents move the container. Now let the ribs move the organs, the container move the contents.
- ❍ Let's do this again, but this time you can feel both the movement of the rib cage and of the internal organs, moving together.
- ❍ You can try lengthening one arm up, feeling the support of your lungs as you lift your arm. Then lift the other arm, as you breathe in, and feel the support of your lungs again. *(Fig. 15.3.)*
- ❍ Now move around just as you want, exploring this on your own. *(Pause while students explore this.) (Fig. 15.4.)*

Discussion

- What did you experience? What movements occur in your body when you breathe? How does your rib cage respond when you inhale? exhale? What is responsible for this movement? Where is your heart located? How do the lungs move when you breathe?
- Could you feel your contents and your container when you moved? What did you notice? How did it feel to lift and move your arms? Was this any different than when you were moving at the beginning? Could you feel the support of your lungs?

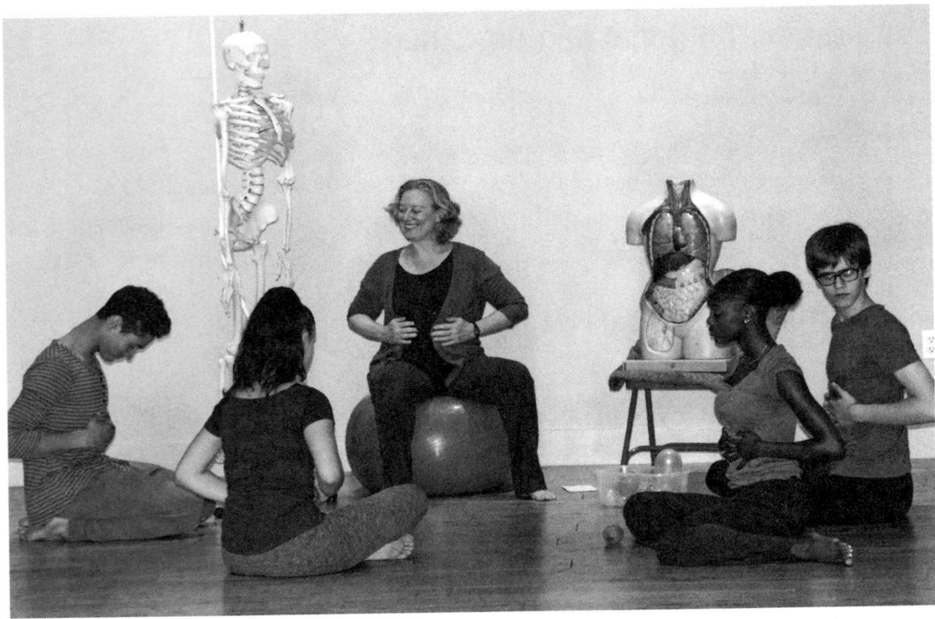

Fig. 15.2. Teens explore moving from the contents and container, first, with a focus on the ribs and then on the lungs and heart.

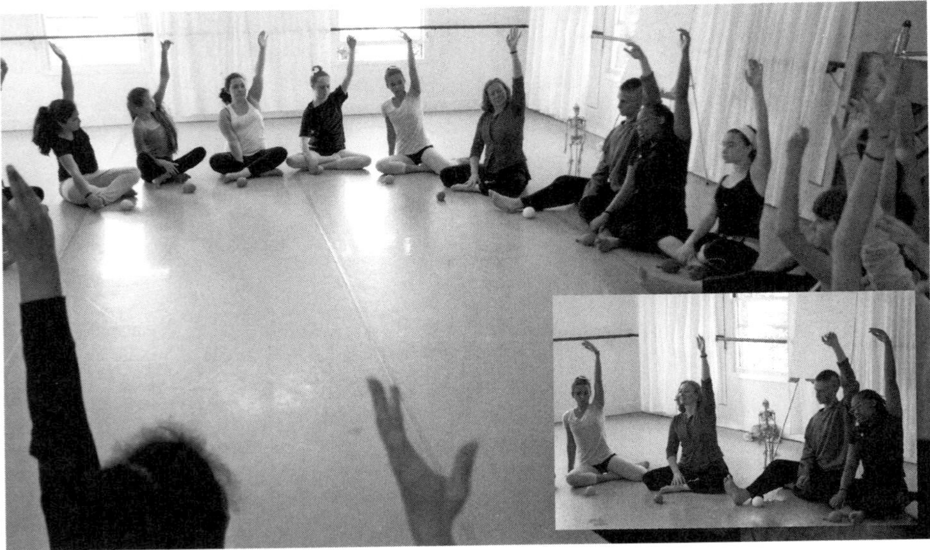

Fig. 15.3a, b. Teens discover how it feels to "reach from the lungs"; this often brings a feeling of inner support, expands their breathing, and gives them a more three-dimensional sense of their upper bodies.

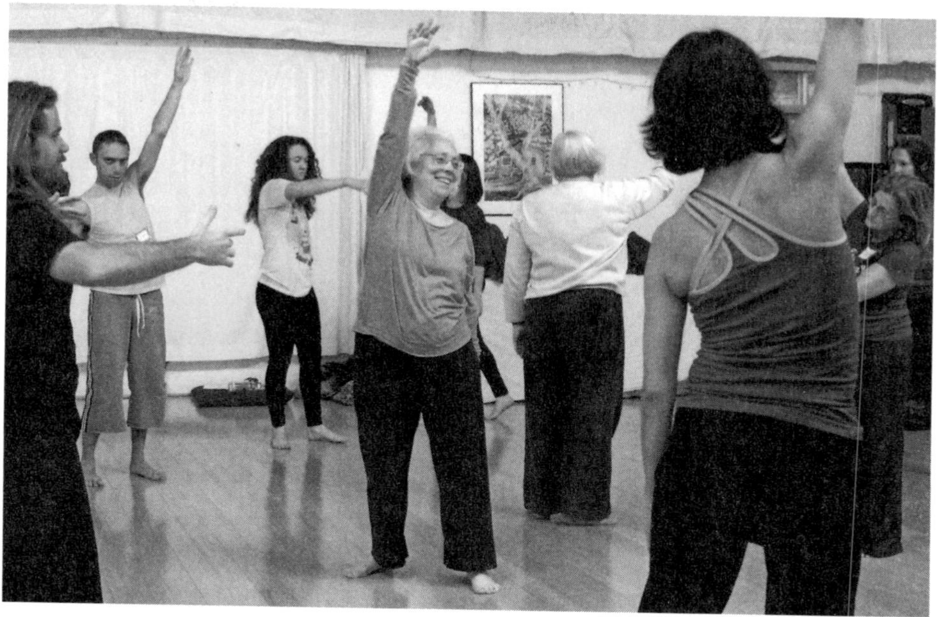

Fig. 15.4. Guest faculty Bonnie Bainbridge Cohen leading a group of educators in exploring organ support and expression in the Embodiment in Education training, California.

Exploration: Hug of the Lungs and Heart

(15–20 minutes)

PURPOSE. To experience the relationship of the lungs and heart; to increase awareness of the three-dimensional support of the lungs around the heart; to integrate this awareness into your movement.

Activity

Have your students do this activity in partners, sitting or standing facing each other.

First review the anatomy of the heart and lungs using a drawing or an organ model first to show the way the lobes of the lungs, two on the left and three on the right, embrace the heart three-dimensionally so students have a clear visual image of this relationship. If you have a skeletal model, you can also use balloons placed inside the rib cage to demonstrate this, with a red water balloon to represent the heart and lighter-colored air balloons to represent the lungs on either side. *(Fig. 15.5.)* Then begin the partner activity.

- *(Partner One)* Put one arm out and make a fist. You are the heart.
- *(Partner Two)* Take your hands and gently embrace the "heart" with your own hands on either side. You are the lungs.
- *(To the full group)* Feel your hands together. Feel how the lungs are hugging the heart, and how the heart is being embraced by the lungs. Close your eyes. Rest here a moment. *(Pause.) (Fig. 15.6.)*
- Now release your hands from your partner, and place them on your own body, one hand on your heart and one somewhere on your ribs/lungs. Still keep your eyes closed.
- Take a few deep breaths and feel this in your own body. Your lungs hugging your heart, your heart beating and pulsing within the embrace of your lungs.

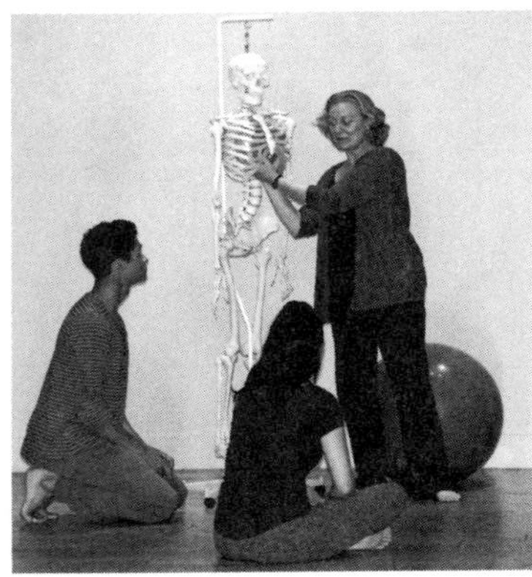

Fig. 15.5. Using a combination of air-filled balloons (to represent the lungs) and a water balloon (to represent the heart) helps teens to visualize the organs in their own bodies, and understand where they are situated in relation to their rib cage.

- You may want to move your hands to feel this in different parts of your rib cage/ lungs, since your lungs extend in the front, sides, and back as well. You can also move around as you do this. Notice what you experience. Then rest.

End here, or partners can switch roles and repeat. Partners can take a few minutes to talk together, or move to the large group discussion.

Variation

When partners have their hands together, those who are representing the heart with their fists can be asked to "start beating," by pumping the fist slightly in rhythm with their pulse, while those who are representing the lungs can gently expand and contract their hands in rhythm with their own breath. This gives more of a sense of the visceral movement of the "massage" of the lungs around the heart.

Discussion

- What did you experience? What did you discover? Were there any surprises? How did you feel from doing this activity? Did anyone have a different experience? What questions do you have?

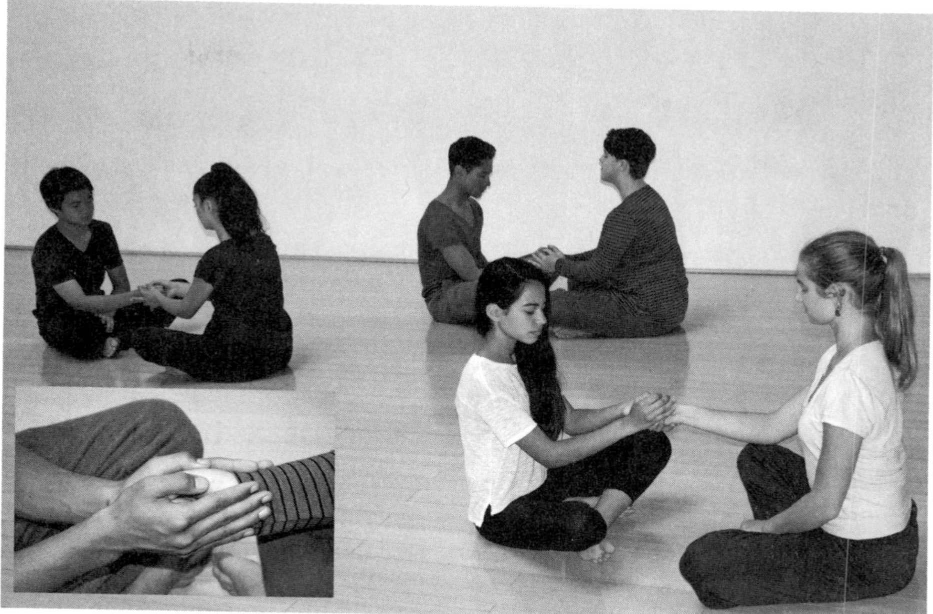

Fig. 15.6a, b. The Hug of the Lungs and Heart exploration allows teens to work in partners to feel the intimate relationship between the lungs and heart in their own bodies (a and b). They then place their hands on their own torsos, to reinforce this image from within.

Exploration: Awakening the Back

(20 minutes)

PURPOSE. To experience the three dimensions of breathing; to increase awareness of the back surface of your body in breathing; to integrate this awareness into your movement.

Activity

Have your students do this activity in partners, sitting together back to back.

- Sit back to back with your partner. Allow your weight to relax back into your partner's back. Close your eyes. Feel your breathing through the back surface of your body.

- ❍ Feel the breathing of your partner as your rib cage responds to the inhale and exhale of your breath.
- ❍ Without talking about it, see if you can allow your breathing to take on a common rhythm, so you are each inhaling and exhaling at the same time. Feel the massage of your back from the movement of your breathing with your partner.
- ❍ Place your hands on your front surface, perhaps using one hand on your belly and one on your sternum. Feel the front and back surfaces of your body, as you breathe in. *(Fig. 15.7.)* Can you feel the fullness between your front and back surface as your breath fills your lungs? And then how the volume inside gets smaller as you exhale? *(Pause.)*
- ❍ Repeat this again, but now place your hands on your sides. Feel the breathing in both the front, back, and side surfaces of your body. *(Leave several minutes of silence for students to experience this.)*
- ❍ Now take a deep breath, in and out, simultaneously with your partner. Take another breath in, releasing any sound or sigh on your exhale. Take another breath now, and on the exhale you can gently separate your back surface away from your partner.
- ❍ As you sit on your own, notice your breathing, still with your eyes closed ... then again with eyes opened. Get up when you are ready and take a walk. Notice how you feel. *(Leave a few minutes for students to walk around the room.)* You might even try some stretching with your arms or any other movements to see how it feels to move now.
- ❍ When you are ready, rejoin with your partner and take a minute to each talk about what you each experienced.

Discussion:

- *(In the full group)* What did you experience? Could you feel your partner's breathing through your back? How is it possible to feel the movement of breathing through the back surface of your body? Could you find a common rhythm of breathing? How did that happen? What did it feel like? When you placed your hands on the front of your body (sternum and belly) were you aware of both the front and back sides of your body at once? Could you feel movement in the sides of your body? In how many directions do the lungs expand?
- How did this feel when you did it on your own? Was there a difference with your eyes closed or your eyes opened? What did you notice as you walked around the room? How did it feel to move? Did you notice the back surface of your body more than usual? Did anyone have a different experience?

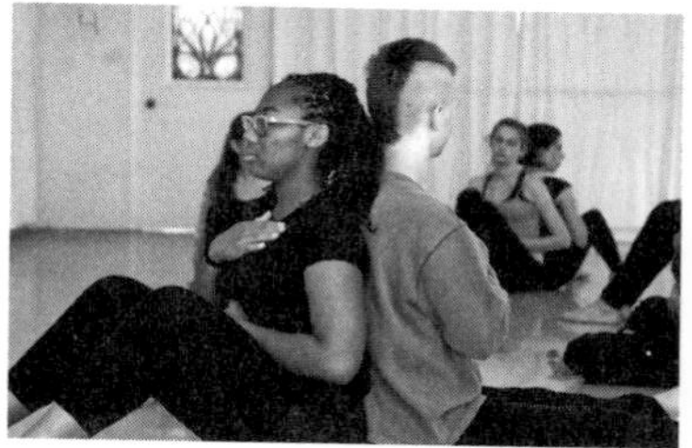
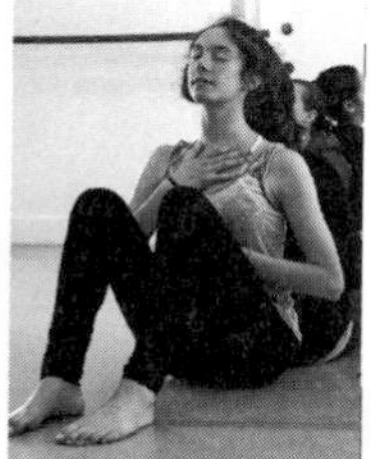
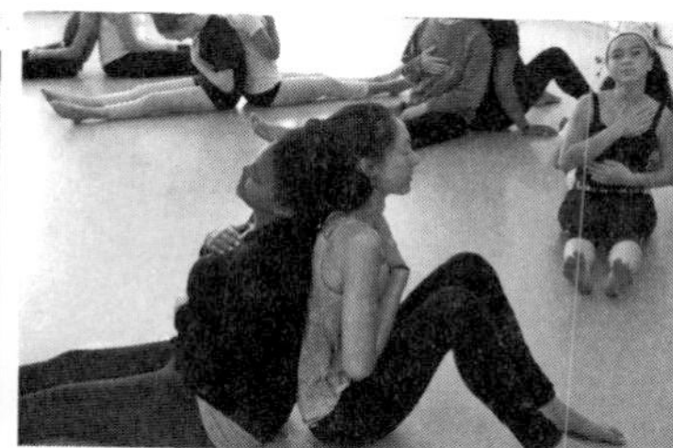

Fig. 15.7a, b, c. The Awakening the Back exploration enlivens students' experience of breathing as they sit back to back and place their hands on their sternum and belly. This awakens awareness of the expansion of the lungs in both the back and front sides of the body. Working together in partners, they also experience the common rhythm of their breath.

Tips for Teachers

- If you don't think it best to have your students do this activity in partners, it can be done with each student sitting against a wall. Students can also use an exercise ball (physioball) braced up against a wall, which gives a more responsive surface to lean against to allow them to feel their breathing through the back surface of their bodies.

Exploration: Rib Cage, Lungs, and Diaphragm

(20 minutes; 30–50 minutes with variations)

PURPOSE. To understand and experience the mechanics of thoracic breathing; to feel and visualize the movement of the diaphragm in inhaling and exhaling; to physicalize your learning; to understand the movement of the diaphragm related to your thoracic and abdominal cavities.

Activity/Discussion

Have your students do this sitting or in Constructive Rest.

- Place your hands on the either side of the ribs, so that your fingers are facing into your center. *(Demonstrate this.)* Close your eyes now, and breathe in and out. How do your hands move as you breathe? *(Your fingers will spread apart on the inhale and come together on exhale.) (See Figs. 15.8a, b.)* Feel the movement of both the rib cage and the lungs under your hands.
- Place your hands on the back of your rib cage, so your fingers face the center of your back, with your thumbs at the sides of your rib cage. Now close your eyes and take another few deep breaths. How do your hands move now as you breathe? *(Your fingers will spread apart on the inhale and come together on exhale.) (Figs. 15.8c, d.)*

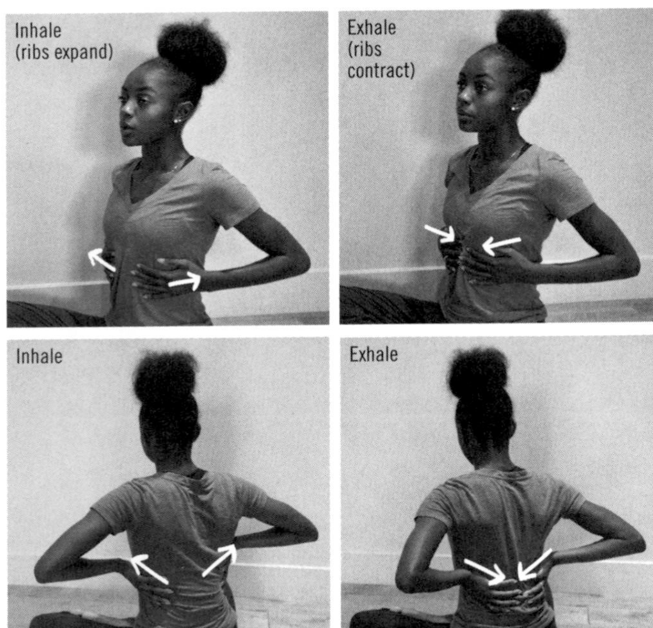

Fig. 15.8a, b, c, d. Students can use their hands to feel the movement of the rib cage in both the front and back when breathing (a–d).

- What about the diaphragm; how does it move? Use your fingers to reach gently under your lower ribs. *(Fig. 15.8e.)* Now take a moment and cough, just once or twice. What do you feel under your hands? Can you feel the downward pressure of your diaphragm? Now see if you can reproduce that movement without coughing.
- Then relax your arms back down and take a deep breath. Can you feel your diaphragm move as you breathe in?
- Now you can use your hands to make a dome shape at level of your diaphragm. *(Demonstrate by using your hands in a curved position with your fingers touching and facing inward. Refer to skeletal model or photo/drawing.)* Now as you inhale, flatten your hands out and down, letting your fingers interlace further as you move them down; and as you exhale, curve your hands again and let your fingers separate again as your hands move up again. *(Fig. 15.8f,g.)* This shows the movement of your diaphragm as you breathe. *(Try this together a few times. Then have students close their eyes again if they have opened them, and let students try this on their own.)*
- Now relax your arms at your sides and rest here for a moment; then open your eyes when you are ready.

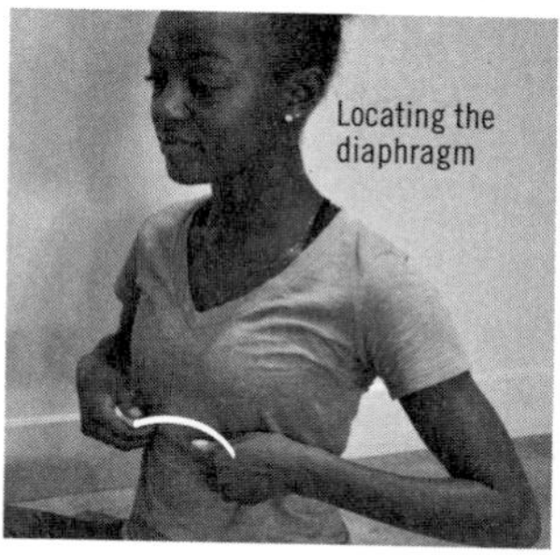

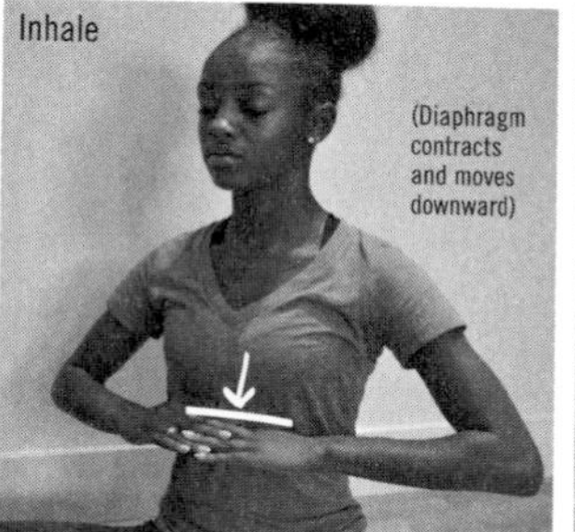

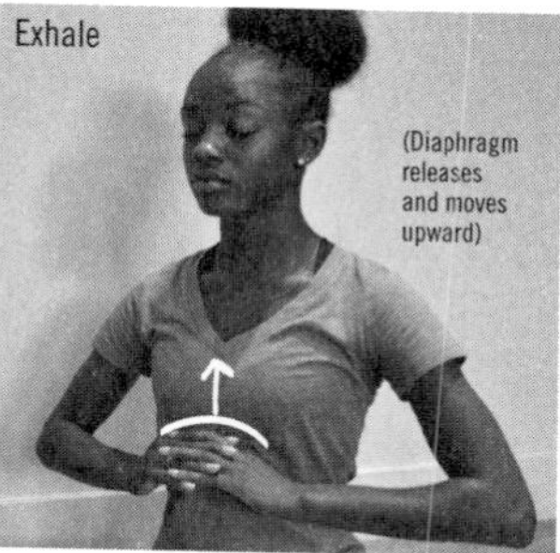

Fig. 15.8e, f, g. Students can use their hands to locate the diaphragm (e), and use their hands to simulate its movement when inhaling and exhaling (f and g). By taking the time to identify and isolate these various aspects of the process of breathing, teens find that this simple activity allows them to breathe more deeply.

Variation: Group Movement Models

Using Props: Students can use a large cloth or parachute to demonstrate the movement of the diaphragm. If you are using several pieces of cloth, you can divide into small groups of three to five students for them to try this.

If you have a large parachute, you can work as one group. Standing in a circle and holding onto the ends of the cloth, they can move the "diaphragm" down on the inhale, and lift it up for the exhale *(Fig. 15.9)*. With a parachute this can be done on its own; with a smaller cloth a few students can be underneath and lift it up into a dome shape.[3]

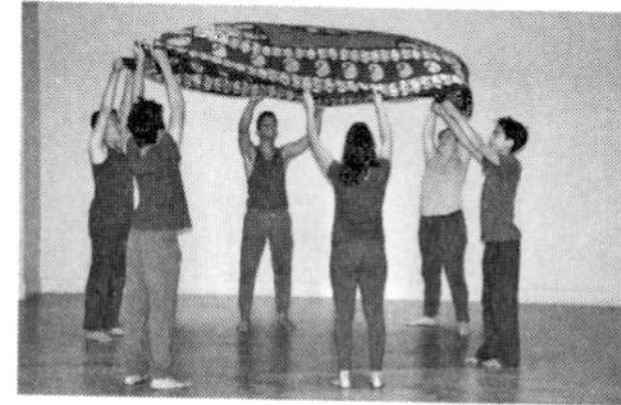
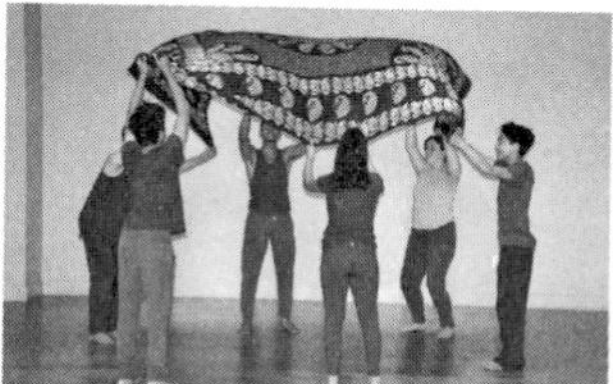
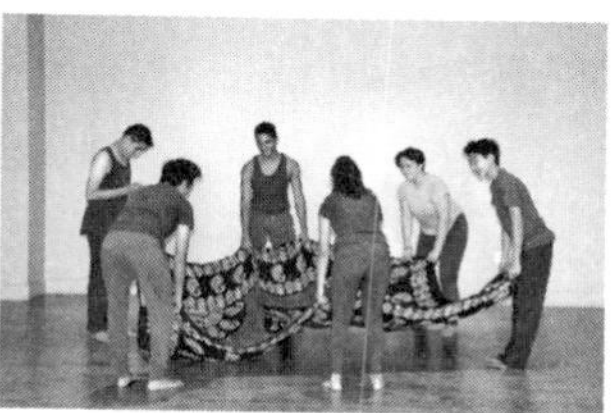

Fig. 15.9a, b, c. Variation: using a parachute to simulate the movement of the diaphragm can be a fun way to reinforce the anatomy and movement of our breathing.

Discussion

- Could you feel your diaphragm moving? Could you feel it move downward when you coughed? What did it feel like? Could you move your diaphragm on your own initiative, without coughing? How did you do that? What is the function of the diaphragm? Where does this muscle attach?

Review the shape and attachment points of the diaphragm with students using a skeletal model, organ model, or anatomy drawing.

- Which images or activities helped you most in understanding the movements involved in breathing? Do any of the images confuse you still? Can anyone help explain this image? Could you feel both actions, of the rib cage and thoracic diaphragm, happening at the same time? What did you discover? Were there any surprises? What questions do you have?

Exploration: Full Breathing

(20 minutes)

PURPOSE. To experience an unrestricted flow of breathing, such that the thoracic and abdominal cavities are free to respond to the movement of the lungs and diaphragm; to integrate the previous learning.

Activity

Have your students do this in Constructive Rest.

- ❍ Take a few deep breaths. Your belly can respond to the flow of your breath, in and out—as your diaphragm moves down as you breathe in, and then releases back up as you breathe out. You can place your hands on your belly to feel this movement. *(Pause.)* Now relax your arms at your sides and continue this until it feels smooth and effortless.
- ❍ Now focus on breathing into the thoracic cavity. Place your hands on your ribs and feel the rib cage respond to the flow of your breath, in and out. Feel the movement of the sides and back of the rib cage as well, as the lungs respond to your breathing. *(Pause.)* Now relax your arms at your sides and continue until this feels smooth and effortless.
- ❍ Focus on your upper chest, the top of the thoracic cavity. Place your hands just below your clavicles and feel the upper ribs respond to your breathing. Allow your clavicles and shoulders to widen as you breathe. *(Pause.)* Again, relax your arms at your sides and continue to breathe into the upper chest.
- ❍ Now you will be focusing on all of these areas, breathing first into your abdomen and progressing up to your upper chest. You may want to use the image of pouring

a glass of water and allowing it to fill up from the bottom first to help you feel this. First, exhale completely. Now slowly inhale, allowing the abdomen to expand first, then the rib cage, then the upper chest.

- Slowly exhale, releasing first in the abdomen, then in the rib cage, then in the upper chest. If you are having difficulty feeling your breath in any one area, go back to using your hands as a gentle reminder.
- Repeat this a few times until you begin to feel the flowing, steady movement of your breathing. *(Pause for several minutes.)*

Discussion

- What do you feel from doing this? Was it easier for you to breathe into certain areas than others? Were you able to feel the breathing in each area? What helped you to do this? Could you feel the clavicles move as you were breathing? Why would they move in response to breathing? *(Refer to the skeletal model.)*
- Were you able to feel your breathing like a glass filling up, starting from the bottom and progressing up to your chest? Did the image help you? What other images might help you to feel this?
- You may have heard this idea of taking a deep breath called *belly breathing*. Why do we use that term? Do you actually breathe in your belly area? Why do you feel movement there when you breathe?

Tips for Teachers

- Activities that encourage "breathing into" parts of the body, such as in this and the previous exploration on Breathing and Sound can be somewhat confusing. Since your lungs are in your thoracic cavity, or rib cage, you don't actually inhale into your abdominal cavity or belly area, as in the term belly breathing; rather, this term refers to the fact that when the diaphragm descends, the belly expands, giving the *sensation* that it is becoming fuller and therefore that you are "breathing" there. Clarifying this for students helps them understand the term "belly breathing" in the context that it is meant, rather than being taken literally. You can also clarify the difference between *actual lung breathing* and using *the image of the breath* to open or "breathe into" certain parts of your body, which can be an effective visualization technique.

Breathing Our Earth Body

Breathing is a key moment in time, one of true interdependence. With each breath we can realize that we are not separate from nature: the very air we breathe is part of our outer environment, becomes us, and sustains us. Simultaneously, our exhaled breath sustains the life around us, feeding trees and plants with carbon dioxide. We receive and we give, millions of times a day, in this interconnected web of life. We can experience this dynamic exchange within our own body, and reflect on the reality of our interdependence with each other and with all of nature.

Teen environmental activist and rapper Xiuhtezcatl Martinez, director of Earth Guardians and author of the book *We Rise,* emphasizes that as a culture we've fallen out of love with our planet, and with our own humanity. But he also has a hopeful vision for our future, and encourages youth to reconnect with the earth as their home:

> It's my human duty to protect the Earth.... Regardless of the color of our skin or the God that we believe in, we are all indigenous to this earth.... We come from the same earth, breathe the same air, and drink the same water—and we've got one planet!... What we gotta shift is the way we see ourselves in relationship to this Earth.[4]

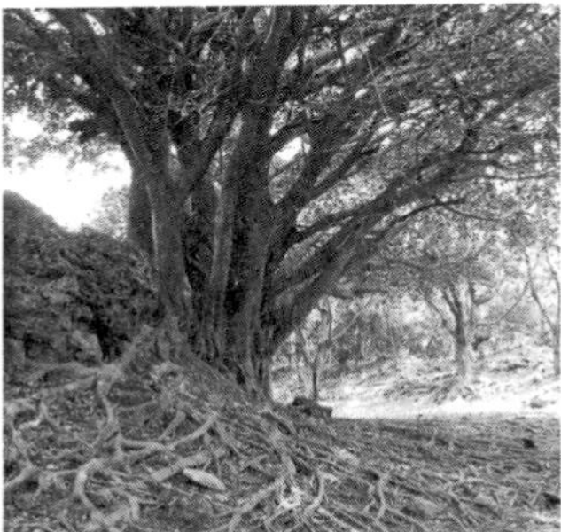

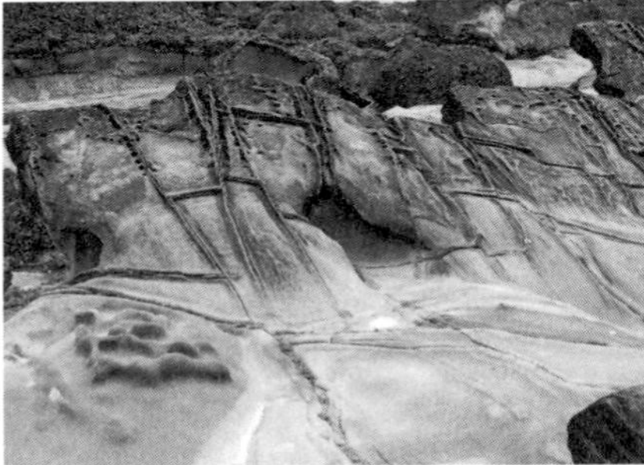

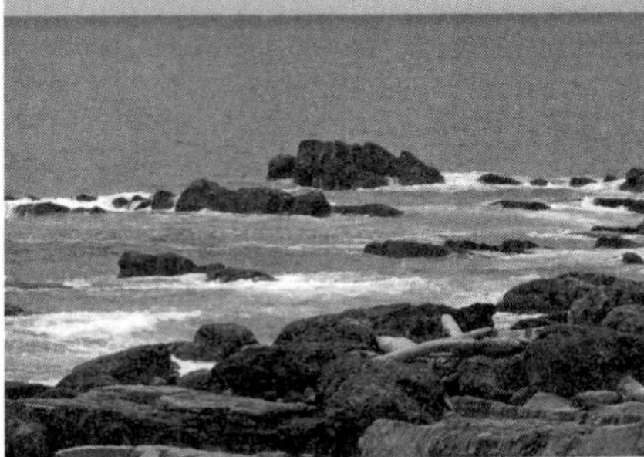

Fig. 15.10a, b, c. Our bodies and the elements of nature are in symbiotic relationship: the trees with their deep roots provide us oxygen and reflect our lungs and capillaries; the minerals of the earth are the same as those in our bones; and the waters of the sea are similar to the fluids in our bodies. Reflecting on this invites us to celebrate the power, complexity, and mystery of nature of which we are a part.

In the exploration called The Breath of Life, students reflect on this interdependence by focusing on the interchange of oxygen and carbon dioxide in the process of breathing. A variation of this activity then guides students to become aware of all the beings on the planet who are also involved in this amazing process—reflective of a practice from the Buddhist tradition called *Metta,* meaning loving-kindness. During *Metta* meditation, you practice sending loving-kindness to oneself first, then begin to extend this loving-kindness outward: for instance to one's immediate friends and family, then to one's "enemies," then to the whole country, to all countries, and finally to all sentient beings. Similarly, in the Breath of Life exploration, students reflect on the way in which their own breathing process relates with that of others and the environment. In this way, we experience ourselves as part of the breathing whole—what I call "the Earth body."

Exploration: The Breath of Life

(20–30 minutes)

PURPOSE. To introduce (or review) the process of cellular breathing; to bring awareness to the reciprocal relationship between plants and humans related to breathing; to heighten awareness of the intimate interconnection of our bodies and the natural world around us; to inspire awareness of our interdependence with others; to inspire loving and responsible stewardship of our planet.

Activity

Have your students do this sitting up or lying in Constructive Rest; ideally this activity would be done outdoors, in which case students can each sit up against a tree or lie down on the earth. This activity draws on embodied anatomy knowledge from previous explorations.

Part 1: (15 minutes)

- Close your eyes and bring your awareness to your breathing. Feel the air coming in your nose and mouth, feel it pass down the trachea in your neck to fill your lungs. Oxygen is transferred from this air in your lungs through the many capillaries in the lungs to your bloodstream to nourish all the cells of the body. Simultaneously, carbon dioxide is released from each cell, and then taken back to the lungs to be released back out. Each cell in your body is revitalized and energized as you breathe. Take a few moments to breathe and feel the energy seep into each cell in your body. Place one hand on your sternum and one on your belly if you like.
- Now take a deep breath in; where does this life-giving oxygen come from?

- Take another deep breath in, and then exhale as fully as you can. As you feel your exhale, imagine the carbon dioxide releasing from your lungs. Where does this go?
- Imagine yourself lying in a forest, with many trees shading you from the hot sun. *(Or, if you are outdoors: Now feel the trees around you, listen to the rustling of their many leaves in the wind; or, feel the bark of the tree against your back, and the strong support of its tall trunk with deep roots, etc.)* As these trees "breathe in," they take the carbon dioxide from your exhale—it is the substance they need to live, like you need their oxygen.
- And as these trees "exhale," they give off the oxygen you need to breathe. Of course, there is both oxygen and carbon dioxide in our atmosphere, but if we didn't have the plants and trees, we wouldn't have enough oxygen to breathe. They replenish the atmosphere, giving us life through our breath.
- Take a moment to feel yourself breathing in coordination with the trees and plants around you. You can even take a moment now to appreciate them for this gift, and appreciate your lungs for accepting this gift, and working so well to release the carbon dioxide you no longer need, while "feeding" it back to the plants.

You can end there, or add this next section. You may also repeat the activity above on a subsequent day, and then add in part 2 at that time.

Part 2: (10–15 minutes)

- Now take a moment to feel yourself lying down *(or sitting)*. Feel the weight of your body, and the movement of your lungs, ribs, and diaphragm as you breathe.
- Bring your awareness to the others in the room, also lying *(or sitting)* on the earth next to you. Feel the room breathing, as each person inhales—bringing oxygen into their lungs—and exhales—releasing carbon dioxide back into the environment around you.
- This air we breathe is all the same. Feel all of us breathing as one. Feel yourself as part of this breathing unit.
- Imagine all the other people around you, also breathing and sharing this vital air we all need.
- Imagine all the plants and trees around you. *(Or if outdoors: Bring your awareness to all the plants and trees around us.)*

Continue to guide students to expand this awareness incrementally to include the full neighborhood they are in, then the state they are in, then the country, the oceans, other countries, our entire planet, and so on.

- Feel yourself as one part of this interconnected web, with your own lungs breathing with all the living beings around us. Even the animals are breathing, taking in oxygen and releasing carbon dioxide to give back to the plant life.
- This air we breathe supports life on earth. For you, your family, the animals, the community. Our world.
- Now relax and notice where you have arrived to in yourself, how you feel now as you just rest here for a few moments.

Discussion

Part 1

- How do you feel after doing this? Do you notice any difference in your body? In your breathing? In your mood or feelings?
- What did you notice while you did this? What did you experience? What did it remind you of? What did you learn from doing this?
- What do you know about plants and how they breathe? Would anyone be interested to learn more about that?

Part 2

Repeat discussion from part 1; in other words, focus on the experiential aspect first. This discussion can then go in various directions; here are a few suggested possibilities.

- What happened when you tried to expand your perception to include the other people around you, all breathing the same air? Could you feel yourself as part of this?
- Were you able to imagine the rest of the world or just the people around you? What happened when you tried to expand your imagination to the rest of the world? Could you feel yourself as part of this?
- Do you feel you have clean air to breathe? Why or why not?
- Do you have any ideas for what we could do to protect our air? Would anyone be interested to research this further?

Tips for Teachers

HOME PRACTICE

- Students can explore this practice at home, keeping a log in their body journals about their experience during the week.

HOME PROJECTS

- Students can design individual or group research projects related to any of the human and plant anatomy and physiology topics that emerged in the discussion, as well as to any related environmental issues that are of interest to them or may be particularly relevant to their communities.
- Once familiar to them, students can also teach this breathing activity to others, such as introducing it to their parents, a group of teachers, or a group of younger or older students in their school or community group.

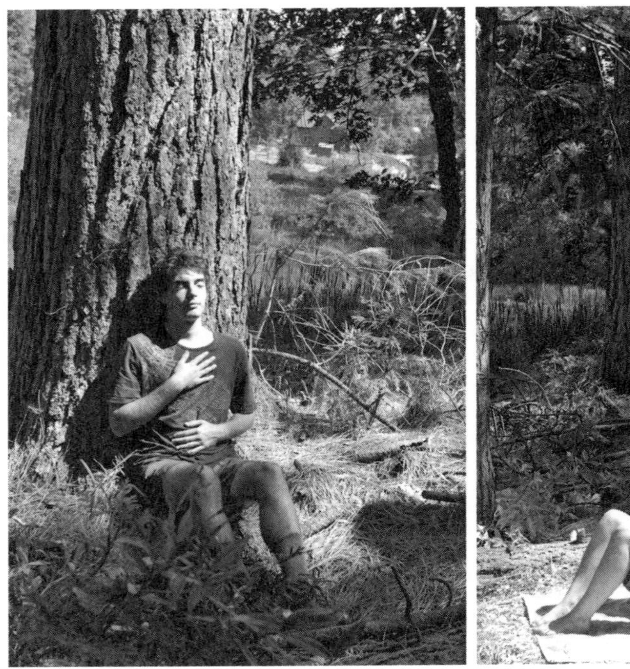

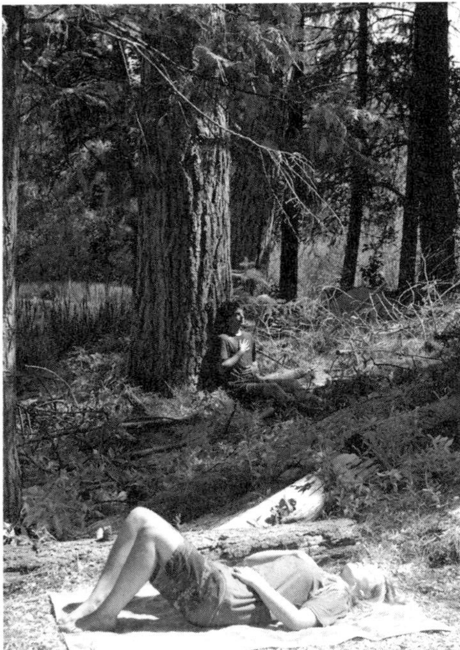

Fig. 15.11a, b. Teens practicing The Breath of Life.

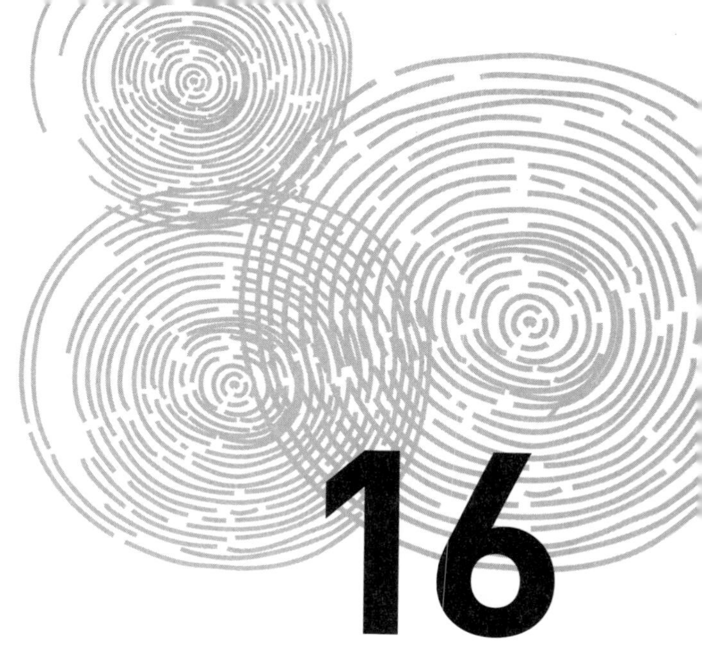

16

A Somatic "Warm-Up": A New Approach to an Everyday Practice

After having engaged in the activities in this curriculum, students will have gained an increased knowledge of their bodies and myriad means of moving with greater somatic awareness. Much of this newfound kinesthetic intelligence permeates their experiences in other aspects of their lives, yet may not necessarily translate into their more codified movement routines without some guidance. For example, when students perform warm-ups before a sport or physical activity, they often fall into habitual movement patterns. Similarly, many of us have been taught a certain way to "warm up" back in grade school, and have continued with much the same routine ever since. Often when we exercise, we treat ourselves like purely functional instruments, moving in a repetitive and mechanical manner.

This chapter explores the concept of "warm-up" in this conventional sense, and presents an alternative method that integrates all of students' previous learning in the curriculum into principles and practices for a somatically sound warm-up. Bringing more conscious awareness to their movement choices helps students formulate a healthier approach to warming up that supports their health and vitality—whether preparing for another physical activity or simply as a daily practice. For, although in Physical Education terms, warm-up is understood to precede physical activity such as in the definition, "low-intensity exercises that prepare the muscular/skeletal system and heart and lungs (cardio respiratory system) for high-intensity physical activity,"[1] we can benefit from a movement "warm-up" for its own sake as well. As students learn, a somatic warm-up such as presented here provides a healthy means to begin the day, or to get moving during the day, as well!

Perceptions of Warm-Up

To explore their perceptions of warm-up, the first exploration allows students to discover what they already do, reflect on that by writing in their journals, and then share this in a discussion. In this activity, you start by asking students to take ten minutes to warm up and then watch what they do. In class after class, students generally repeat a similar scenario: they sit on the floor, stretch over one leg then the other; they stand and bend one leg backwards while holding on to their foot; they bend down to touch their toes; they pull one arm back over their head with the other—all movements they have learned to stretch their muscles. While they are doing this, they look around the room, watch each other, and perhaps even talk with each other. Often, this is because they either don't know what to focus on or they don't understand the purpose of the movements they are doing. *(See Fig. 16.1.)*

Rather than telling students that what they have done is right or wrong, you can discuss with them their present perspectives about warm-ups and how these have been formed. Often they have learned most of what they do as a warm-up from someone else (a coach, friend, sibling, parent) or by watching what others do. By discussing what they do, they discover concepts that underlie their present practice of warming up. Students can then review the body systems they have studied and discuss which systems they are currently focusing on in their warm-up. This begins a dialogue about what it means to warm up, and what a healthy warm-up might actually mean.

Exploration: What Is a Warm-Up?

(30–40 minutes)

PURPOSE. To encourage awareness of your present beliefs and practices of warming up; to reflect on how this relates to previous learning about mind-body awareness and principles of anatomy and physiology.

Activity

MATERIALS

- Journal and writing supplies

Students can place their journals to the sides of the space so they can get them easily after the movement portion of the activity.

Explain to students that they will have ten minutes to warm up, and that they should do whatever that means to them.

At the end of the ten minutes, invite them to return to their journals and make a list of what they did in their warm-up, and then to reflect on how they chose what to do, or perhaps where they learned what they did. You may also just proceed to the discussion, rather than having students write about this first.

In either case, students can discuss this together in partners or small groups, or you can proceed directly to the group discussion.

Discussion

- What did you do to warm up? Why?
- What does "warm-up" mean? Where did you learn the things you did to warm up?
- How did you choose what to do? *(You might choose certain activities that you observed and ask why they did these, such as jumping or stretching in a particular way.)*
- What were you focused on while you were warming up? What were you thinking? Were you talking?
- Were your eyes opened or closed for most of the time? If you closed your eyes, why was that? If you had them open, why do you think you kept them opened?
- What was your relationship to weight? To space?
- Which body systems did you focus on in your warm-up?
- What systems are involved in moving? What functions are necessary in your body for you to actively move?

Tips for Teachers

- When students are asked to warm up, they may ask some clarifying questions, such as "What do you mean by warm-up?" or, "Like, warm-up for *what?*" These are very good questions—tell them that—but say that for the purposes of this activity you actually aren't going to answer them yet. Later, in the discussion, you can revisit these questions to see how they relate to the topic of warm-up.

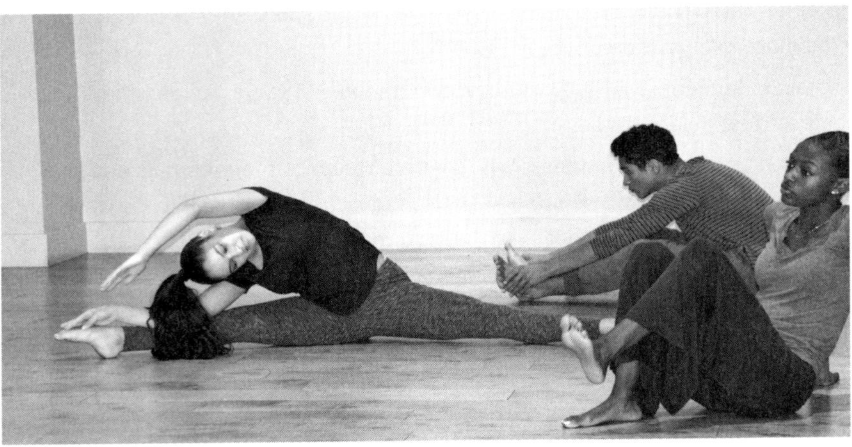

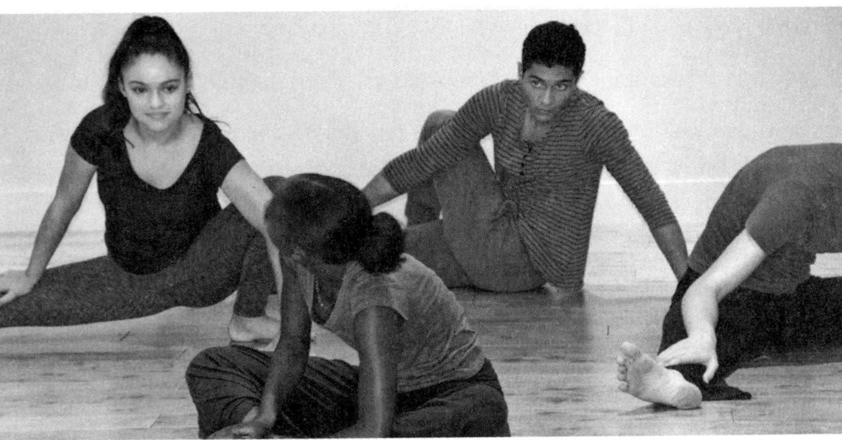

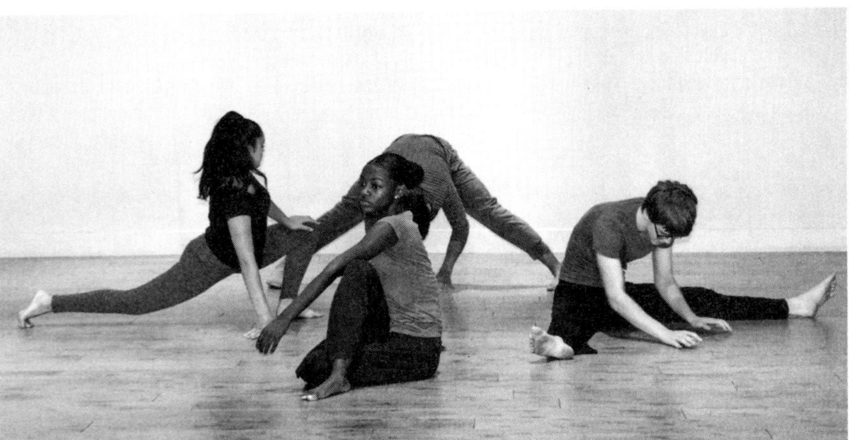

Fig. 16.1a, b, c. Teens warm up in their usual way, and then reflect on what they generally do. This often includes repeating habitual patterns of movement, such as stretching in various ways, as well as looking around at one another to see what someone else is doing.

A Somatic Warm-Up for Health and Vitality

When warming up in a repetitive way, we often lose both our motivation and the kinesthetic awareness of the movement we are doing. Motivation and kinesthetic awareness are essential elements in fully embodying our movement, in effectively warming up, and in establishing a healthy body-mind relationship. We each embody our physical selves in our own unique way. As you move, you can learn to respond to your particular needs in both warm-up and exercise activities by engaging both body and mind. To quote somatic educator Irene Dowd: "If the self is fully engaged in the performance of the movement, then one is effectively preparing (to move)."

Rather than teach a prescribed series of exercises as a warm-up, here we *redefine* warm-up as a series of four principles upon which to base your movement:

1. Aligning intent and action
2. Integrating use of all body systems, beginning with the deepest layers first
3. Balancing both sensory and motor experience
4. Maintaining motivation through a combination of improvisational and structured activities

Whether warming up as a daily practice or for an athletic competition, dance class, or some form of exercise, if students understand these basic principles they can stay fully engaged in their activity, expand their potential for movement, and decrease their chances of injury.

Alignment of Intent and Action: Check-ins

Alignment of your attention with your movement is a first step in developing kinesthetic awareness and in improving movement quality. One of the purposes of a warm-up is to create this type of focused awareness, described earlier as "body listening." Bonnie Bainbridge Cohen refers to this body-mind awareness as active choice, presensory motor focusing, or sensory planning, which she sees as directly related to motivation: "In ourselves we see this presensory motor focusing as motivation, desire, attention, and discriminating awareness. We can see the absence or repression of it in boredom, resistance, and difficulties in learning."[2] The lack of presensory motor focusing, which often feels like you are "going through the motions," can cause you to become disinterested and increase your chance of injury as well. As Irene Dowd explained in a workshop for the National Dance Association, "avoidance of boredom is the best injury preventative."[3] Dowd notes both repetition to the point of inattention and fatigue as clear factors in many overuse injuries such as tendinitis, muscle strains, and stress fractures.[4]

To introduce this topic of the need to align intent and action in a warm-up, you can discuss the metaphor of tuning a guitar with your students. Tuning a guitar requires a series of practices involving awareness (listening), initiating movement (tuning the chords), and then further awareness (listening again to hear if the scale has improved). First, the guitar player plays the instrument and listens to the sound of the strings. Then, based on what is heard, the guitarist changes the pitch of each string by tightening or loosening the strings. Finally, all the strings can be played again to hear if the tones are more harmonious. Because the guitar responds to many factors in the environment such as heat and cold, the strings must be tuned each time the guitar is played. Imagine what would happen if you were to tune the guitar without ever listening to the sound of the strings first? You wouldn't know whether to tighten each string or loosen it, for instance.

Similarly, many students begin to stretch without any sense of the present state of their bodies! Yet our bodies are continually responding to factors in our physical environment—not unlike the guitar, our bodies respond to heat and cold—as well as to our previous level of physical activity and to the internal state of our thoughts and feelings. To adapt to these variations, warm-ups should involve essential awareness practices so that students are actively engaged in listening to their bodies, rather than responding mechanically. As preparation for warming up, students therefore learn to use several "check-in" activities as a first stage in warming up. These activities provide them with a few moments to check in with how they are feeling and with what their bodies may need on a particular day. Then, similar to the guitar player who must strum the guitar after tuning it to be sure the tuning has worked, they repeat whatever check-ins they choose at the end of the warm-up, for purposes of comparison.

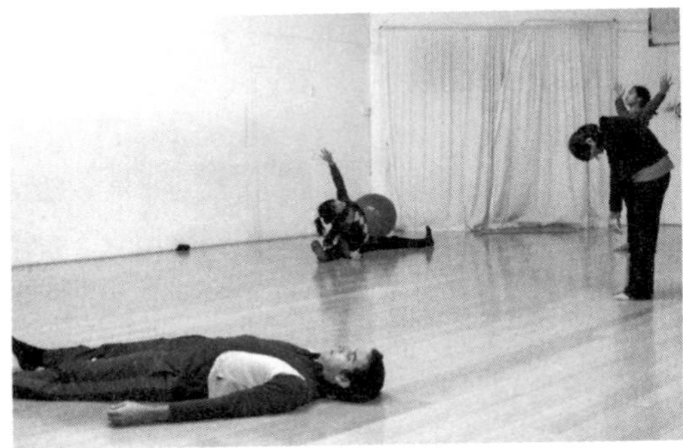

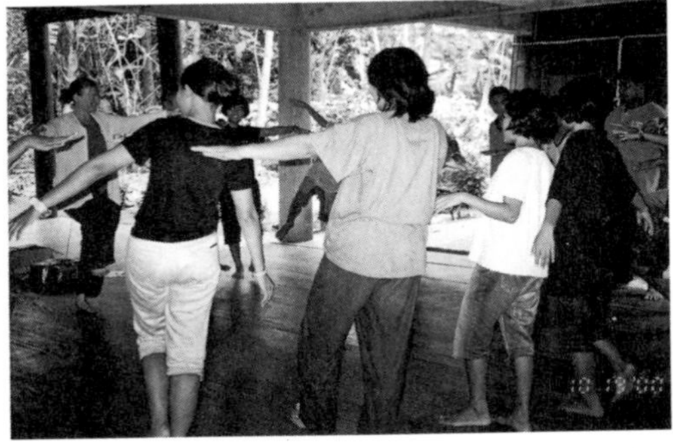

Fig. 16.2a, b. Check-ins help students to gauge the present state of their bodies, as well as their more psychophysical state, both before and after moving: participants in the Embodiment in Education training adapting various check-in activities (a); teens in Thailand practicing balancing on one leg and then the other as one of their check-in activities (b).

As an initial check-in activity, for example, students might use body scanning while in Constructive Rest, focusing on their breathing, weight, or body alignment. Other check-ins they can use include standing with eyes closed to feel their alignment through body scanning, or checking their flexibility by using some familiar activity, such as standing spine curls or sitting and reaching over to each side. They might also try standing on one leg and then the other to check their balance, or even do this with their eyes closed, which requires even more reliance on the proprioceptive senses. Generally students choose a variety of these, such as using two or three check-ins each time.

Self-Directed Movement: Responsive Moving

After these initial check-ins, students are guided to use a method of warm-up that encourages learning to follow their own movement needs in a practice I call "Responsive Moving." This is another way they learn to focus within and "check-in" with themselves. Through this method, you start in stillness and follow your impulses to move as a gentle way to begin warming up. In contrast to the typical stretches in which students tend to mechanically follow a pre-prescribed order, such as stretching to one side and then the other side, this allows them to move in a more spontaneous way. Students can recall, for instance, how it feels to yawn: often we are yawning before we even realize it is happening! To get used to this way of moving, students are encouraged to close their eyes and focus on their bodies. Moving with eyes closed helps them to move without the self-consciousness that can come from being aware of being watched by others.

Throughout the process, encourage your students to be nonjudgmental about their movement and to move for the *sensation* of moving, rather than to produce a certain result like stretching a muscle or creating an interesting shape. By following their impulses to move without consciously directing the movement, they find the movement they need. Although we each have the same basic body structure, each person's body is also unique. By paying attention, students can begin to identify their particular needs as well as to appreciate the uniqueness of their own bodies. This experience also helps students develop an inner "nonjudgmental witness" to support them while moving. Especially in adolescence, when self-consciousness can lead to strong self-criticism, teens benefit from taking time to notice and "repattern" their inner voice, much as they begin to repattern their movement. After completing the previous explorations in the curriculum, students are more prepared for this type of free-form movement practice, as they have generally become less judgmental and more comfortable with an inner-directed focus, as well as having established a sense of trust among the group.

When they practice this initially, students' experiences vary widely. On one end of the spectrum, some teens discover that they can quite easily feel what movement they need as they begin to pay closer attention, as expressed in this journal response from a ninth-grade student:

> *Moving like this was really different! It made me notice where I was tight in my body, and get to move around a bit to feel more at ease there.*

Another eleventh-grade boy also enjoyed the experience, and said that he felt like his body "just seemed to know what to do, and I could just let my movement happen."

Other students find this process more difficult and feel that they simply don't know how to do it, such as a tenth-grade girl named Abby expressed in her journal:

> *During the Responsive Moving exploration, I felt my body doing the same poses over and over again, just out of habit. It was hard to find new poses, even though there are so many options out there.*

And another student noted:

> *As a dancer I typically just do the move, I don't think about what my body needs to do in order for me to actually carry the move out. I guess I don't even really consider what my body needs.*

Similarly, many students—especially those with extensive previous training in a particular movement form, such as gymnastics, martial arts, or yoga—find themselves drawing upon a familiar repertoire of movements, and then similarly try to consciously "find new poses" as they think about what else they might do.

Eventually, as students share these various responses and we discuss them together, they begin to discover that there are *many* ways to initiate movement. They may be consciously directing the movement with their minds in order to move in a specific way, or they may be mindlessly following patterned sequences that have been previously established in their nervous system. Another approach—often less familiar to many of them—is to begin to shift their attention within to their *sensory perceptions,* and allow their movement to unfold from within as they *feel* what they need. Making these distinctions helps students to understand the difference between their own approach and this potentially new one that encourages a more free-flow, "responsive" process. With time to explore the practice over time, teens begin to discover a more internally directed basis for their movement that can be freeing and expressive.

Exploration: Responsive Moving[5]

(20–25 minutes)

PURPOSE. To become aware of your habitual way of moving and invite another approach; to experience following inner impulses for movement rather than following conscious directives or predetermined exercises; to introduce this as an aspect of warm-up.

Activity:

Give a brief introduction to this form, referring to this as another method of listening within, like with the check-in activities, again referring to the guitar metaphor described previously. You can also use the metaphor of yawning, as a way to explain the spontaneous nature of movement that is not mentally pre-planned. In this way students can begin to see the Responsive Moving activity as related to, though different from, the previous predetermined check-in activities.

Students should also be reminded that although they will be moving with their eyes closed, they should open their eyes a little if they want to move fast, such as walking or swinging their arms, to avoid bumping into anyone else. They should also be told how long the movement time will last. You might provide approximately 10 minutes for a first exploration.

- Begin by finding a spot in the room where you would like to be. Find a comfortable position and close your eyes. *(Students can begin lying on the floor, in any position they choose.)* Take a few breaths, in and out, and feel your weight being supported by the floor. Which parts of your body are supporting your weight?
- Now begin to change your position. As you do this, notice the parts of your body touching the floor in this new position. Now pause in this position and let your weight be supported by the floor. Feel the shape you are in, the parts of your body touching the floor, and the areas that are surrounded by air.
- Now change your position again. Pause. Where is your weight supported in this new position? Feel this new shape you are in, and how it feels to be in this position.
- Now we're going to change again, but this time as you shift, use this same attentive awareness you've been bringing to the *shape* you were in, and bring it to your *movement* as you move to the next shape. How does it feel? Where is your weight? Then pause in your new shape.
- Now change again, feeling each aspect of your movement, as you move to your new position. Then pause.
- Continue to change your position and to pause on your own timing now. Feel the massage your body gets from the floor as you move and change positions. You might try to let each part of your body get that massage, and let go of the pauses now if you like, so you can just move freely.

- ❍ Continue to move, allowing your body to lead you, moving just as you need to, just as your body wants to move at this moment. You don't have to think about it, just notice what you do. It's as if you are picking up a thread and following where it leads. *(Give students a few minutes to explore this before continuing.)*
- ❍ If you find you aren't feeling any impulse to move, or that you keep directing your movement, let yourself pause until some part of your body wants to move. Remember as you are moving you are awakening your body and bringing fresh oxygen to all your cells. Let that feeling of energy opening up throughout your body guide your movement.
- ❍ Let yourself move to sitting if you want to, or even to standing. There is no right or wrong way to do this; just let your movement unfold in any way in this moment. If you find you are judging yourself or thinking about how the movement looks, notice that too, and then try to let those thoughts go and keep following impulses from your body. *(Again, give time for students to explore this without any directions or suggestion.)*
- ❍ Now take a few more minutes to make sure you've found just what your body needs. Slowly begin to find an ending to your movement, or let an ending find you. You don't have to decide how to end, but let it feel just right.

Students can share about their experiences in partners first, or proceed to the group discussion.

Discussion

- What did you experience as you did this?

This question may be enough to get the conversation going. Here are some further suggestions that can be interjected along the way as appropriate.

- What kind of thoughts went through your mind? Were you able to let your body lead? What does that mean to you? How is that different from deciding how to move and then doing it? Is there a difference?
- What did you find was your favorite moment in what you did? Why do you think you remember that movement/moment? Were there any surprises?

Then you can relate this back to their warm-up formula.

- How does this relate to warm-up? When might you do this as part of a warm-up? Is this different from what you have been doing? How?

Tips for Teachers

- ◆ After you have led the Responsive Moving activity once, or a few times so students can get a feel for it, they can explore it without your verbal directions.

For example, students can take 10 minutes for Responsive Moving at the start of the class, to give them time to arrive and settle in to themselves. In such cases, I often ring a bell at the beginning, which gives students a cue to begin to focus within, and again at the end to provide a clear delineation for the activity. They can also practice Responsive Moving as a break from more structured activities during the class. You can gauge for yourself when this is needed, or ask students directly if they would like to do a next activity, or have time for Responsive Moving first.

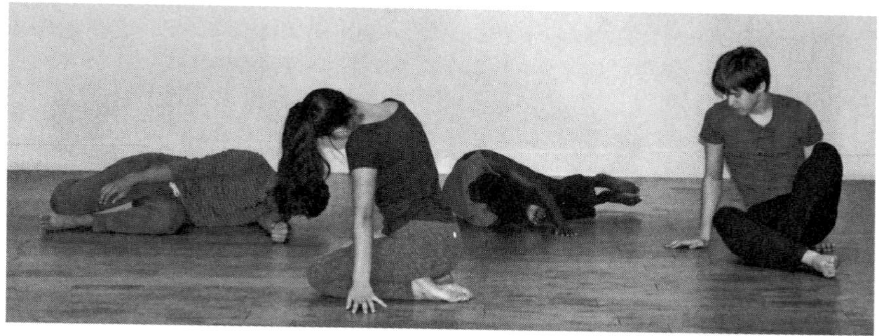

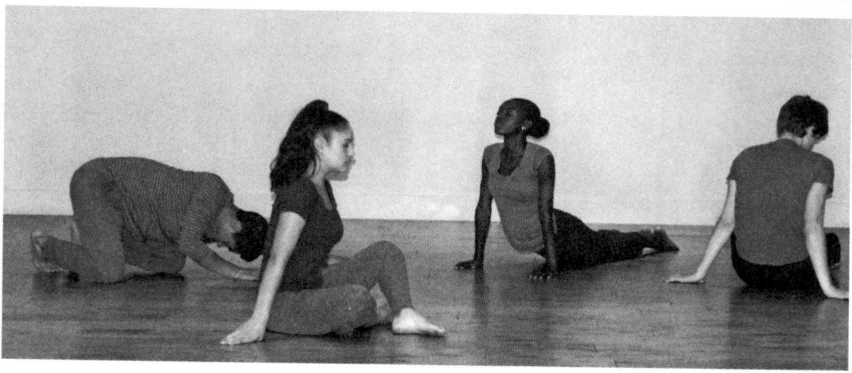

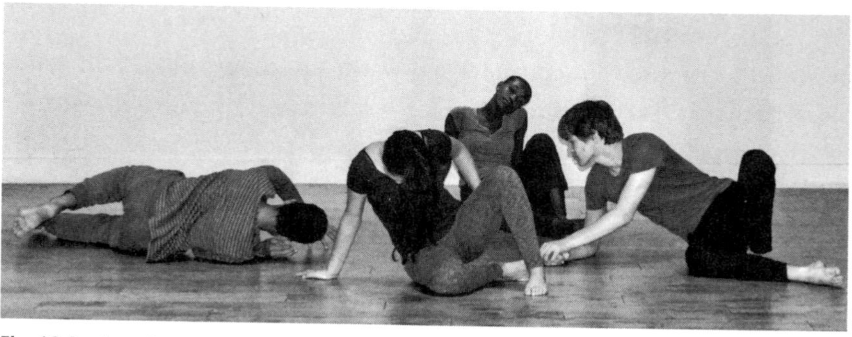

Fig. 16.3a, b, c. Responsive Moving 1: In practicing Responsive Moving, teens begin to move beyond their habitual movement routine, as their movement evolves with more variety and subtlety. Compare this series of photos, for example, with those in the previous exploration on warm-up *(Fig. 16.1)*.

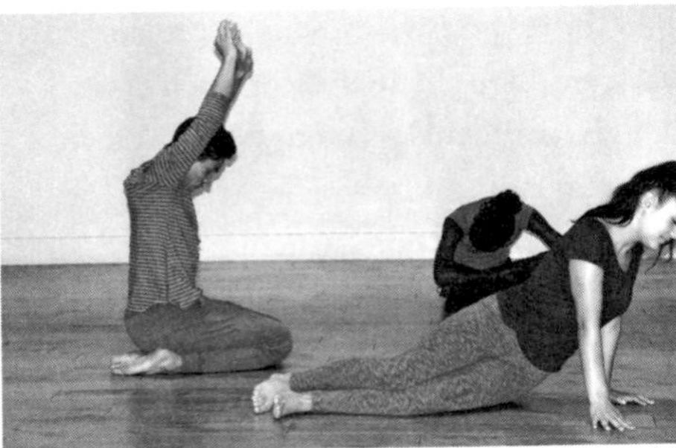
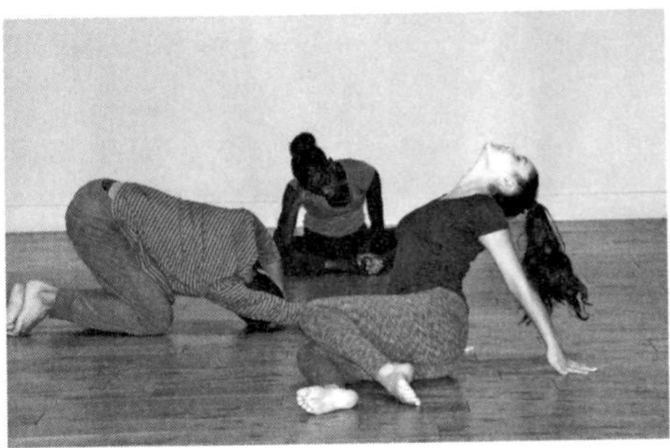

Fig. 16.4a, b. Responsive Moving 2: With experience in this new way of moving that is more self-directed, teens gain confidence in their own movement and enjoy the process of finding the movement that feels good to them in the moment with less self-consciousness about how they might appear.

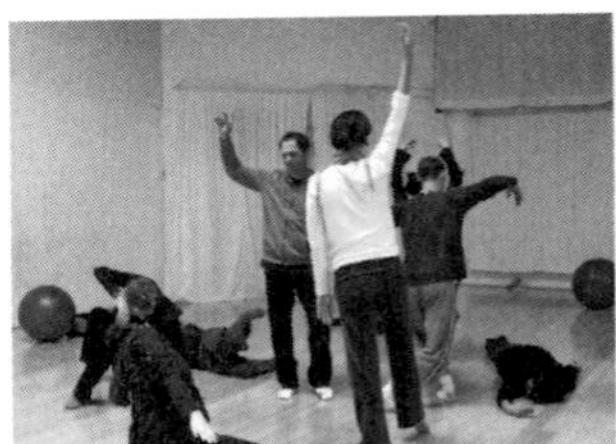
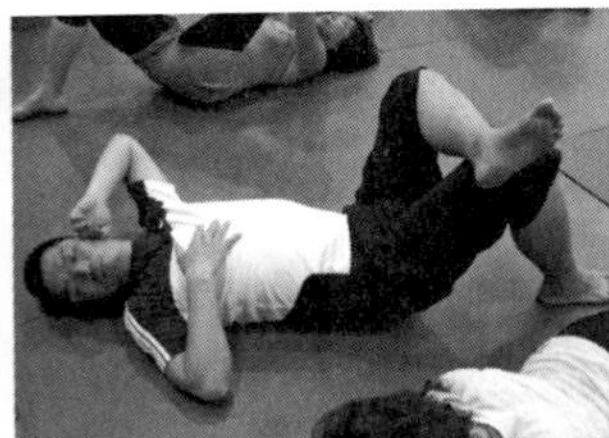
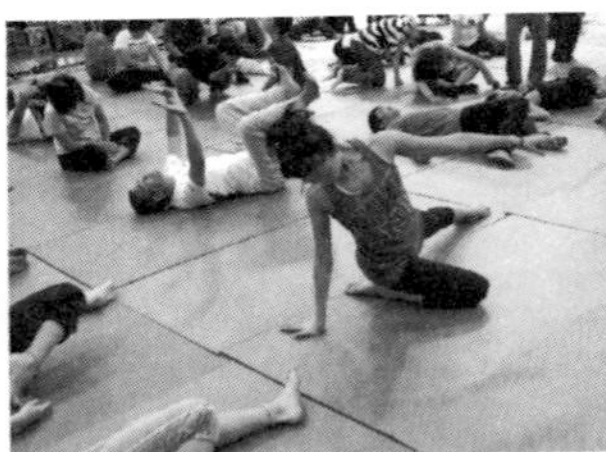

Fig. 16.5a, b, c. Responsive Moving 3: Moving with eyes closed and with no music to direct the movement can also be unfamiliar to adults. Here teachers practice Responsive Moving for the first time: participants in Embodiment in Education in California (a), and a group of physical educators, physical and occupational therapists, and dancers at a conference workshop in Taiwan (b and c). (Photos b and c courtesy of the Somatic Education Society of Taiwan.)

Integrating All Body Systems

As students begin to discover, conventional warm-ups tend to focus on certain body systems, primarily the skeletal and muscular systems, and often begin with stretching the muscles. Yet *movement* actually needs to precede stretching to increase blood flow and warm-up the synovial fluid, muscles, and other tissues at the joints; for maximum effect, a warm-up should begin at the deepest level of the body and move outward. A full warm-up, in fact, should activate all of the body systems. To introduce this idea to students, you can compare this to needing a balanced diet with foods from a variety of categories. Although students often know that they need to stretch their muscles before an activity, they don't consider the complexity of the body and the need to activate all of the body systems—not just the muscles.

Understanding joints, muscles, proprioception, and organ support through previous explorations helps students broaden their perspective of warm-up to include a wider variety of movement. As they realize that by moving they increase blood flow to the muscles, prepare the synovial joints to absorb shock, and increase their ability to sense their position in space, they begin to recognize the complexity and interrelationship of the body systems.

As Bonnie Bainbridge Cohen explains, dance and athletic warm-ups are often limited in that they are often structured to precede particular dance styles or athletic skills, rather than to activate our full movement potential:

> The support and articulation of the major body systems and our early developmental patterning are the basic foundations of all our movement, ranging from everyday activities to the more skilled and complex movements of the dancer and athlete.... Yet, dance warm-ups often tap into only a few body systems or developmental patterns—usually the ones that support a particular dance style and mood.[6]

Providing an improvisational warm-up based on the various body systems helps students to break out of habitual patterns and broaden their functional and expressive range. As an element in warm-up, exploration of the body systems through movement helps students to more fully embody their movement in a personal sense, as they discover their own relationship to these systems and their qualities. In fact, they will learn that it is the complex weaving together of the systems that gives movement its subtlety and personal distinctions.[7] Activities such as Responsive Moving, along with the following explorations, encourage a broader range of movement qualities and inspire students to incorporate new ways of moving into their practice of warming up.

Balancing Sensory and Motor Experience

A balance of sensory and motor experience allows for the integration of new movement patterns, from the basic skills we acquire in infancy to the more complex skills of the dancer or athlete. As in all explorations presented so far, warm-up activities should encourage both sensory and motor experience to create a balance of these two modes.

Walking, for example, is a simple and familiar way to begin moving. As a first stage in warm-up, walking serves several purposes. It activates blood flow, nourishing the cells with fresh oxygen and bringing this oxygenated blood to the muscles. It stimulates proprioceptive responses and synovial fluid production in the joints. For the purposes of warm-up it also can be combined with imagery, such as imagining walking in sand to ground through the feet or using the crayon image to lengthen the spine. Walking serves as a bridge from a more external awareness (of one's surroundings) to a more internal awareness (of one's inner sensations), as students have experienced throughout the curriculum thus far.

Another method of warm-up is based on shifting positions to encourage supporting weight on different parts of the body, as in the exploration called Shaping, drawing on the previous exploration students engaged in as a means to learn about proprioception. As they also learned when studying the organs, bearing weight on different surfaces of the body stimulates the proprioceptive and interoceptive senses throughout the body. Students can also do the activity with a partner. Through supporting weight with a partner, students balance the previous, inner-focused explorations—that were more sensory in nature—with playful interaction. All of these activities bring about a more enlivened, embodied presence.

Exploration: Walking

(15–20 minutes)

PURPOSE. To increase your cardiovascular activity, to warm up your body tissues and synovial fluid, to mobilize your joints, to use imagery to transition from a more outward focus to an internal one.

Activity

The following is an example of one variation of this activity. Many variations can be developed based on bringing awareness to specific aspects of movement as demonstrated below.

- Start walking around the room. Take a few minutes to notice each other, to say hi to each other. *(Fig. 16.6.)*
- Now as you are walking by someone, notice the color of his or her eyes. Keep going until you've seen each person.
- Now as you are walking look around the room, start to focus on the spaces in between people. As you see a space, walk through it. *(Add variations such as changing speed, i.e., walk faster or run through the space. Also vary spacing, e.g., make the spaces smaller, spread out and increase the space between people, and so on.) (Fig. 16.7.)*
- Now as you walk notice the temperature of the floor against your feet, feel the texture of the floor.
- Pause. Close your eyes. Take a breath, in ... and out. Notice your weight through your feet. Is your weight more on one foot than another? More on your toes or your heels? Now open your eyes and continue walking. *(Repeat several times, shifting the focus to various parts of the body.)*

- Now begin to feel the weight shift on your feet as you walk. You may want to imagine yourself walking in sand. *(Continue suggesting various focuses and/or images, such as letting your shoulder girdle hang freely, noticing your breathing, growing the crayon from the top of the head, or whichever images have helped students most.)*
- Now as you walk, you can start to shake your hands and arms, then your shoulders. *(Continue through the torso, hips, legs, and feet. As well as shaking and giggling, explore the movements of flexion, extension, rotation, and proximal to distal successive joint movements. Students may need to stop walking to explore some of these, such as successive joint movements in the legs.)*
- Continue walking at your own speed. Now begin to slow down your walk. Allow your walk to slow down until you come to a stop; just let the momentum of your movement gradually come to an end.
- Stand with your eyes closed for a moment and take a moment to do your body scan from your feet to the top of your head.

Discussion

- What did you experience from doing this? What did you notice as you did your body scan just now? Which felt more natural or easier for you—to focus outwardly (as in looking at each other or what was in the room) or to focus inwardly (as in noticing your weight on your feet or using the imagery)? How does each affect your movement?
- How does this relate to warm-up? What systems does walking activate? At what stage in your warm-up might you add walking? Why?

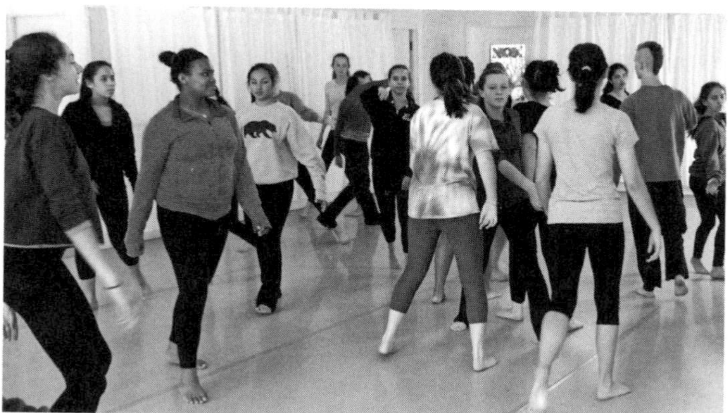

Fig. 16.6. Walking is a healthy way to begin warming up and can also help students to shift from an external to internal focus.

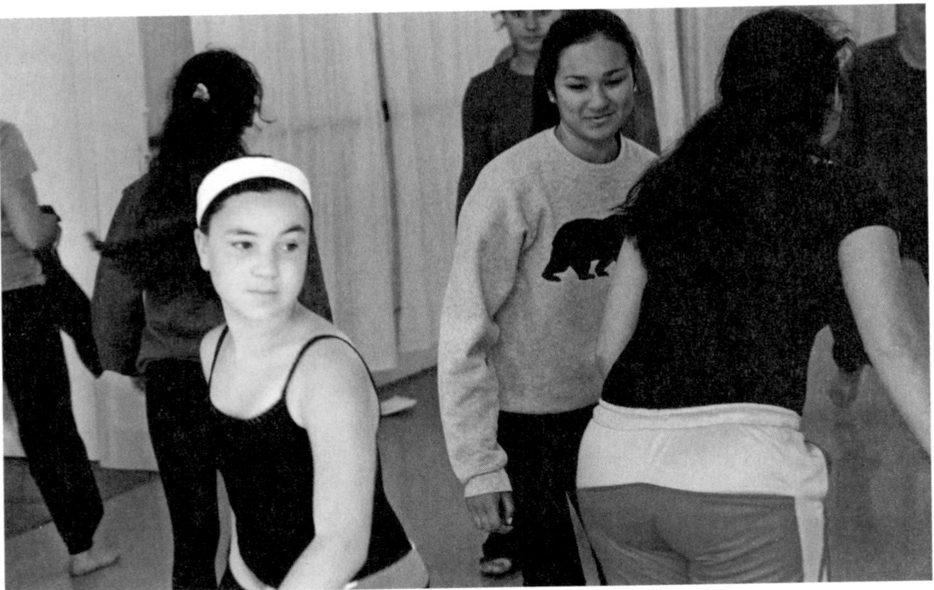

Fig. 16.7. Students enjoy moving through the spaces between each other as they walk, while maintaining an inner awareness that guides their movement.

Exploration: Shaping

(10–15 minutes)

PURPOSE. To activate the proprioceptive sensors; to encourage awareness of the need for variety and playful spontaneity in a warm-up to avoid boredom and injury.

Activity

For this activity students can be guided to change their shape either on the cue of a clap, a drum, a "go" signal, or do this more spontaneously based on their own timing. They can also use physioballs to move on, helping them to move in various new shapes and "off-balance" positions. (See variations.)

- Find a spot in the room to begin in so you have plenty of space around you to move and sit in that spot.
- Now freeze just as you are sitting. Close your eyes. Notice the shape you are in. When I clap, change the way you are sitting. Change again. Now open your eyes and keep changing your position on your own timing.

- Now start to add lying down shapes to the sitting ones. Alternate between lying down on your back, on your stomach, sitting up, kneeling ... notice what parts of your body are supporting your weight. Now see how else you can support your weight—on your head, on two hands and one leg, on both legs and one arm, on the arms and legs. Shift the weight from one part of your body to another. Now add some balance shapes, balancing on different parts of your body.

End here or add the variations below.

Variations

With Physioballs: Students can use physioballs during this activity to provide further means to shape their bodies and balance in various positions. This also adds a fun element of momentum and unpredictability to the activity. *(Fig. 16.8a,b.)*

In Partners: Students can work with a partner to find balance shapes together. Here is one way to facilitate this:

- Find a partner as you are moving and find ways to balance with your partner. Go slowly and see if you can help each other to support your weight. Try back-to-back shapes, hands to hands, head to head, etc. Go slowly enough as you move so that you can stay together when you change shapes. Play with this for a few minutes without talking to each other. Experiment and see what you discover.
- Now move on your own again, shifting weight and changing your shape.

Discussion

- What did you experience? Was this fun? Why do you think that is? Why might you do this as part of a warm-up? How does it relate to proprioception?
- *(For variation in partners)* What did you experience with your partner? Were you able to work with your partner without talking about it? Could you balance together? What did you discover?

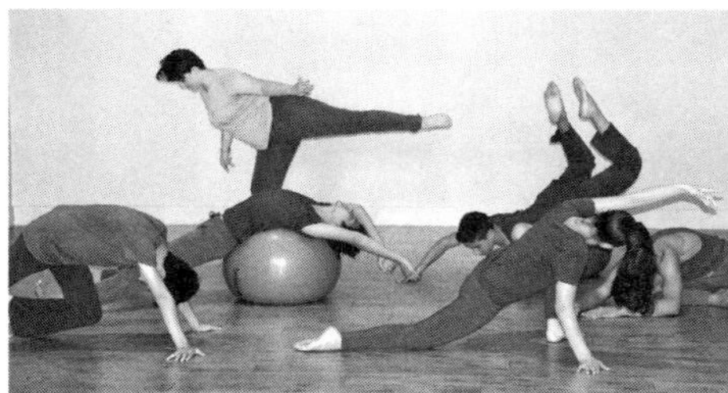

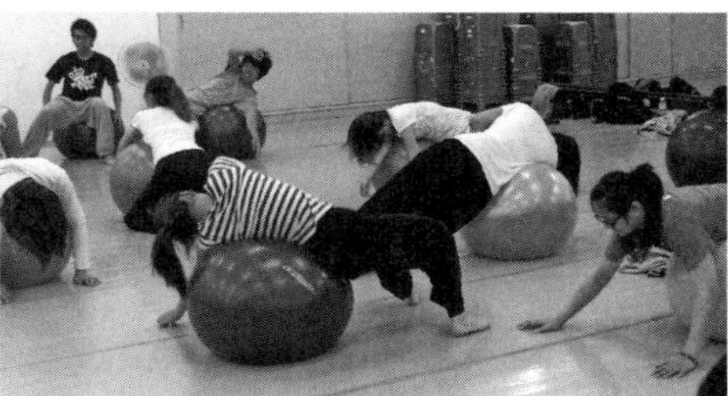

Fig. 16.8a, b. Waking up the proprioceptive senses with the Shaping activity provides students with a fun and more spontaneous way to move as part of a warm-up; using physioballs also allows students to explore new positions and orientations to gravity. (Photo b courtesy of Somatic Education Society of Taiwan.)

Full Body Integration: Structured Movement Sequences

While many of the previous explorations described have been improvisational in nature, structured movement sequences can also provide a familiar sense of stretching often associated with warm-up. Keeping a balance of improvisational and structured activities helps to provide an inspiring experience of both spontaneity and disciplined practice, as well as to avoid the boredom that can lead to injury. Structured activities included here help students to stretch through the large muscle groups of the body. Many activities can be used for this purpose, such as the Sun Salutation yoga sequence previously discussed; or you may want to draw on other yoga poses or martial arts activities.

In the sample activity I provide here, an exploration called Starfish Cross-Stretch,[8] you lie down in an "X" or starfish shape, and then reach and roll from your back to your belly and back again. This activity initiates spinal rotation and successive movement initiation through the core body and limbs. This helps you develop an awareness of when certain joints may be "locked," or not as free to respond to movement as it travels through your body. By freeing these pathways, you gain more ease of movement. This activity also helps to begin to experience all six "limbs"—arms, legs, and head and tail—equally radiating from your core. A further variation focuses on integrating movement of the musculoskeletal system with the support of the internal organs to encourage integrated and injury-free movement.

With older students, and those with more experience with these somatic practices, the Starfish activity can also be done in partners. This helps students gain experience in perceiving movement patterns in themselves and others, as well as learn to facilitate more easeful movement for their peers. It also helps the student doing the movement to receive the guided movement and touch, which enhances their proprioceptive senses and focuses their spatial intent while moving.

This level—of facilitating the movement for others—is more advanced, and can be used after students have had time to practice it for themselves first. Groups that have successfully understood and physically integrated the movement for themselves can then learn to guide the movement with others.

Exploration: Starfish Cross-Stretch

(20–30 minutes; 50–60 minutes with variations)

PURPOSE. To clarify the experience of "levering" through the bones; to develop an awareness of when certain joint(s) may be "locked" or not as free to respond to movement as it travels through your body; to encourage integrated, cross-lateral movement; to explore spinal rotation and core/distal initiation; to improve your ability to sense and perceive movement initiation and movement patterns in yourself and to perceive it in others; to integrate awareness of the skeleton (container) and organs (contents) as an aspect of integrated and injury-free movement (variation).

Activity

Demonstrate this movement pattern first, moving from your back to your belly, and then back again by leading through your hands and arms on the way over, and initiating the movement with your feet and legs on the way back. Then lead students in the movement as follows. Slow down and speed up your verbal instructions as needed so that you speak at the appropriate time to coordinate with students' movement.

Have students begin lying down on their backs in a starfish position, i.e., arms and legs out to the side in an "X" or starfish position, with the arms and legs opened to the sides *(Fig. 16.9a)*.

- ❍ As you lie in this "X" position, you can feel yourself like a starfish, reaching and radiating out from your core, through each of your six limbs at once—your two arms, two legs, your head, and your tail.
- ❍ Now you are going to begin to initiate your roll from your back to your belly by reaching with your fingers *(Fig. 16.9b)*, and allowing the movement to lever through all your joints and bones so the rest of your body glides along easily as you roll. You might imagine a wave has come along, and is gently guiding you over on to your belly—fingers to hands, to wrists to your arms, to your clavicles, to your ribs, to your spine, and down to your pelvis, and then to your legs and feet—as you turn over onto your belly.
- ❍ Then rest here on your belly, and be sure you are back in your "X" position. *(Fig. 16.9c.)*
- ❍ Now begin to roll back over to your back, by initiating the movement in your foot, *(Fig. 16.9d)* and levering through the bones, again easily shifting back over to your back: foot to your leg, to your pelvis, to your ribs, to your spine to your shoulder girdle, to your arms and hands and fingers.
- ❍ Then rest here on your back, and be sure you are back in your "X" position. *(Fig. 16.9e.)*
- ❍ Try this on your own a few times. See if you can use the least amount of muscular effort to turn over, so that you are letting the momentum of the turn travel easily through all of your joints.

Have students try this several times, rolling from back to front and front to back, changing sides each time so they have done this in both directions.

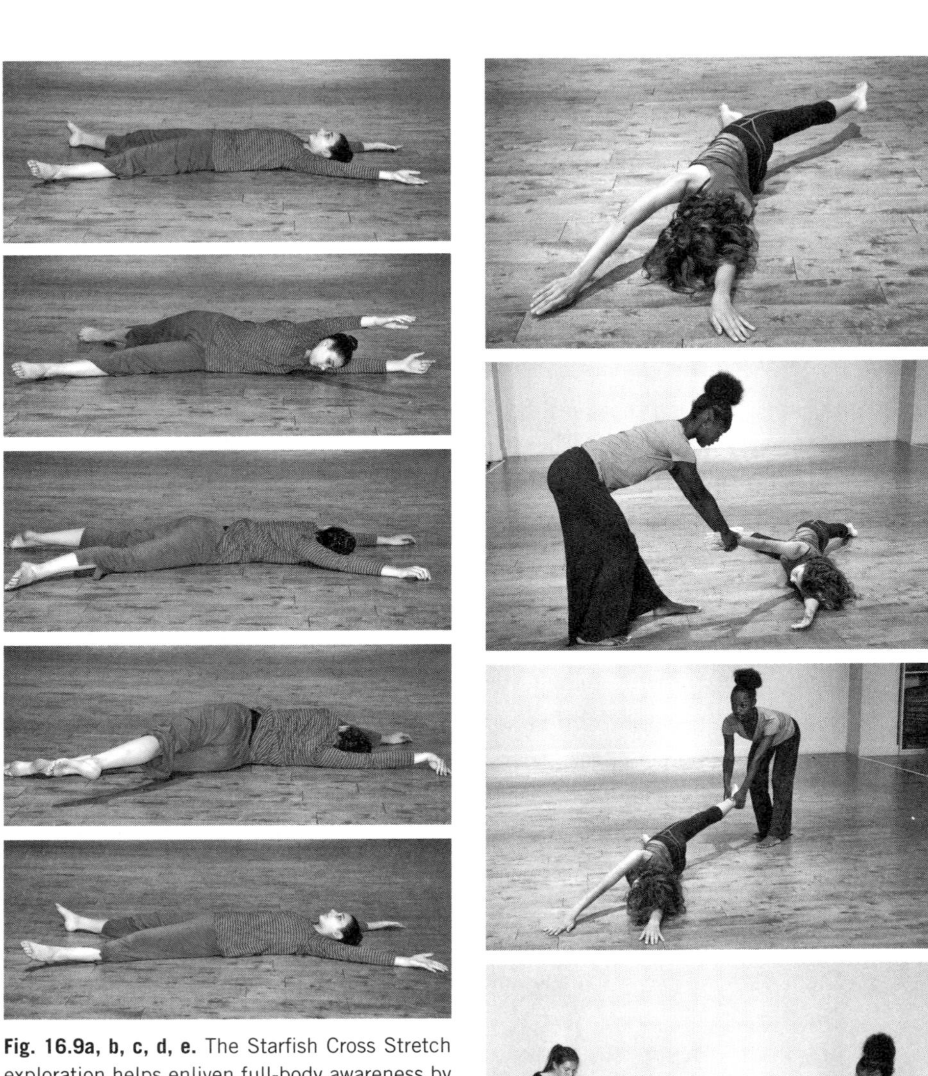

Fig. 16.9a, b, c, d, e. The Starfish Cross Stretch exploration helps enliven full-body awareness by experiencing all six "limbs"—arms, legs, and head and tail—radiating out from the core. This activity also helps students to find fluid, cross-lateral connectivity throughout their bodies as they move.

Fig. 16.10a, b, c, d. Starfish Cross Stretch variation. After gaining experience with this activity in their own bodies, students can help each other by facilitating the movement in partners. One student first does the movement on their own (a) while the other observes, then the movement can be facilitated in partners (b and c), or in groups of three (d).

Variations

You can demonstrate with a few students after they have had a chance to try this. For each student, you can have the group discuss what they notice, as you help to facilitate clear levering in the movement.

In Partners: Students can work in partners, with one person lying and moving while the other person observes *(Fig. 16.10a)*. Then the person observing can help to facilitate the movement as you have demonstrated, by leading the person with their hand or arm on the way over, and with their foot or leg on the way back *(Fig. 16.10b and c)*.

In Small Groups: Students can work in groups of three, with one moving and two facilitating. This helps to get the full-body diagonal stretch, as one person facilitates the upper body and the other the lower body *(Fig. 16.10d)*.

With a Focus on the Organs: You can also repeat this with a focus on initiating the movement from the organs, then on integrating both skeleton and organs, to encourage full inner-supported movement.

Discussion

- What did you notice? Were you able to feel the movement travel through your body? Was there anywhere that felt "stuck"? Did it get easier as you tried it a few times? What did you feel? Did anyone have a different experience?

Tips for Teachers

- When students are engaging in cross-lateral movement that initiates an extreme rotation in the spine, as in this activity, be sure they are using abdominal support to protect the lower back area. This is especially important when they work in partners or groups, due to the added momentum from the lengthening of their arms and legs provided by the facilitator(s).

Practice with Using the Warm-Up Formula

Once students have experienced each of these elements of the somatic warm-up "formula" separately through the previous explorations, they can try this method of warming up on their own. To review, the formula consists of the following six elements:

1. **Check-ins** to take stock of how you are feeling on any given day; to note the current state of the body-mind; to quiet the mind and become present in the moment (Check-in activities may include Constructive Rest, followed by a movement that

measures flexibility, such as rolling down the spine or leaning over one leg and the other, or to measure balance, such as standing on one leg and then the other.)

2. **Responsive Moving** to allow time to follow your own sense of what your body needs on any given day; to respond to your impulses to move rather than directing your movement consciously.
3. **Walking** to begin to increase blood flow to the muscles and to increase the amount and temperature of the synovial fluid in the joints; can be combined with shaking of the various joints.
4. **Shaping** to encourage full proprioceptive feedback and further awaken the body from within by taking weight on various parts of the body.
5. **Structured sequences** to activate core connection and full body movement (Starfish activity, Sun Salutation, or another familiar movement phrase.)
6. **Check-in** (repeated) to notice the effect of the warm-up; to measure presence, body-mind awareness, and flexibility as compared to the previous time when these check-in activities were done at the beginning.

These elements are meant to be explored in an improvisational manner, such that the order can vary each day as needed, allowing students to choose what order feels best each time. For instance, after their initial check-ins they may want to start by walking, then doing the more intentional Shaping activity, then transitioning to the more free-form Responsive Moving, and so on. On another day, after their check-ins they may want to begin on the floor and ease into Responsive Moving, then progress into Shaping, then walking, and so on. In any case, the more structured sequences should come *last,* followed by a final check-in.

This type of warm-up may be all that is needed to feel more vibrant and "present" in yourself—and can be beneficial *on its own* as an aspect of maintaining a healthy lifestyle and increasing your vitality on a daily basis. As students discover, after engaging in this warm-up process they generally feel more centered, grounded, and flexible. Giving students time to practice the warm-up formula on their own is an important step and concluding activity in the curriculum. Students can create a movement sequence that fits their individual needs each day—giving them a sense of independence—using the many tools they have learned to attend to their body-mind health.

Using Additional Warm-Up Activities

Beyond using this method of warm-up as a daily personal practice, at the end of a general warm-up such as this, students are more prepared for any additional movement or stretching needed to meet the specific physical challenges of their activities. These can include specific practices to improve mobility, strength, flexibility, endurance, or the performance of specific motor tasks. When warming up for a specific activity, then, students can design the rest of their warm-up to meet the goals of the particular activity by choosing which of these areas are important to be focused upon. For example, a marathon runner will want to focus on endurance, while the gymnast might want to focus on developing flexibility and mobility, and the soccer player will need to prepare for running, leaping, and quick, reflexive responses to change direction and speed. To help students understand this basic premise you can begin by discussing each of the following concepts related to the musculoskeletal system, by first pooling students' knowledge of them each:

- Mobility—the range of motion of a joint based on the shape of the bones at that joint
- Flexibility—the range of motion at a joint based on the mobility and resilience of the surrounding tissues
- Strength—the ability of a muscle or muscle group to function against resistance
- Endurance—the ability of a muscle or muscle group to function over time

In addition to these factors, depending upon the nature of the activity, you may need more of an internal focus, or more of an external focus. For example, inner sensing is an essential part of yoga or t'ai chi, while an external awareness is in the foreground for team activities like basketball or soccer. In fact, you often need a combination of the two: a dancer who is performing a group piece or a rock climber who is navigating a steep cliff will use both. As students begin to analyze what is needed for any given activity, they can extend their warm-up to include any other elements that are necessary to adequately prepare for an upcoming movement activity, as in the more traditional definition of "warm-up." Learning about these types of warm-ups may also be covered more extensively in other areas of their education through specific physical trainings, and need not be the main focus in this curriculum. Students will find, however, that they can bring this somatic approach to warm-up—and their newfound somatic awareness—to bear on movement practices in many areas of their education, such as in their sports or dance training. This will support them in these activities as well and help them improve in those areas.

Finally, whether engaging in movement as a daily personal practice, such as in this somatic warm-up, or doing any other type of movement activity, you can remind students of the concept of dedicating their practice, as described in chapter 8. This can be done individually or as a group. Keeping this in mind helps adolescents move away from the idea of movement performance as competition—in the sense of somehow needing to prove themselves—and instead supports the experience of movement as a personal practice, an aspiration to do one's best, and an offering to the self and the larger community.

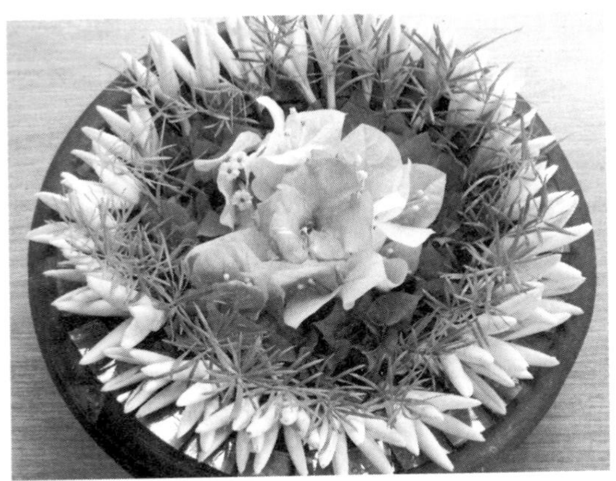

Flower Offering, Bali, Indonesia

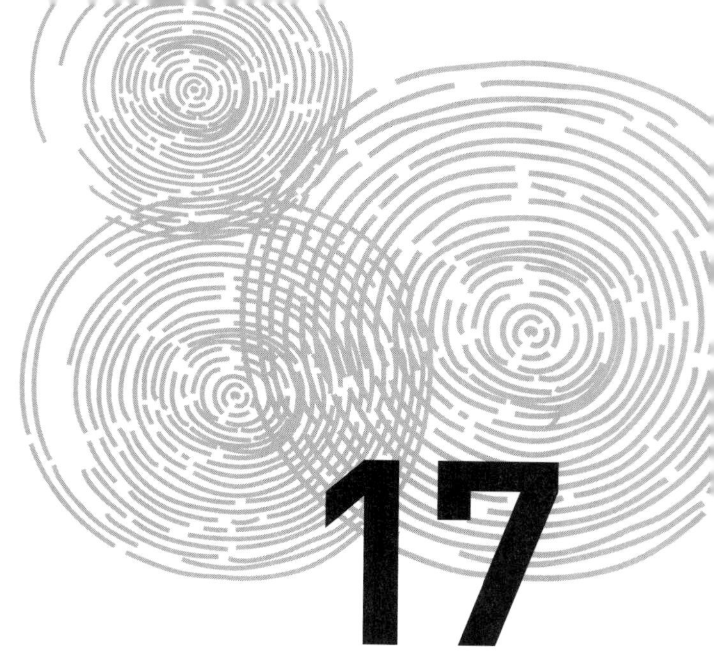

17

Coming Full Circle

Perceiving is about one's personal relationship to the incoming information. We all have sense organs, which are similar, but our perceptions are totally unique. Perception is about how we relate to what we're sensing. Perception is about relationship—to ourselves, others, the Earth, and the Universe.

—Bonnie Bainbridge Cohen

In these classes, although all students engage in similar activities, each of their responses is unique. What is meaningful to them is what they discover about their own movement patterns, their body-mind relationship, their lifestyles, their feelings, their connection to themselves and to others. Rather than accumulating a standard set of learned facts or predetermined physical skills, learning occurs as students become aware of their personal responses to changes in their own internal and external environment. The range of students' perceptions speaks for itself in the following student journal entries.

Today we did some standing relaxation exercises. We did a mental picture of our bones. I concentrated really well and saw it ... and I examined it. I became aware of the weight of my bones and their structures, and then it was like I saw and felt it in my own body, not just in my mind.

Then we did some illustrations of what we thought we saw. I think I have finally found the secret to great figure drawing. A person must not just look at the human figure and draw them, but they must first feel their own and draw their own. I liked my quick sketches and was pleased with the way class went today.

Also, I can feel my concentration level getting better because of those few fifteen-to-thirty-minute blocks during class everyday. It helps me to relax and helps me with my other studies, too.

—Anna, grade eleven (from daily journal of semester course)

When we first began the class, the things we did I thought were funny and I couldn't notice any difference from the exercises. I did think the Constructive Rest was comfortable, though. Then I began noticing I was very stiff most of the time and had an automatic arched back. This was probably from years of horseback riding where you have to sit with an arched back and pinched nerves in your neck. It felt like I was slouching when I stood in alignment. Most of the other kids seemed to have the opposite problem, of slouching and trying to stand up straighter.

In the Constructive Rest at first I'm very stiff, but when we're done, I don't feel stiff at all and it's easier to get into better alignment. Now, at the end of the course, none of the stretches are difficult, I don't come into class as stiff, and my alignment is much better.

—Diane, grade seven (from final course evaluation of six-week PE unit)

Now I am more aware of what is in my body and how it works. There is an overall good feeling that I have about myself. I feel like my athletic abilities have gotten better, and my coach has noticed it too. I think this class has given me a better awareness and knowledge that I can keep forever.

—Bryan, grade eleven (from final course evaluation of six-week PE unit)

In the beginning of the course, my body as I saw it was a five foot three structure of complex stuff! Now I can visualize the differences in the systems of the body. I can feel the bones of the body and how they are connected. It feels really nice to really know something solid about yourself that is factual and important.

Over the time of the class I think I have come to understand my body in a much clearer way. I was interested in and curious about the construction and function of my own body and it has been a very informative class for me, one that I can honestly say I have learned a lot from, and most importantly retained a lot of. Everyone, no matter who, should learn as much as they can about their bodies—your body is with you forever.

—Sarah, grade twelve (from final course evaluation of semester course)

Today was a bad day. A lot of things happened in short amounts of time so, consequently, I had my mind full of troubling things. By the time it came for our class, I got really excited to get there. I thought, "Great, I'll be able to clear my mind and just observe my body in my mind's eye." It wasn't that easy but it did help. I really emptied my mind while walking around the room.

However, when we stood still in one spot I began concentrating on my balance. Balance made me think of my balance between relationships and friends and a good "balanced" diet. I kept thinking of all these balances in my life that are lacking. So I tried to use the time to get to the bottom of these problems of the day.

—Stephanie, grade twelve (from daily journal of semester course)

Through experiential study of their bodies, students' learning becomes active *discovery*. They gain valuable insight into ways in which their lifestyles affect their bodies and may begin to integrate activities learned in class into their daily lives, helping them to improve patterns or habits that could otherwise lead to strain and/or injuries. Some students experience increased concentration as the class progresses, helping them with their academic subjects; others notice increased physical ability in myriad movement forms; some overcome their fears of their bodies as the silence about the body is broken and some of the mysteries of their internal worlds are addressed; and still others gain insight into their lives through the many metaphors the body teaches as we learn to listen.

As these stories illustrate, we don't know how individual teens will relate to this material or how this work will influence their lives. But clearly, it is time to open up this doorway. By engaging in this curriculum, adolescents can gain some of the valuable tools necessary to assume responsibility for the quality of their lives now and into adulthood. Perhaps nothing attests to this better than this final journal entry from one of my students:

I've been rather stressed and anxious recently. I know from experience that I tend to feel kind of out of my body at these times, like the ground is shaky and shifting. I feel like I just need something solid to grasp. There's no talking myself out of this experience with logic. So, this time, I began to imagine my skeletal structure instead, quite without intending to. I sat on the bus, anxious and tight, and just began to sink in internally. Now there isn't quite as much mystery involved in my body scan as there was the first time we tried it in class, so as a result it was a quite calming and centering process. I also did some of the bone tracing with my arms. I thought, "OK. Here I am." Then, I felt ready to step off the bus and walk into class.

As educators, we can offer students experiences that help them feel more at home with themselves and increase their self-understanding and resilience. The way we relate to others and our environment is a reflection of this primary relationship to ourselves. By nourishing students' primary relationship to themselves, we cultivate their broader relationships with others and with the environment. This connection to ourselves, to each other, and to the earth forms the circle of our lives.

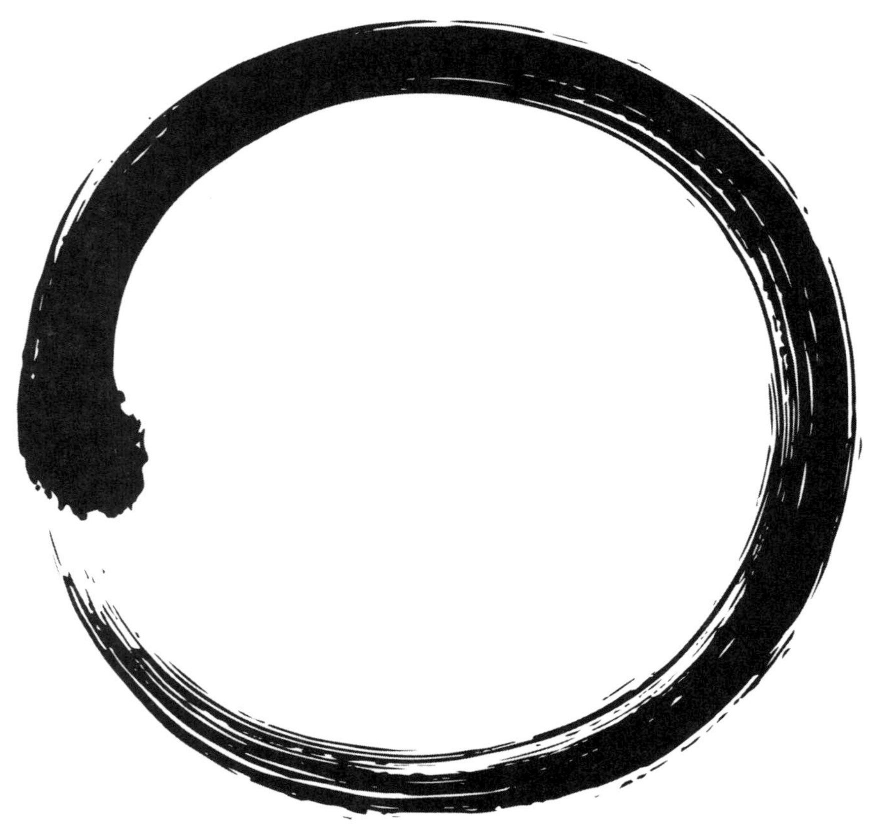

Afterword: Envisioning the Future of Somatic Education

Being confronted with the impossible makes us ask unexpected questions.

—Emilie Conrad

By this point, I hope you have gained a vivid sense of the ways in which somatic movement education can be taught with teenagers and the many concrete benefits it affords. Including somatic education as a core component of education for adolescents is still a revolutionary idea in the early twenty-first century. While it has the potential to be a burgeoning addition to programs for youth, both directly in our schools and through multiple educational contexts, there is still a lot of work ahead to bring this vision to fruition, with many questions left to be answered. Yet as our ideas and beliefs evolve, so do our cultural practices. With dedicated effort, what seems strange today can become the norm tomorrow. I have become particularly aware of this when teaching abroad, where what are considered "best practices" in both education and the culture at large can vary widely.

For instance, during a three-day workshop I recently gave at Taitung University in Taiwan, as part of our first morning together I taught the Constructive Rest Position. We also discussed the many physiological benefits of even a short time resting in this position. After our lunch break, upon returning to the studio I was surprised to see that the lights were out, and all forty or so of the students were lying down—many of them in Constructive Rest. Of course I thought, "What great students, already practicing what they've learned!" But when I asked the program director about it, to see if the students had initiated this on their own or if it had been her suggestion, she looked confused. "We do this *every day,*" she responded. "This is just how we rest after lunch before the next activity."

In educational contexts in the United States, "nap time" has traditionally only been included in preschool, and is otherwise generally considered a superfluous amenity we should leave behind in our preteen, teenage, and adult years. However, from a somatic perspective, recuperative activities—be it a nap or a walk or otherwise—could be similarly woven into the fabric of our education, and thus our daily lives. In fact, many corporate organizations—and even some airports in the U.S.—have begun to include specific rooms for yoga, napping, or fitness; other businesses have added standing desks and walking meetings. With education comes change. As more people become attuned to the benefits of somatic practices, our bodily intelligence becomes more of a concern and a priority. The notion of "embodiment" will then come more to the forefront and begin to inform our cultural practices.

Consider, for instance, the trajectory of yoga in our schools. As the practice of yoga became more mainstream and its benefits more broadly acknowledged and supported by research, educators began to consider yoga—albeit a secularized and sometimes over-simplified version—as a viable method of "physical education." Due to the pioneering work of inspired and committed individuals and organizations, now many public and independent middle and high schools offer yoga programs. This shift, along with the expanding presence of programs in both mindfulness and social-emotional learning, goes a long way in indicating that the body-based approach to developing somatic awareness advocated in this book is a natural fit for twenty-first-century education! Somatic education also aligns well with programs that emphasize more interactive project-based learning, which is becoming established as a best practice in schools in many countries. Once understood and *experienced* by more of the general population—including administrators, educators, parents, and teens themselves—programs in somatic education will find a ready welcome among those proponents who want to move adolescent education toward a more holistic model.

Essentially, if we want systemic change we need to begin with the *individual,* with each of us gaining our own embodied experience with inner somatic awareness. As Deane Juhan has noted, "the problems of the individual and society are no more separable than are those of the body and mind."[1] We can each take time to realistically assess where we are in our own process of cultivating and applying somatic awareness. In our own lives, we might then decide to add or alter practices in our daily routine to help us reconnect with our inner resources. For example, some people find that adding a practice of movement and meditation to their morning routine gives them greater vitality; to their surprise, some even find it helps them give up caffeine as a means to get going for the day. In our role as educators, taking a next step could mean a group of teachers who take a somatic-related workshop and then begin to explore the material together on their own, or advocate for further training in somatics as part of their professional development. Or this might translate into a high school teacher who can add a simple practice like bone tracing to a human anatomy class, or it could be outdoor educators who add ecosomatic activities to their teen programming.

To offer independent somatic education programs, we will also need trained and knowledgeable teachers. Presently many professionals have undergone extensive in-depth training in various somatic disciplines and can become further engaged in working with youth. Over the past thirty years, the field has continued to thrive in and around the world, and although there are somatic educators who have worked with groups of adolescents, nevertheless few actual programs have been created for teens and been included in schools.[2] To get there, we need creative, somatic curricula like this one that is student-centered and responsive to the needs of developing adolescents. Athletic trainers, dance teachers, science teachers, physical educators, health and wellness teachers, and other educators can also increase their skill in and knowledge of somatics to create more body-based approaches and curricula. Further, and perhaps most importantly, the training and degree programs for educators in these fields can include somatics. Through such initiates, a larger population of children and adults can increasingly benefit from this growing field. All of these steps, however small or large, can have a significant impact on creating the large-scale cultural shift needed to establish a value system welcoming of such programs within our schools, dance studios, outdoor education, and other community programs for youth.

In addition to somatic education programs becoming more prominent in schools at the middle and high school levels, significant changes can be made in school-wide programming at the national level to help our youth learn more holistically—in a way that respects their bodies and their need for movement. For instance, as a start the Centers for Disease Control and Prevention now recommend at least one hour of movement for adolescents each day.[3] Teens now get PE as part of their school day in 78 percent of school districts in the United States.[4] Yet with an article distributed by the American Heart Association estimating that only 3.8 percent of elementary, 7.9 percent of middle, and 2.1 percent of high schools provide daily physical education or its equivalent for the entire school year,[5] clearly there are more hurdles to jump to achieve this CDC standard for our youth.

On a more positive note, in response to recent studies that demonstrate adolescents require more sleep than they routinely get—due to a variety of factors including biological changes in sleep associated with puberty, along with lifestyle choices and academic demands—some middle and high schools have begun initiating later start times to the school day, thus accommodating the physiological reality of adolescence.[6] And although prioritizing the body may be a new frontier, I've seen promising evidence of change in many schools and organizations over the past ten years that aspire toward a more holistic education for young people.

For example, many of the individual educators who have been participants in my programs have been developing creative somatic-related curricula for youth. This includes a health and wellness director who integrated somatic practices into a yoga unit for teen students at her school, a dance teacher who created an experiential anatomy component in her middle school dance program, and a mindfulness teacher who created a more movement-based, somatic approach to his workshops with teens. Another participant, who works with youth as a coach and continued to pursue extensive study in somatics, developed his own approach to teaching tennis.

Other middle and high schools have also been making substantial changes to their programming, such as changes to the school day, classroom design, and curricular offerings. Adaptations schools can consider include longer movement classes; more periodic breaks during the day (in which students can choose an activity that would best serve them at the time); options like physioballs along with chairs in the classroom setup; and including various movement forms such as yoga, t'ai chi, and aikido.[7]

These are just some examples of the kind of creative and responsive program designs that can evolve when individual educators and organizations commit to learning that includes body-based activities that promote somatic awareness. As these examples demonstrate, along with offering a specific somatic program, somatic *principles* can be incorporated into school programming at all levels. Increasing the time spent in nature in outdoor curricular activities—with time to play and explore—can also help teens to cultivate a more vibrant and sensory-based perceptual base. Engaging directly with the natural world through activities like hiking, cooking, gardening, and other horticulture practices can also be integrated into our education. Ecosomatic education, outdoor play, and hefty doses of daily movement contribute to a healthy lifestyle and a much more vital and sensible educational model.

Given the current state of our educational systems in the United States and elsewhere, where and how can somatic programs be implemented? Ideally somatic education would serve students from a wide range of economic neighborhoods and diverse populations, yet this will take a concerted effort on the part of educators to realize this goal. As Martha Eddy notes:

> [T]o enhance somatic education there needs to be more time, space, and quiet. These provide the conditions necessary for supporting body-mind learning and somatic action. Unfortunately, time, space, and quiet have become expensive.... Long enough periods of time would be needed during the day or at school to learn about the body, relax, learn from the body and practice new habits ... [and yet] may be exactly what we need to address a host of educational quandaries and even contribute to societal balances.[8]

This brings up the issue of who can afford such programs, and the risk that poorer schools may not have access to such practices. Until the benefits of somatic movement education are more widely understood, it may be that such programs offered within the school day may initially become more widespread in the independent sector—through public charter schools, home-schooling, and private middle and high schools—as these programs may already uphold a model of education that is explicitly student-centered, and thus align well with the values inherent in somatic movement education. Here key administrators and educators may be more readily welcoming of such a curriculum. Sometimes private or charter schools may also already have alternate movement spaces or the financial means to support new programming.

While it is beyond the scope of this book to deal extensively with this grievous inequity, there are several approaches to inclusivity that I have found effective and can offer as initial suggestions. One way to ensure a broader range of student access to programs in somatic movement education—particularly within public schools and related after-school contexts—may be to pursue grant funding. Although this may sound counterintuitive, since grants can be so difficult to come by, in my experience grants are likely to be more available to support programs for underserved and poorer populations, whether in rural or urban areas. As the benefits of somatic movement education become more broadly appreciated, it is possible that these communities can be most widely served in the long term through such grant-funded initiatives.

For instance, in one case I worked with a nonprofit organization[9] with an extensive after-school program, including weekly dance classes and educational services, offered free of charge to middle and high-school students from low-income families. In addition to their work with me, together we were able to craft a successful grant application to fund further professional development for their dance faculty in a variety of somatic disciplines.

Expanding the participant diversity in training programs for somatic movement educators can also be a primary goal, which would then provide a more diverse population of teachers for a curriculum such as this one. This is essential in reaching a broader student base, since any one teacher will not necessarily be the right fit for a particular teen population—in which having an adult figure with whom students can relate as a role model is especially important. In my own case of the Embodiment in Education training, I reached out to diverse communities to create a group with a variety of racial backgrounds, physical abilities, and sexual and gender orientations, as well as to international students from various countries. I also partnered with a nonprofit organization called Dancers' Group in San Francisco as a fiscal sponsor in order to raise scholarship funds.

Over several years, all of these efforts resulted in a much more diverse group of participants. This felt especially crucial to the efficacy of these professional development workshops, which include opportunities for participants to share ideas and concerns as colleagues to learn from our collective experience. The more voices we can hear from about adapting and creating effective curricula to meet the needs of a variety of students—with differences in race, religion, gender, physical capacity, or socioeconomic status—the better for us all. As the saying goes, "it takes a village," and it will take many educators championing a similar vision to meet the needs of a range of educational contexts and diverse communities.[10]

Fortunately, training opportunities in somatics have also begun to flourish, with many independent programs offered through ISMETA, as well as several universities offering advanced degrees in somatics and somatic-related studies in the United States and abroad. Somatic practices are also increasingly being integrated into the teaching of subjects such as dance and movement by dance educators trained in specific somatic disciplines. Other developments internationally include the first undergraduate program in the world with a degree in somatic movement education, offered at Taiwan's Taitung University in their somatics and sports leisure department. As a next generation becomes more versed in somatic practices, a new model of education that includes such practices becomes even more viable.

Finally, suggesting that we include somatic practices in adolescent education also brings up the important question of who gets to design and control the embodiment techniques—and the values they transmit that enculturate our youth. As educators, we need to be conscious of the values underlying our body pedagogies, and aware of our own biases, as well as of the efficacy of our programs. As somatic educators know and as research suggests, people's identities are integrally related to the forms of embodied education they receive, steering the development of people's capacities in certain directions.[11]

The curriculum we offer students both reflects and can create the culture from which they come. When crafted with awareness and sensitivity, somatic education programs can contribute to empowering adolescents with newfound awareness and choice. As dancer and dance anthropologist Cynthia Novack has noted, "Culture is embodied… To the degree we can grasp the nature of our experience of movement, both the movement itself and the context in which it occurs, we learn more about who we are and about the possibilities for knowingly shaping our lives."[12]

We can support adolescents' development from within—to help them experience an embodied sense of self and develop their own interests. We can also encourage them to cultivate holistic perspectives and become leaders with responsible, compassionate views. Teen environmental activist Xiuhtezcatl Martinez notes that many of today's teens are disconnected from themselves and from each other, compounding the many problems they inevitably face in our complex world. His words, from a keynote speech in 2016, are a powerful testament to the need to work with youth in a way that helps them to reconnect with themselves, each other, and the Earth, which empowers them to make their own individual contributions:

> What we gotta shift is the way we see ourselves in relation to this Earth. People are like, "Oh, what are the solutions?" "How do you fix the world?" And I'm just like damn, I'm sixteen, I'm tryin' to figure it out too! People are always like, "Oh, you are the future, young people are so important." But what I've come to understand is that the intergenerational movement that needs to be created is more important than anything.... The innovation, the creativity, and the *passion* that young people have is amazing, it's so powerful. When our voices are given the attention they need—when we are told that our voices have power, that we can be leaders—young people rise to the top![13]

Somatic education can provide an essential component to providing teens with an education that encourages and prioritizes the creative developmental process of each individual. Adding curriculum in somatic movement education can support teens as they navigate the volatile physical and emotional challenges they face during this vibrant, transformational stage of life. Giving our youth the opportunity to explore *themselves* and what it is to be a human being, embodied and living sustainably on this planet, is essential to a twenty-first century education.

This is the call of our times: to learn to care for ourselves, for each other, and for the planet. Such a generation of embodied teens will be best equipped to develop to their fullest potential—empowered to live healthy and meaningful lives.

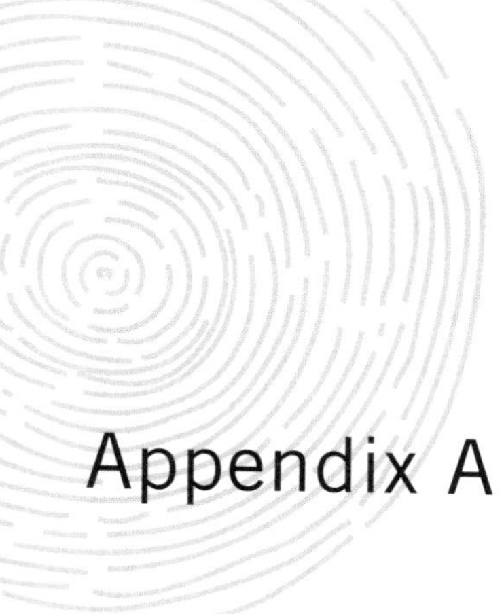

Appendix A

Summary Sheet of the Eight Pedagogy Principles

Eight Key Pedagogy Principles for Teaching Somatic Movement Education to Teens

1. OBJECTIVE AND SUBJECTIVE EXPERIENCE

Core Principle: To facilitate a somatic experience requires an approach to the body and movement that is inclusive of both objective information and subjective experience.

While *information* can be learned, true *knowledge* comes from one's own lived experience. To offer knowledge, then, we must offer *experience.* By focusing on students' own sensations and perceptions, we include their subjective experiences in the learning process. This is the *soma,* the body experience from within—the lived experience.

2. STUDENT-DRIVEN CURRICULUM

Core Principle: Start with what students already know, and build on their interests from there.

When students are given a chance to *discover what they already know* and *share that knowledge collectively,* they gain confidence from progressing from where they actually are, rather than measuring themselves against some outside standard of what they believe they should already know or have experienced.

3. BALANCE OF SENSORY AND MOTOR EXPERIENCE

Core Principle: Create a balance of activities that provide both quiet inner sensing and active physical movement to keep each class engaging.

Motor activities can provide teens with an essential bridge to more inner sensory work. Motor activities stimulate the *sympathetic nervous system* (outer-oriented action), while sensory activities stimulate the *parasympathetic nervous system* (inner-oriented sensing). It is the balance of rest and activity—or inner and outer focus—that is truly healthy and revitalizing.

4. PROPRIOCEPTION AND ORIENTATION

Core Principle: Teach about proprioception (our "self-receiver cells") and its relationship to learning new skills and movement patterns. This helps students develop patience with the process of kinesthetic learning, often new to them, which may include initial periods of disorientation as they "unlearn" old patterns in order to learn new ones.

Help students to understand the process of somatic learning by teaching about proprioception and kinesthetic sense. Allow for *disorientation* (and various comfort levels with new material) that is a precursor to inviting new learning—hold the "big picture view" for your students as they gain comfort with the process.

5. LAYERED LEARNING APPROACH

Core Principle: Teach using a layered learning approach to help students to experience some level of proficiency and ease without being overly challenged. This also allows you to add new material that builds on previous experience to keep students engaged.

When using a layered approach, the activities become familiar without being merely repetitive, as the new information and challenges keep students engaged, while reinforcing previous knowledge. This provides some measure of comfort in which new body learning can occur.

6. CREATE A SAFE CONTAINER AND BUILD A SENSE OF COMMUNITY

Core Principle: We learn best when we are respected and approached with love and compassion. Create a community of mutual respect and kindness as a foundation for growth and learning.

To facilitate the focused environment needed for somatic work, establish *clear directions and boundaries* in all activities (particularly those that involve touch). Finding an appropriate balance of structure and spontaneity is also an important aspect of creating a safe container for teens to enjoy these embodiment activities. Teach with love. We demonstrate our caring for students as human beings by *valuing their opinions and experiences as part of the educational process.*

7. TIME FOR INTEGRATION OF NEW MATERIAL AND EXPERIENCES

Core Principle: Include a motor activity at the end, such as walking, to help integrate the more inner-directed parasympathetic activities often explored in somatic exercises and to help students reorient as they prepare to move on to whatever activity follows your class or session. Leave time for a final discussion section as a further way to help students integrate their experiences that day.

Stay aware of and monitor the amount and type of movement and/or processing time that may be needed to provide adequate closure to each class. When facilitating somatic work, it is especially important to remain flexible to keep the priority on adequately meeting the needs of the moment.

8. TEACH FROM WHAT YOU KNOW AND HAVE EXPERIENCED IN YOUR OWN BODY; TRUST YOURSELF.

Core Principle: Remember that you are teaching by transmission through your own movement, as well as by the structured activities you are offering. Be willing to demonstrate that you are *both* a "student" and a "teacher" in this process.

In teaching embodiment practices, your physical presence will speak louder than your words. Your own embodied experience—past and present—is central to your ability to facilitate the material. Remember that you are *teaching by "transmission" through your own body/movement,* as well as by the structured activities you are offering. At the same time, remember that we are all students in the process of embodiment.

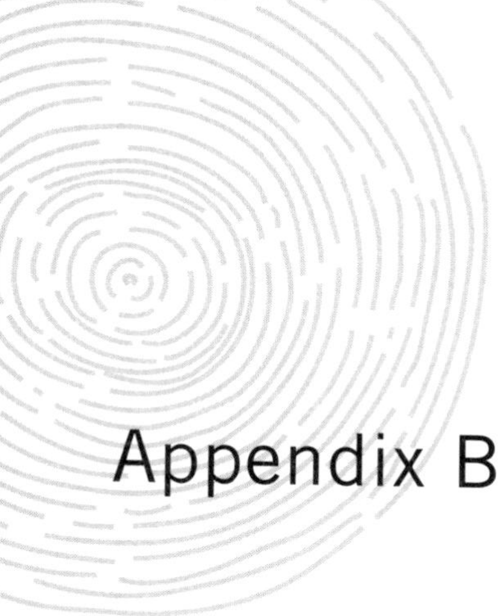

Appendix B

Summary Sheet of Four Guidelines for Teaching Intentional Touch

As discussed in chapter 6, you will want to be sure that there is adequate support within the school or program—among teachers, parents, and administrators—for including touch in the curriculum. This begins by clarifying the purpose and scope of the activities ahead of time (related to self-touch or partner touch) with all those involved in the decision-making process. Once touch-based activities are well established as a part of the curriculum, these pedagogy guidelines can help you to responsibly include touch for your students.

1. BEGIN WITH SELF-TOUCH

Core Principle: Introduce self-touch activities first, so students can become familiar with basics of touch for body awareness and learn self-care skills.

Once familiar, self-touch activities—like tracing the bones of the feet, for instance—give students easy and effective self-care tools to do on their own. Self-touch is also an essential aspect of embodied anatomy in that you can discover distinctions in form and function in your own body through touch and movement, which increases proprioceptive awareness and allows you to move with more ease.

2. GIVE SPECIFIC GUIDELINES IN EACH TOUCH-BASED ACTIVITY

Core Principle: Use clear guidelines and be specific as to the goal and type of touch to be used.

Set the stage for *intentional touch,* that which has a stated purpose and method, by telling students directly: 1) the purpose of the activity, 2) the type of touch to use, and 3) why that type of touch is being used. Using clear guidelines also helps students learn about and distinguish between various types of touch. This also helps them to feel more comfortable, in both self-touch and in partner activities, as they have a clear context and purpose for the activity.

3. WORKING WITH PARTNERS: SET AN EDUCATIONAL CONTEXT FOR TOUCH-BASED ACTIVITIES

Core Principle: Be clear to set an educational context, rather than a therapeutic one, especially when working with touch as a group or with a partner.

When working in partners, establish an educational context for students in which both students—the one touching and the one being touched—are seen as active learners. To do this, first bring awareness to their assumptions about touch. The stereotypical assumption is that the one touching is going to be "fixing" or "working on" you, and often that they know more about what your body needs than you do. Discussing this, you can then reframe the touch activities to put students on equal ground as participants in the experience. Another important aspect to shifting toward a more educational context is to explicitly invite verbal feedback from each partner, particularly from the one who is receiving touch.

4. WORKING WITH PARTNERS: ESTABLISH A PROTOCOL OF CONSENT AND COMMUNICATION

Core Principle: Set the stage for touch-based activities done in partnership by creating a system of establishing consent and appropriate communication between individuals, while keeping the main focus on sensory experience.

In all touch-based activities, you should establish a protocol of consent—but keep it simple. Derive a formula that works best for you for this process, such as having a student simply ask the partner, "Are you ready?" with the other person responding, "Yes, you can start now," or simply "Yes." Clear and specific communication establishes trust and safety, allowing students to feel more relaxed and able to focus on the activity at hand.

Illustrations

CHAPTER 8

Fig. 8.5 Sun Salutation: Shutterstock, Baleika Tamara

CHAPTER 9

Fig. 9.3b Pelvis; Shutterstock, Sebastian Kaulitzki

Fig. 9.5 Forearm; Shutterstock, Sebastian Kaulitzki

Fig. 9.7 Skeleton; Shutterstock, Sebastian Kaulitzki

Fig. 9.9d Foot; Shutterstock, Sebastian Kaulitzki

CHAPTER 10

Fig. 10.1 Synovial Joint, Marghe Mills-Thysen

CHAPTER 11

Fig. 11.6 Figures, with Skeleton and Organs: Michael Ridge, courtesy of Bonnie Bainbridge Cohen

CHAPTER 14

Fig. 14.1 Side View of Spine and Torso: Shutterstock, Sebastian Kaulitzki

Fig. 14.14 Vertebrae Drawing: Marghe Mills-Thysen

Figs. 14.15 b and d Vertebrae Drawings: Marghe Mills-Thysen

CHAPTER 17

Circle Drawing, Shutterstock, Sewonboy

Photo Credits

Dedication photo by Kiera Brodsky Chase

Author biography photo by Shinichi Iova-Koga

Outdoor photos on pages 115 and 286 by Yve St. John

Nature photos on pages 282 and 310 by Susan Bauer

Photos taken during the Embodiment in Education training by Susan Bauer or workshop participants.

All other photography courtesy of Monica Xu and Danny Yugen, unless otherwise noted in the captions.

Drawings on photos by Susan Bauer, with thanks to Emma Cofod for technical assistance.

Special thanks for photography permission granted from the Somatic Education Society of Taiwan.

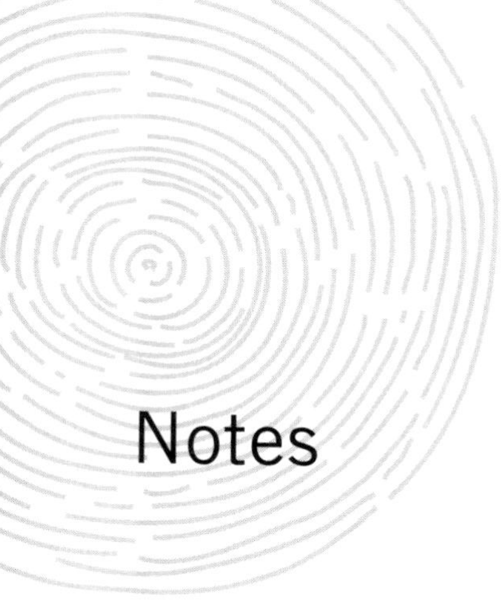

Notes

Introduction

1 Paus, Keshavan, and Giedd, "Why Do Many Psychiatric Disorders Emerge during Adolescence?" quoted in Broderick, *Learning to Breathe,* 177.
2 Much of this course has now been documented in Olsen, *BodyStories.*
3 From personal email communication to the author, September 22, 2017, used with permission.
4 For more information, see Alexander, *Constructive Conscious Control of the Individual.*
5 Moo Baan Dek ("Children's Village") was founded in 1978 to provide orphans and underprivileged children with free education and accommodations. For more information, see http://www.ffc.or.th. My teaching there was organized and sponsored by the Thai nonprofit organization Spirit in Education Movement (SEM), with founding patrons including Thich Nhat Hanh. For more information, see http://www.sem-edu.org.
6 The first version of this program that I designed was offered at Moving on Center School in 2006, where I served as program director from 2006 to 2009. Then called Somatics in Education, the program included guest faculty Caryn McHose and Deane Juhan.

Chapter 1

1 Steinberg, *Age of Opportunity,* 148.
2 Association for Mindfulness in Education, Mindful Education Map; for more information see http://www.mindfuleducation.org/mindful-education-map/.
3 CASEL website, Partner Districts; for more information see http://www.casel.org/partner-districts/districts/.
4 Some more progressive programs in PE do include additional movement forms, such as yoga or martial arts, as discussed further in the final chapter in this book.
5 Caldwell, "Mindfulness and Bodyfulness," 80.
6 Ogden et al., "Trends in Obesity Prevalence," quoted in Centers for Disease Control and Prevention, "Child Obesity Facts."
7 "Childhood Obesity."
8 Porges, *The Pocket Guide to the Polyvagal Theory,* 222.
9 Ibid.
10 Bainbridge Cohen, *Sensing, Feeling, and Action,* 114.
11 Schwartz, "Creativity and Dance," 9.
12 Gardner, *Frames of Mind,* 206.

13 Whitehouse, "Creative Expression in Physical Movement Is Language without Words," 35.
14 McHugh, "Restoring Original Grace," 16.
15 Juhan, *Job's Body*, 338–39.
16 From a lecture given by Deane Juhan in the Embodiment in Education workshop, 2012; used here with permission.
17 Tsabary, *The Awakened Family*, 2016, 12.
18 Claxton, *Intelligence in the Flesh*, 290.
19 Ibid., 290–91.
20 In 1964, Marion Diamond produced the first scientific evidence to demonstrate that we can develop increased connections between neurons in the brain over time as a result of stimulating environments. In fact, Diamond was particularly interested in education and conducted many of her experiments in schools with youth, as she passionately set out to improve our models of education.
21 Claxton, *Intelligence in the Flesh*, 274.
22 Haase et al., "When the Brain Does Not Adequately Feel the Body."
23 Singh, "Physical Activity and Performance at School," 2012.
24 Eddy, "Somatic Practices and Dance."
25 "National Health Education Standards," Center for Disease Control and Prevention, updated August 18, 2016, https://www.cdc.gov/healthyschools/sher/standards/index.htm.
26 Ibid.; see also "Health Education Content Standards for California Public Schools," updated March 2008, https://www.cde.ca.gov/be/st/ss/documents/healthstandmar08.pdf.
27 For further information, see https://www.casel.org.
28 Gutman, *The Impact of Non-Cognitive Skills*, 4.
29 Steinberg, *Age of Opportunity*, 121.
30 Ibid., 162.
31 From lecture given in the Embodiment in Education Workshop, 2013. Deane Juhan refers to sensory awareness and methods of experiential learning through movement that build sensory intelligence as being the first of three essential stages to self-development: self-awareness, self-regulation, and self-adaptation. For more information, see https://www.jobsbody.com/resistance-release-and-re-coordination-the-deane-juhan-method/.
32 See Merleau-Ponty, *Phenomenology of Perception*.
33 Kabat-Zinn, "Father of Mindfulness on What Mindfulness Has Become."
34 Steinberg, *Age of Opportunity*, 16.
35 For further information, see https://www.mindandlife.org.
36 The secular mindfulness practices often introduced in education are based primarily on the innovative work of Jon Kabat-Zinn, who developed his technique for mindfulness-based stress reduction (MBSR) at the University of Massachusetts Medical Center in 1979—versions of which are taught in hospitals and schools worldwide. Such programs, primarily based in meditation, have been highly researched and shown to provide myriad health benefits, such as reduced anxiety and improved attention. There are also cases in which mindfulness practices may be contraindicated, as other research has revealed, so educators will need to consider both the teaching context and the specific population of students when determining best practices.
37 Kabat-Zinn, *Mindfulness for Beginners*, 1.
38 Eddy, *Mindful Movement*, 264.
39 Kee et al., "Mindfulness, Movement Control, and Attentional Focus Strategies."

40 This "mindful body" approach of teaching stillness with children can be seen in the methods used by Mindful Schools; see www.mindfulschools.org and the video titled "K–5 Curriculum Demo: Class One—Mindful Bodies and Listening 1st Grade," available at http://www.mindfulschools.org/resources/explore-mindful-resources/ (accessed Sept. 26, 2017).

41 Caldwell, "Mindfulness and Bodyfulness," 79. Noting the lack of an appropriate word is primarily because we can't name something that we don't regularly know how to feel or that isn't important to us or that we actively marginalize, she even proposes the word *bodyfulness* to name this embodied state.

42 Kabat-Zinn, *Mindfulness-Based Stress Reduction (MBSR),* 21.

43 As an example, even in the popular mindfulness curriculum called Learning to Breathe, used worldwide to cultivate "emotion regulation, attention, and performance," there does not seem to be any mention of the diaphragm in the book. Broderick, *Learning to Breathe.*

44 Martinez et al., "School Climate in Middle School," 3, referencing Zins et al., *Building Academic Success on Social and Emotional Learning.*

45 Ibid., 6, and Dweck, Walton, and Cohen, *Academic Tenacity,* 27.

46 Dweck, Walton, and Cohen, *Academic Tenacity.*

47 For more on the growth mindset vs. fixed mindset theory, see the work of Stanford University psychologist Carol S. Dweck, PhD, in her book *Mindset: The New Psychology of Success.*

48 Rosenthal, "Some Dynamics of Resistance," 361.

Chapter 2

1 Murphy, *Future of the Body,* 38.

2 Johnson, *Body,* 154.

3 See www.ISMETA.org.

4 Eddy, *Mindful Movement,* 27.

5 Ibid., 25.

6 Personal communication with the author, used with permission, September, 2017.

7 Eddy, *Mindful Movement,* 192. As Eddy also notes, along with improvements in physical skill, Kleinman's research showed that students in these programs also had improved grades and focus, demonstrating both cognitive and physical growth as a result of such programs.

8 Berland, *Sitting,* 22.

9 See www.bodymindcentering.com.

10 Dowd, *Taking Root to Fly,* 7–8.

11 Mulder, in Berland, *Sitting,* 24.

12 Dowd, *Taking Root to Fly,* 8–9.

13 See www.bodymindcentering.com.

14 Bainbridge Cohen, *Sensing, Feeling, and Action,* 2.

15 Ibid., 2–3.

16 Hartley, *Wisdom of the Body,* xxviii.

17 A plethora of books on the enteric nervous system emerged in the late 1990s; see *The Second Brain* by Michael Gershon, 1998; *The Gut, Our Second Brain* by Jackie D. Wood, and *The Mind-Gut Connection* by Emeran Mayer, among others.

18 Enghauser, "Quest for an Eco-Somatic Approach to Dance Pedagogy."

19 For more about Somatic Expression, see www.somaticexpression.com.

20 Bauer, "Dancing with the Divine," 401.
21 For more information, see www.workthatreconnects.org.
22 I was first introduced to dance anthropology in a course with Cynthia Jean Cohen Bull (AKA Cynthia Novack) at Wesleyan University in 1995, followed by study with Joann Kealiinohomoku at UCLA in 1998.
23 Eddy, *Mindful Movement,* 233. In fact, in her article "Somatic Practices and Dance: Global Influences," Eddy posits that the separation of mind-body studies from cultural influences was originally reflected in the writings of Thomas Hanna, which she critiques as proposing an ethnocentric and male construct of somatics devoid of emotion and cultural context (46–62). In this sense, social somatics attempts to reclaim a broader view of the human experience.
24 Eddy, *Mindful Movement,* 234; Carol Swann, quoted in Leguizaman et al.
25 For more on Contact Improvisation see Cynthia J. Novack, *Sharing the Dance.*
26 After Whitehouse's death, Adler formed the Mary Starks Whitehouse Institute in Northampton, Massachusetts, in 1981 to continue the study and practice of Whitehouse's "movement in depth" or "authentic movement." Adler now calls her approach the Discipline of Authentic Movement; for more information, see www.disciplineofauthenticmovement.com.
27 See Adler, *Offering from the Conscious Body.*
28 See Olsen, "Being Seen, Being Moved," 47. In my own teaching, I have often called my workshops in Authentic Movement "Mindfulness in Motion," and have long experienced the practice of Authentic Movement as a way to cultivate greater mindfulness of body, speech, and mind.
29 The philosophies of Authentic Movement were also influenced by the Jungian concepts of the unconscious and the collective unconscious. Authentic Movement is often seen as a way to gain access to these aspects of ourselves, and requires specific guidelines to ensure a safe container for this deeply personal process. To clarify, Authentic Movement is not part of the curriculum and, in general, I would not recommend you offer it for teens in an educational context, though it may be appropriate in certain therapeutic contexts.

Chapter 3

1 Biermeier, "Inspired by Reggio Emilia," 74.
2 Steinberg, *Age of Opportunity,* 5.
3 I also give students an evaluation form at the end, which we also discuss, though an ongoing discussion about how students are doing is the best method of evaluation and should not merely be left until the end.
4 I facilitate most small group activities based on the theories of an educational approach called "Cooperative Learning." This method utilizes group experiences to foster student interaction and positive interdependence, as well as to maintain accountability for individual participation. I have especially drawn on the Learning Together model presented by Johnson and Johnson. A summary of this model can be found in Kapitan, *Cooperative Learning in the Classroom,* though more recent cooperative learning models may now be available.

Chapter 4

1 Bainbridge Cohen, *Sensing, Feeling, and Action,* 64.
2 Weber, "Integrating Semi-Structured Somatic Practices and Contemporary Dance Technique Training," 2009.

3 Dweck, Walton, and Cohen, *Academic Tenacity*, 26–28.
4 Steinberg, *Age of Opportunity*, 161.
5 Neff, *Self-Compassion.*
6 Jinpa, *A Fearless Heart*, 156–57.
7 Ibid., 158–59.
8 Gutman and Schoon, "Impact of Non-Cognitive Skills on Outcomes for Young People."
9 Steinberg, *Age of Opportunity*, 140.
10 Sroufe et al., quoted in Broderick, *Learning to Breathe*, 9.
11 Broderick, *Learning to Breathe*, 9.
12 Ibid.

Chapter 5

1 Olsen, *BodyStories*, 122; for further discussion of Olsen's perspective on the use of the terms *visualize*, *imagine*, and other similar terms, see 121–23.
2 Bonnie Bainbridge Cohen espouses this perspective as well, noting that in embryology, the supporting structure of the bones develop *first*, before the muscles attach to create movement. From workshop notes, used with permission.
3 Hartley, *Wisdom of the Body*, xxxii.
4 Ibid.
5 Bainbridge Cohen, *Sensing, Feeling, and Action*, 11.
6 Ibid., 12.
7 Ibid., 13.
8 Ibid. Bonnie Bainbridge Cohen also mentions that her intention in teaching in this way is that the person may later "discover" the material more consciously on their own in time, providing more self-agency than if the information had just been given to them.

Chapter 6

1 Hartley, *Wisdom of the Body*, 16.
2 Juhan, *Touched by the Goddess*, 42–43.
3 Field, "Touch for Socioemotional and Physical WellBeing," 2010.
4 Field, "Violence and Touch Deprivation in Adolescents," 2002.
5 Juhan, *Touched by the Goddess*, back cover.
6 Juhan, from a lecture given in Embodiment in Education workshop, 2013; used by permission.
7 For a chapter on experiential anatomy curriculum focused on sexuality, see Olsen, *BodyStories*, 141.
8 Chadwick, *To Shine One Corner*, 78.

Chapter 7

1 The term *Body Listening* was also used by Andrea Olsen and Caryn McHose in *BodyStories*, in relation to the nervous system. See Olsen, *BodyStories*, 119–25.
2 Todd, *Thinking Body*, 175–79.
3 For further discussion on the best ways to enact this position and the resulting physiological and mental benefits, see Sweigard, *Human Movement Potential*, 215–21; further descriptions of

CRP can be found in Dowd, *Taking Root to Fly* (description and drawings of energy lines, pp. 2, 3, 8, 15), and Olsen, *BodyStories* (description and activity, p. 13).

4 McHose and Frank, *How Life Moves,* 2006, 2, 7.

5 This concept of "yielding" is a basic principle discussed in Body-Mind Centering. See Bainbridge Cohen, 1993, and Hartley, 1995.

Chapter 9

1 The movement portion of this exploration was inspired by an activity led by Anna Halprin, in which we similarly worked in partners (sitting one behind the other with our hands on our partner's back) to explore movement of the spine. *(See Fig. 9.11.)*

Chapter 10

1 McHose and Frank, *How Life Moves,* 95–96.

2 Bainbridge Cohen, *Sensing, Feeling, and Action,* 11.

3 For Mabel Elsworth Todd's description of these activities, see Todd, *Thinking Body,* 175–79.

Chapter 11

1 Berland, *Sitting,* 68.

2 For a more in-depth description of "bellital alignment," see Olsen, *BodyStories,* p. 91.

3 Hartley, *Wisdom of the Body,* 191.

4 Ibid., 184–88.

5 McHose and Frank, *How Life Moves,* 29–31.

6 Ibid.

7 For further description, see Bainbridge Cohen, *Sensing, Feeling, and Action,* 10, which presents an interview with Bonnie Bainbridge Cohen in which she discusses the concept of contents and container in relation to movement initiation.

8 In the Body-Mind Centering system, the organs are defined as one "body system," even though they may be technically classified within various body systems in the Western anatomical sense of the term. While each of the organs has particular movement qualities and associated emotional expression and can be embodied individually, you can also embody the organs in a more generalized way, such as in the explorations in this book, to evoke physical qualities of fullness and three-dimensionality. Balloons are often used to represent the organs and evoke these qualities.

9 Personal communication with the author, used with permission.

10 The concept of "contents and container" is a primary theory of Body-Mind Centering.

Chapter 12

1 For further discussion of touch and intention, see Dowd, "Use of Intentional Touch."

2 Rolf, *Rolfing,* 39. For further discussion, see the chapter on fascia, 37–43.

3 The idea of movement initiating various emotional states is a primary theory of Body-Mind Centering.

Chapter 13

1 Whitehouse, "Creative Expression in Physical Movement Is Language without Words," 35.

Chapter 14

1 For Steve Paxton's description of the Small Dance see Paxton, "Transcription."
2 In addition to these four curves of the spine, Bonnie Bainbridge Cohen also refers to the curve of the occipital bone of the skull as another curve, thereby including the cranium along with the spine in functional use. From workshop notes, used with permission.
3 For this version of the activity, see McHose and Frank, *How Life Moves,* 64.

Chapter 15

1 Use of the hissing sound was first described in Todd, *Thinking Body,* 290–92.
2 The concept of "contents and container" is a primary theory of BodyMind Centering.
3 This activity of using a parachute to simulate the movement of the diaphragm was introduced to me by educator Jessica Cerrulo, who created it as part of our "professional application lab" in the Embodiment in Education training, though it may be used in other somatic methods as well.
4 Martinez, "What Are We Fighting For?" 2016.

Chapter 16

1 California Department of Education, "January 2005 Physical Education Model Content Standards for California, Public Schools, Kindergarten Through Grade Twelve," 55.
2 Bainbridge Cohen, *Sensing, Feeling, and Action,* 117.
3 Dowd, "Biomechanically Sound but Aesthetically Pleasing Warm-up," 1.
4 Ibid., 2.
5 I developed this exploration, Responsive Moving, inspired by my practice of Authentic Movement. The philosophies of Authentic Movement were influenced by the Jungian concepts of the unconscious and the collective unconscious, and the practice is often seen as a means to gain access to these deeper layers of consciousness. For the purposes of this curriculum, I do not use it in this way, and this activity is not meant to be a simplified version of Authentic Movement. In fact, Authentic Movement would not be recommended as a practice for adolescents in this type of educational context.
6 Bainbridge Cohen, *Sensing, Feeling, and Action,* 14.
7 Ibid.
8 This activity is adapted from a Bartenieff Fundamentals exercise emphasizing cross-lateral connectivity. For more detailed descriptions and alternate methods of facilitating this movement sequence, see Peggy Hackney's account in *Making Connections,* pp. 189–193 called "Turning Over Using Diagonal Connections." Here Hackney notes that although this movement sequence is complex, Bartenieff did not hesitate to use it with beginners. In my version, "Starfish Cross Stretch," I draw on the starfish image and also incorporate a focus on organ support as well as muscular engagement and fluid, sequential movement at the joints.

Afterword

1 Juhan, *Touched by the Goddess,* 15.

2 A few prominent educators who have been instrumental in working with youth in schools in the US include Martha Eddy, Anne Green Gilbert, Eleanor Criswell Hanna, Paul Linden, and Beth Riley, among others; for the purposes of this brief chapter I have only discussed those educators with whom I have worked directly in my programs and professional consultations.

3 Centers for Disease Control and Prevention, "Youth Physical Activity Guidelines Toolkit."

4 American Heart Association, "Teaching America's Kids."

5 Ibid.

6 American Academy of Pediatrics, "Let Them Sleep."

7 As a few examples of innovative programs I am aware of locally in California that include some of these adaptations see www.lwhs.org (high school), www.milleniumschool.org (middle school), and www.theberkeleyschool.org (middle and elementary school).

8 Eddy, *Mindful Movement,* 242.

9 When I worked with this organization it was under the artistic direction of Melanie Rios Glaser, who also had participated in the Embodiment in Education program and was instrumental in spearheading a somatic approach for her students. For more information on this program, called the Wooden Floor and under new direction, see www.thewoodenfloor.org.

10 Making any substantial headway into creating a more diverse professional field in somatic education will require a broad and extensive community endeavor to be successful. Moving on Center, established in 1994 in Oakland, California, with its tagline of "bridging the somatic and performing arts for social change," has been one strong proponent. New programs such as the Institute for Somatics and Social Justice in Philadelphia—founded in 2017 with the express mission to expand diversity and access to somatic education in the United States—are also an inspiring indication that such advocacy efforts are indeed on the rise.

11 Shilling, *The Body,* 58.

12 Novack, *Sharing the Dance,* 8.

13 Martinez, "What Are We Fighting For?"

Bibliography

Adler, Janet. *Offering from the Conscious Body.* Rochester, VT: Inner Traditions, 2002.

Adolescent Sleep Working Group, Committee on Adolescence, and Council on School Health. "School Start Times for Adolescents." *Pediatrics,* August 2014. http://pediatrics.aappublications.org/content/early/2014/08/19/peds.2014-1697.

Alexander, F. Matthias. *Constructive Conscious Control of the Individual.* London: Methuen, 1923.

American Academy of Pediatrics. "Let Them Sleep: AAP Recommends Delaying Start Times of Middle and High Schools to Combat Teen Sleep Deprivation." Press release, August 25, 2014. https://www.aap.org/en-us/about-the-aap/aap-press-room/pages/let-them-sleep-aap-recommends-delaying-start-times-of-middle-and-high-schools-to-combat-teen-sleep-deprivation.aspx.

Amritanandamayi Devi, Sri Mata. *Cultivating Strength and Vitality: An Address by Sri Mata Amritanandamayi Devi.* Translated by Swami Amritaswarupananda Puri. Kerala, India: Mata Amritanandamayi Mission Trust, 2010.

Aposhyan, Susan. *Natural Intelligence: Body-Mind Integration and Human Development.* Baltimore, MD: Williams & Wilken, 1999.

Aston, Judith. *Moving Beyond Posture: In Your Body on the Earth.* With Kimberly Ross and Kimberly Ruess Bridgeman. Self-published by Amazon Digital Services, 2007.

Bainbridge Cohen, Bonnie. *Sensing, Feeling, and Action: The Experiential Anatomy of Body-Mind Centering.* Northampton, MA: Contact Editions, 1993.

Bartenieff, Irmgard. *Body Movement: Coping with the Environment.* With Doris Lewis. New York: Gordon and Breach Science, 1980.

Bauer, Susan. "Body and Earth as One: Strengthening Our Connection to the Natural Source with Ecosomatics." *Conscious Dancer,* Spring 2008, 8–9.

———. "A Body/Mind Approach to Movement Education for Adolescents." Master's thesis, Wesleyan University, 1994. [Reprinted by the author 2005, 2008.]

———. "Dancing with the Divine: Dance Education and the Embodiment of Spirit, from Bali to America." In *Dance, Somatics and Spiritualities: Contemporary Sacred Narratives,* edited by Amanda Williamson, Glenna Batson, Sarah Watley, and Rebecca Weber, 375–416. Bristol, UK: Intellect, 2014. Distributed by University of Chicago Press.

———. "Find Your Position: An Embodied Approach to Movement and Daily Life." In *Embodied Lives: Reflections on the Influence of Suprapto Suryodarmo and Amerta Movement,* edited by Katya Bloom, Margit Galanter, and Sandra Reeve, 211–20. Axminster, UK: Triarchy Press, 2014.

_____. "Finding the Bone in the Wind: A Journey with Prapto Suryadarmo in Bali, Indonesia." *A Moving Journal,* 12, no.3 (Fall/Winter 2005): 14–20.

_____. "Must to the Mountain: A Journey with Sardono Kusumo at UCLA." *Contact Quarterly*, 23, no.2 (Summer/Fall 1998): 21–37.

_____. "Oracles, Authentic Movement and the IChing." In *Authentic Movement, Moving the Body, Moving the Self, Being Moved*, A Collection of Essays, Volume Two, edited by Patrizia Pallaro, 364–67. London and Philadelphia: Jessica Kingsley Publications, 2007.

———. "Somatic Movement Education: A Body/Mind Approach to Movement Education for Adolescents, Part 1." *Somatics Journal* 12, no. 2 (Spring/Summer 1999): 38–43.

———. "Somatic Movement Education: A Body/Mind Approach to Movement Education for Adolescents, Part 2." *Somatics Journal* 12, no. 3 (Fall/Winter 1999/2000): 40–47.

_____. "Welcome to City of Nice People: Cross Cultural Dialogues on Authentic Movement in Thailand." *Contact Quarterly* 32, no.1 (Winter/Spring 2007): 48-55.

Berland, Erika. *Sitting: The Physical Art of Meditation*. Boulder: Somatic Performer Press, 2017.

Biermeier, Mary Ann. "Inspired by Reggio Emilia: Emergent Curriculum in Relationship-Driven Learning Environments." *Young Children* 70, no. 5. http://www.naeyc.org/yc/node/324.

Broderick, Patricia C. *Learning to Breathe: A Mindfulness Curriculum for Adolescents to Cultivate Emotion Regulation, Attention, and Performance*. Oakland, CA: New Harbinger, 2013.

Caldwell, Christine. "Mindfulness and Bodyfulness: A New Paradigm." *Journal of Contemplative Inquiry* 1 (2014): 77–96. https://www.naropa.edu/documents/faculty/bodyful-art-joci-2014.pdf.

Centers for Disease Control and Prevention. "Child Obesity Facts." Updated January 25, 2017. https://www.cdc.gov/healthyschools/obesity/facts.htm.

———. "Youth Physical Activity Guidelines Toolkit." Accessed September 2017. https://www.cdc .gov/healthyschools/physicalactivity/guidelines.htm.

Chadwick, David, ed. *To Shine One Corner of the World: Moments with Shunryu Suzuki*. New York: Broadway Books, 2001.

"Childhood Obesity." Harvard T.H. Chan School of Public Health. Accessed September 23, 2017. https://www.hsph.harvard.edu/obesity-prevention-source/obesity-trends/global-obesity-trends -in-children/.

Claxton, Guy. *Intelligence in the Flesh: Why Your Mind Needs Your Body Much More Than It Thinks*. London: Yale University Press, 2015.

Dowd, Irene. "The Biomechanically Sound but Aesthetically Pleasing Warm-up." Paper presented at the National Dance Association Symposium on the Science and Somatics of Dance, Salt Lake City, 1991.

________. *Taking Root to Fly: Ten Articles on Functional Anatomy*. Northampton, MA: Contact Editions, 1990.

________. "The Use of Intentional Touch." *Contact Quarterly* 16, no. 1 (Winter 1990): 21–29.

Dweck, Carol S. *Mindset: The New Psychology of Success*. Rev. ed. New York, Ballantine, 2016.

Dweck, Carol S., Gregory M. Walton, and Geoffrey L. Cohen. *Academic Tenacity: Mindsets and Skills That Promote Long-Term Learning*. Seattle: Bill and Melinda Gates Foundation, 2014. https://ed.stanford.edu/sites/default/files/manual/dweck-walton-cohen-2014.pdf.

Eddy, Martha. *Mindful Movement: The Evolution of the Somatic Arts and Conscious Action*. Bristol, UK: Intellect. Distributed by University of Chicago Press, 2016.

________. "Somatic Practices and Dance: Global Influences." *Dance Research Journal* 34, no. 2 (2002): 46–62.

Enghauser, Rebecca. "The Quest for an Eco-Somatic Approach to Dance Pedagogy." *Journal of Dance Education* 7, no. 3 (2007): 80–90.

Feldenkrais, Moshe. *Awareness Through Movement.* New York: HarperCollins, 1972, 1977.

Field, Tiffany. "Touch for Socioemotional and Physical WellBeing: A Review," in *Developmental Review,* 30, no. 4 (2010): 376–83.

_______. "Violence and Touch Deprivation in Adolescents. Retrieved December 17 2017 from https://www.thefreelibrary.com/Violence+and+touch+deprivation+in+adolescents.-a097723210.

Gantz, Judy. "Cultivating Body Knowledge." *Somatics Journal* Vol XVII no. 3, 2015.

Gardner, Howard. *Frames of Mind: The Theory of Multiple Intelligences.* New York: HarperCollins, 1985.

Goleman, Daniel. *Emotional Intelligence: Why It Can Matter More Than IQ.* New York: Bantam Books, 1995.

Gutman, Leslie Morrison, and Ingrid Schoon. "The Impact of Non-Cognitive Skills on Outcomes for Young People: Literature Review." London: Institute of Education, 2013.

Haase, Lori, Jennifer L. Stewart, Brittany Youssef, April C. May, Sara Isakovic, Alan N. Simmons, Douglas C. Johnson, Eric G. Potterat, and Martin P. Paulus. "When the Brain Does Not Adequately Feel the Body." *Biological Psychology* 113 (January 2016): 37–45. http://www.sciencedirect.com/science/article/pii/S030105111530079X.

Hackney, Peggy. "Remembering Irmgard." *Contact Quarterly* 18, no. 1 (Winter/Spring 1993): 13–20.

________. *Making Connections: Total Body Integration through Bartenieff Fundamentals.* London: Gordon & Breach, 1998.

Halprin, Anna. *Moving Toward Life, Five Decades of Transformational Dance.* Middletown, CT: Wesleyan University Press, 1995.

Hartley, Linda. *Wisdom of the Body: An Introduction to Body-Mind Centering.* Berkeley, CA: North Atlantic Books, 1989, 1995.

H'Doubler, Margaret N. *Dance: A Creative Art Experience.* Madison: University of Wisconsin Press, 1957.

Jinpa, Thupten. *A Fearless Heart: How the Courage to Be Compassionate Can Transform Our Lives.* New York: Hudson Street Press, 2015.

Johnson, Don Hanlon. *Body: Recovering Our Sensual Wisdom.* Berkeley, CA: North Atlantic Books, 1983.

Johnson, Rae. *Embodied Social Justice.* New York: Routledge, 2018.

Juhan, Deane. *Job's Body: A Handbook for Bodywork.* New York: Station Hill Press, 1987.

———. *Touched by the Goddess: The Physical, Psychological, and Spiritual Powers of Bodywork.* New York: Station Hill Press, 1994, 1995, 1996, 2002.

Kabat-Zinn, Jon. "The Father of Mindfulness on What Mindfulness Has Become: An Interview with Jon Kabat-Zinn, Creator of Mindfulness-Based Stress Reduction." By Drake Baer. Thrive Global, April 12, 2017, https://journal.thriveglobal.com/the-father-of-mindfulness-on-what-mindfulness-has-become-ad649c8340cf.

———. *Mindfulness-Based Stress Reduction (MBSR): Authorized Curriculum Guide, 2017.* Worcester, MA: Center for Mindfulness in Medicine, Health Care, and Society, University of Massachusetts Medical School, 2017.

———. *Mindfulness for Beginners: Reclaiming the Present Moment—and Your Life.* Boulder: Sounds True, 2012.

Kabat-Zinn, Myla, and Jon Kabat-Zinn. *Everyday Blessings: The Inner Work of Mindful Parenting.* New York: Hyperion, 1997.

Kapit, Wynn, and Lawrence M. Elson. *The Anatomy Coloring Book.* New York: Harper & Row, 1977.

Kapitan, Roxanne, ed. *Cooperative Learning in the Classroom.* Massachusetts: Regional Alliance for Education Reform, 1993.

Kee, Ying Hwa, Nikos N. L. D. Chatzisarantis, Pui Wah Kong, Jia Yi Chow, and Lung Hung Chen. "Mindfulness, Movement Control, and Attentional Focus Strategies: Effects of Mindfulness on a Postural Balance Task." *Journal of Sport and Exercise Psychology* 34, no. 5 (2012): 561–79.

Leguizaman, Sea, Sam Grant, Carol Swan, and Martha Eddy (n.d.). "Key Principles of Social Somatics," http://www.carolswann.net/socialsomatics/principles/. Accessed October 2014.

Levine, Peter. *Waking the Tiger, Healing Trauma.* Berkeley, CA. North Atlantic Books, 1997.

Macy, Joanna. *Coming Back to Life: Practices to Reconnect Our Lives, Our World.* Canada: New Society Publishers, 1998.

Martinez, Lorea, Susan Stillman, Ilaria Boffa, and Tommasso Procicchiani. "School Climate in Middle School: What Are Students Telling Us about Their Experience in Schools?" Paper presented at the AERA Annual Conference, Washington, DC, April 2016.

Martinez, Xiuhtezcatl. *We Rise: The Earth Guardians Guide to Building a Movement That Restores the Planet.* Emmaus, PA: Rodale/MacMillan, 2017.

__________. "What Are We Fighting For?" speech given at the Bioneers Conference in Marin, CA, 2016. https://www.youtube.com/watch?v=5OiOpSiWq9Q.

McHose, Caryn, and Kevin Frank. *How Life Moves: Explorations in Meaning and Body Awareness.* Berkeley, CA: North Atlantic Books, 2006.

McHugh, Jamie. "Restoring Original Grace: Movement as Medicine." Unpublished manuscript. 2015.

Merleau-Ponty, Maurice. *The Phenomenology of Perception.* Translated by Colin Smith. London: Routledge & Kegan Paul, 1962.

Miller, Gill, Pat Ethridge, and Kate Morgan, eds. *Exploring Body-Mind Centering, An Anthology of Experience and Method.* Berkeley, CA: North Atlantic Books, 2011.

Montagu, Ashley. *Touching: The Human Significance of the Skin.* 3rd ed. New York: Harper & Row, 1986.

Mulder, T.H. "Motor Imagery and Action Observation: Cognitive Tools for Rehabilitation," *Journal of Neural Transmission,* 114, no. 10 (October 2007): 1265–78.

Murphy, Michael. *The Future of the Body: Explorations into the Further Evolution of Human Nature.* Los Angeles: Jeremy P. Tarcher, 1992.

Neff, Kristin. *Self-Compassion: The Proven Power of Being Kind to Yourself.* New York: HarperCollins, 2011.

Nhat Hanh, Thich. *Peace Is Every Step: The Path of Mindfulness.* New York: Bantam Books, 1991.

Novack, Cynthia J. *Sharing the Dance: Contact Improvisation and American Culture.* Madison: University of Wisconsin Press, 1990.

Ogden, C. L., M. D. Carroll, H. G. Lawman, C. D. Fryar, D. Kruszon-Moran, B. K. Kit, and K.M. Flegal "Trends in Obesity Prevalence among Children and Adolescents in the United States, 1988–1994 through 2013–2014." *JAMA* 315, no. 21 (2016): 292–99.

Olsen, Andrea. "Being Seen, Being Moved: Authentic Movement and Performance." *Contact Quarterly* 18, no. 1 (Winter/Spring 1993): 46–53.

———. *Body and Earth: An Experiential Guide.* Lebanon, NH: University Press of New England, 2002.

———. *BodyStories: A Guide to Experiential Anatomy.* In collaboration with Caryn McHose. Barrytown, NY: Station Hill Press, 1991.

———. *The Place of Dance: A Somatic Guide to Dance and Dance Making.* In collaboration with Caryn McHose. Middletown, CT: Wesleyan University Press, 2014.

Paus, Tomas, Matcheri Keshavan, and Jay N. Giedd. "Why Do Many Psychiatric Disorders Emerge during Adolescence?" *Nature Reviews: Neuroscience* 9, no. 12 (2008): 947–57.

Paxton, Steve. "Transcription." *Contact Quarterly* 11, no. 1 (Winter 1986): 48–50.

Porges, Stephen W. *The Pocket Guide to the Polyvagal Theory: The Transformative Power of Feeling Safe.* New York: W. W. Norton and Company, 2017.

Rolf, Ida P. *Rolfing: The Integration of Human Structures.* New York: Harper & Row, 1977.

Rosenthal, Leslie. "Some Dynamics of Resistance and Therapeutic Management in Adolescent Group Therapy." *Psychoanalytic Review* 58, no. 3 (1948): 353–66.

Saltzman, Amy. *A Still Quiet Place: A Mindfulness Program for Teaching Children and Adolescents to Ease Stress and Difficult Emotions.* Oakland: New Harbinger, 2014.

Schwartz, Peggy. "Creativity and Dance: Implications for Pedagogy and Policy." *Arts Education Policy Review* 95, no. 1 (September/October 1993): 8–16.

Shilling, Chris. *The Body: A Very Short Introduction.* Oxford: Oxford University Press, 2016.

Sing, Amici and Leonie Uijtdewilligen. "Physical Activity and Performance at School: A Systematic Review of the Literature Including a Methodological Quality Assessment," in JAMA Pediatrics, American Medical Association, Jan 1, 2012. Accessed Dec. 17, 2017, https://jamanetwork.com/journals/jamapediatrics/fullarticle/1107683.

Sroufe, L. Alan, Byron Egeland, Elizabeth A. Carlson, and W. Andrew Collins. *The Development of the Person: The Minnesota Study of Risk and Adaptation from Birth to Adulthood.* New York: Guilford Press, 2005.

Steinberg, Laurence. *Age of Opportunity: Lessons from the New Science of Adolescence.* New York: Houghton Mifflin Harcourt, 2014.

Sweigard, Lulu E. *Human Movement Potential: Its Ideokinetic Facilitation.* New York: Harper & Row, 1974.

Todd, Mabel Elsworth. *The Thinking Body*. Brooklyn: Dance Horizons, 1937.

Tsabary, Shefali. *The Awakened Family: A Revolution in Parenting.* New York: Viking, 2016.

Weber, Rebecca. "Integrating Semi-Structured Somatic Practices and Contemporary Dance Technique Training." *Journal of Dance and Somatic Practices 1,* no. 2 (December 2009): 237–54. doi:10.1386/jdsp.1.2.237_1.

Whitehouse, Mary. "Creative Expression in Physical Movement Is Language without Words." In *Authentic Movement: Essays by Mary Starks Whitehouse, Janet Adler, and Joan Chodorow,* edited by Patrizia Pallaro, 33–40. London and New York: Jessica Kingsley, 1999. First time published; written c. 1956.

Zins, Joseph E., Roger P. Weissberg, Margaret C. Wang, and Herbert J. Walberg, eds. *Building Academic Success on Social and Emotional Learning: What Does the Research Say?* New York: Teachers College Press, 2004.

Index

C

D

E

F

G

H

I

J

K

L

M

N

O

P

Q

R

S

About the Author

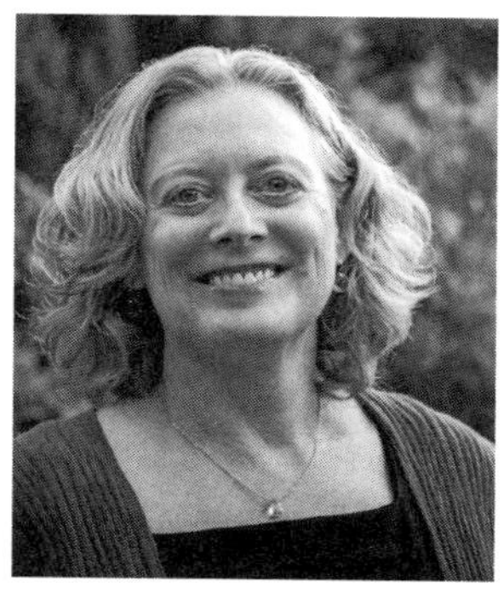

Susan Bauer, MFA, RSME/T, is a teacher, dancer, author, Fulbright Scholar, and somatic educator and practitioner. In her thirty-year career she has taught in middle school and high school, college, and community contexts, and has led teacher trainings and given conference presentations both in the United States and abroad. Her pioneering teacher-training program, Embodiment in Education, is now in its tenth year. She is a Registered Somatic Movement Educator and Therapist with a private practice in the San Francisco Bay Area, and also served on the board of directors of the International Somatic Movement Education and Therapy Association (ISMETA) from 2012 to 2015. Bauer holds an MFA in dance from the Department of World Arts and Cultures at the University of California, Los Angeles, and an MALS in Dance and Movement Studies from Wesleyan University. She is a contributor to the anthologies *Embodied Lives, Authentic Movement (Volume Two)* and *Dance, Somatics, and Spiritualities* as well to the journals *Contact Quarterly, Somatics,* and *Seeds of Peace.*

For more information on her work, including workshops and certification programs for educators, please visit susanbauer.com or embodimentineducation.org, where you will also find free downloads of further educational materials for your use. To inquire about starting an Embodied Teen program at your school or youth program, contact susan@susanbauer.com.

About North Atlantic Books

North Atlantic Books (NAB) is an independent, nonprofit publisher committed to a bold exploration of the relationships between mind, body, spirit, and nature. Founded in 1974, NAB aims to nurture a holistic view of the arts, sciences, humanities, and healing. To make a donation or to learn more about our books, authors, events, and newsletter, please visit www.northatlanticbooks.com.

North Atlantic Books is the publishing arm of the Society for the Study of Native Arts and Sciences, a 501(c)(3) nonprofit educational organization that promotes cross-cultural perspectives linking scientific, social, and artistic fields. To learn how you can support us, please visit our website.